KNOW YOUR FATS

The Complete Primer for Understanding the Nutrition of Fats, Oils and Cholesterol

Mary G. Enig, Ph.D.

Director
Nutritional Sciences Division
Enig Associates, Inc., Silver Spring, MD

2000

Know Your Fats: The Complete Primer for Understanding the Nutrition of Fats, Oils, and Cholesterol is not intended as medical advice. Its intent is solely informational and educational. Please consult a health professional should the need for one be indicated.

c/o Bethesda Press
12501 Prosperity Drive
Suite 340
Silver Spring, MD 20904-1689
U.S.A.
Telephone: 301-680-8600
Fax: 301-680-8100
Website: http://www.bethesdapress.com

Published by Bethesda Press
First Printing April 2000
Second Printing June 2001
Third Printing September 2002
Cover and Book Design: Eric N. Enig

Library of Congress Cataloging-in-Publication Data

Enig, Mary G. (Mary Gertrude), 1931-

Know Your Fats: The Complete Primer for Understanding the Nutrition of Fats, Oils, and Cholesterol / Mary G. Enig -
1st Edition
        p. cm.
Includes biographical references and index.
ISBN 0-9678126-0-7
1. Fats and oils in human nutrition. 2. Fatty acids in human nutrition. 3. Essential fatty acids in human nutrition. 4. Fatty acid metabolism. 5. Cholesterol metabolism. 6. Food and Food Chemistry I. Title.

Library of Congress Catalogue No

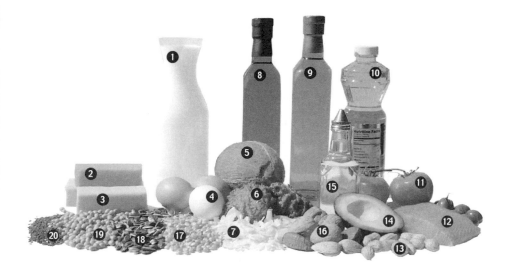

1. milk fat   } sources of anti-infective glycolipids, conjugated
2. cheese   } linoleic acid (CLA), and small amounts of lauric
3. butter   } acid
4. egg - yolk is source of phospholipids, including emulsifier *lecithin,* and phytonutrients *lutein* and *zeaxanthin*
5. whole coconut   } major source of antimicrobial fatty acids
6. coconut macaroons } lauric acid and capric acid; 65% medium
7. desiccated coconut } chain fatty acids
8. extra-virgin olive oil } major source of high omega-9 fatty acids;
9. olive oil   } stable cooking oil
10. safflower oil - omega 6 variety and omega 9 variety
11. tomato - source of important fat-soluble phytonutrients *beta-carotene, lycopene,* and *zeaxanthin*
12. salmon - source of elongated omega-3 fatty acids EPA and DHA
13. peanuts - nearly half omega-9 fatty acid
14. avocado - high omega-9 fatty acid
15. sesame oil - stable cooking oil with nearly equal amounts of omega-9 and omega-6; contains antioxidant *sesamin*
16. mixed nuts - almond, brazil nuts, walnuts
17. corn - omega-6 oil
18. sunflowerseed - both omega-6 variety and omega-9 variety
19. soybean - omega-6 oil with some omega-3 when unrefined
20. flaxseed - high in omega-3 fatty acid alpha-linolenic acid

Table of Contents

Chapter 3

Chapter 4

Chapter 5

Tables

Chapter 3

Appendix D

Credits

Photographs and Graphics
Cover; pages 113, 126: Bethesda Press
Chemical Structures: Author (MGE)

Illustrations
Figures 2.2, 2.3, 2.4, page 133: Eric B. Nicholson 1982 from *The Many Roles of Fat in Our Lives* booklet by Mary G. Enig and Beverly R. Teter , ©1983

Preface

When friends and acquaintances heard that I was writing this book, the comments ranged from "why are you doing that" to "what took you so long to do it."

The answer to "why are you doing that" is because I became increasingly frustrated about being unable to find, (1) a simple, straightforward truthful book about fats and oils and cholesterol written for the general audience, an audience that was in great need of this information, and, (2) an accurate book that I could comfortably recommend to all those who asked for something to answer their questions about fats and oils and cholesterol.

All the books out in the market were either too technical and too expensive *if* they were written by someone who really knew the topic, or they were written by writers who ranged from a number of hucksters who were oil salesmen to those professional writers who had only a glancing knowledge of the subject. And in both instances, their books were filled with inaccuracies. In between, there were some attempts by some good scientists who had combined their efforts with journalists, but the resulting books usually had what I considered to be an inappropriate agenda, the authors frequently repeated some of the standard myths and errors I objected to, and they always lacked the completeness I was looking for.

The "what took you so long" is related to my not being a journalist, but being a scientist whose writing forays in the past had been more or less limited to technical reports. I hope this book on such a technical subject is written in a manner that will make it understandable to most of the people who read and study it in an effort to get a grip on the fascinating subject of fats and oils and cholesterol.

This book actually started out nearly a decade ago as a long report for consumers, which had been requested by the head of an organization. When it was "collaboratively" edited and somewhat shortened, some of the odd errors-of-fact to which I object had crept in. As a result of this, and other similar experiences, this book has been written without the collaboration of a professional journalist and I am hoping it has not suffered for it. Along the way, several "word smiths," including those in my family, have had a go at making sure the usages of the words "which" and "that" were appropriate and that commas were in their rightful places.

I have tried to keep the running commentaries conversational, and I hope the reader comes away from a quick browse or a full reading with the pleasant satisfaction one should have after eating a healthy snack or a good meal of real food. Yes, M. B., it's O.K. to eat bacon sandwiches with good quality mayonnaise.

April 2000   Mary G. Enig
Silver Spring, Maryland U.S.A.

Acknowledgments

I would never have been able to write this book without the cooperation of my family and colleagues, and to all of them I am grateful for their support and collaboration. But most important, I would never have had the knowledge required to do an accurate job without having had the experience of having two superb lipid biochemists as my graduate and post-graduate advisors. To both Dr. Mark Keeney and Dr. Joseph Sampugna, in whose lipids laboratories I learned to love the intricacies of the study of lipids, I owe my gratitude for their roles as teachers *par excellence*.

Introduction

To eat, or not to eat -- fat is the question.
--with apologies to William Shakespeare

The role of fats and oils (technically called lipids) in human nutrition has received considerable attention in recent years. Newspapers and magazines are filled with articles about dietary fat, and radio and television talk shows feature spot announcements about fat. Grocery stores distribute fact sheets about dietary fat, consumer groups discuss the topic of fat in their newsletters, and many internet sites have pages on fats and oils. In addition, enthusiastic writers have produced whole books about fat.

But, almost all of these articles or books have been written by individuals who have no actual scientific training in fats and oils. **And,** unfortunately, too much of what they have written or said is either incorrect or unacceptably incomplete.

Additionally, in current nutrition and dietetics texts and journals, there are many errors, especially about fats and oils. Individually, each can be seen as a careless mistake; collectively they are more insidious. When these mistakes are repeated over generations of students, they lead to a scientifically unsupportable dogma generating dietary recommendations that are false and potentially harmful. This is the sort of thing that has fueled the anti-saturated fat agenda. The fats and oils people who originated this agenda likely never dreamed of its potential effects: their grandchildren and great grandchildren will be the inheritors of the health problems generated by this misinformation.

Know Your Fats: A Complete Primer for Understanding the Nutrition of Fats, Oils & Cholesterol provides the reader with a very broad but also in-depth discussion of the many aspects of dietary fats and oils in our foods and in our bodies. The reader will gain an understanding of the relationship between dietary fat intake and health and between dietary fat intake and disease. The reader will also be able to determine why some information in other books or articles may not be correct.

The book is written broadly enough to appeal to the general public and with sufficient detail to serve as excellent reference to the nutritionist, dietitian and physician. The food/health journalist, who often serves as the intermediary between the researcher and the consumer, should find this book particularly useful. They all should find this book a useful and valuable source of factual information written by an internationally acknowledged expert in the subject. During the writing and editing of this book, individuals in all of the above categories were consulted for ideas, questions, and criticism.

An effort has been made to keep the terminology understandable and in accordance with that terminology used in the numerous reports written for consumers by government agencies. Occasionally, it has been necessary to use technical terms in order to avoid simplistic wording that would sacrifice accuracy. A **General Glossary** of those terms, common to fats and oils in foods and lipids in biological systems, is included at the end of this book for the reader. Technical biochemical terms that require lengthy descriptions are also included in this glossary. Several years ago, the author complained to a food and agriculture bureaucrat about some inaccuracies in some material on fats and oils. The response given by the bureaucrat was that he had no qualms about "lying to keep it simple"; he may not like the more complicated truth presented in this book, but the reader should appreciate the effort.

As we close the second millennium, the prevailing clinical approach from both the nutrition and medical communities in the United States is to condemn a high dietary intake of almost all fats. This emphasis on reducing dietary fat intake has developed from concerns about diet/serum cholesterol/coronary heart disease (CHD) and dietary fat/cancer relationships that have emanated from organizations such as the American Heart Association (AHA), the National Heart Lung and Blood Institute's National Cholesterol Education Program, the National Cancer Institute's Cancer Prevention Program, and the U. S. Department of Agriculture's Dietary Guidelines. Many official and quasi-official articles and publications written for the public reflect this view. Unfortunately for the consumer and the clinician, many of these articles have multiple misstatements about fats, oils, and cholesterol in general, and about the hydrogenated fats and oils in particular. The kindest thing that can be said about the authors of these misstatements is that they are misguided and not sufficiently knowledgeable about the chemistry of fats and oils and hydrogenation. Consequently, they make many substantive mistakes when they try to explain what dietary fats and oils are and what biological lipids are.

Although U.S. government and various private agencies in the U.S. continue to single out dietary saturated fats and cholesterol as the only macro nutrient components in our diet that needs reduction, several governments including the Canadian, British, and Danish have formally recommended that *trans* fatty acids (the unsaturated fatty acids some-times referred to as saturate-equivalents that are formed in partial hydrogenation) should not be increased in the diets of their citizens. The earliest concern about *trans* fatty acids acknowledged by a government agency came from the Canadian government in the late 1980's and proved prophetic because in August 1990 a Dutch study reported that the *trans* fatty acids do have an adverse effect on serum cholesterol. Then, in 1991 the Committee on Medical Aspects of Health (COMA) of the U.K. recommended that *trans* fatty acids be limited to 2% of the caloric (energy) intake. Finally in 1992, an industry-sponsored USDA study, followed by additional USDA studies, verified the 1990 Dutch study, and Harvard School of Public Health researchers reported that both heart disease and breast and prostate cancers are related to increased intakes of *trans* fatty acids. Along the way, European researchers tied the *trans* fatty acids to low birth weight in infants and to the potential compromise of omega-3 status as well as to breast cancer. Most recently, Canadian researchers have verified the concerns of Dutch researchers about the *trans* fatty acids and decreased visual acuity in infants. Importantly, a number of researchers have started to report about the essentiality of some, if not most of the saturated fatty acids found in the natural foods. As this book was being finalized and going to press, the U.S. Food and Drug Administrated announced plans for regulations to label the *trans* fatty acids. This labeling would be mandatory.

The polyunsaturates have also been a recent category of concern, and a decrease in their dietary intake has been recommended. The recommendation to lower intake levels of the omega-6 polyunsaturates came as researchers learned that high levels of these polyunsaturates were not as desirable as originally thought. In addition to the changes in recommendations about polyunsaturates, the monounsaturates have come from their neutral oblivion in the 1970's to a state of prominence in the 1980's, and into questionable worth in the 1990's. As we come to the end of the millenium, there is new emphasis that divides the polyunsaturates into two categories, namely omega-6 and omega-3, with concern about the wrong balance in dietary intakes. Also from some research camps comes the hint that the type of fat may be less important than the amount of total fat, that the saturated fats are not showing up as a problem, and further that low fat intake may be quite detrimental to the health of almost everyone.

All this shifting emphasis over the years has been very confusing to those consumers who tend to pay undo attention to the rhetoric and try to follow the latest recommendation. It is most unfortunate that many in the medical community have become so misled about the relationship of dietary fat and normal physiology. As a consequence many unfounded beliefs have become entrenched.

Chapter 1, Knowing the Basic Facts About Fats explains to the reader the meaning of the following terms: fatty acids, saturated fatty acids, monounsaturated fatty acids, polyunsaturated fatty acids, hydrogenated fats, *trans* fatty acids, the omega-6 family of fatty acids, the omega-3 family of fatty acids, oleic acid, linoleic acid, gamma-linolenic acid, arachidonic acid, conjugated linoleic acid, lauric acid, alpha-linolenic acid, eicosapentaenoic acid, docosahexaenoic acid, and cholesterol. The information in this chapter will give the reader an understanding of the basics, and thus will be very useful to anyone trying to evaluate the writing in, for example, food industry pamphlets, government agency documents, magazine and newspaper articles about fats labeling, and books about diets. This chapter also includes information explaining how fats and oils are processed, including partial hydrogenation.

Chapter 2, Lets Get Physical With Fats is devoted to a review of the role of lipids in normal physiology. The reader will learn that lipids in the body are important parts of cell membranes, are necessary as vitamin carriers, play a pivotal role in producing satiety, form the necessary protective padding for organs, provide efficient energy storage, function as enzyme regulators, are important as hormone precursors, and are necessary for emulsification functions. Some of the lipids required for these functions can be made by many different cells in the body "from scratch" using carbohydrate or excess protein. Some of the lipids come from the food fats and oils, and the body makes certain changes to those fats before using them.

There are so many important roles played by fats (lipids) in the human body, which have been largely ignored in most articles written for the general public. Most of these articles have addressed the known or purported undesirable effects of lipids. Many of the articles written by science writers and journalists for newspapers or magazines are laden with errors and should be "taken with a grain of salt." To an extent, the same is true for the articles written for the general nutrition and medical communities. Whatever the reason, these writers have swamped the literature with a type of information that is detrimental to the public.

The importance of saturated fat to the human body becomes apparent if we think about and understand that the body has developed the ability to synthesize the most important fats even if they are *not* found in adequate amounts in the foods. In other words, the saturated fatty acids and monounsaturated fatty acids that are needed in large amounts for membranes are quite efficiently made by the body. The elongated polyunsaturated fatty acids that are also needed for cell membranes can also be built by the body's special fat-synthesizing machinery using those essential fatty acids that come from the diet as the initial building blocks. When the basic essential fatty acids are in low supply in the diet, the body conserves the elongated forms as long as there are enough of the natural saturated fatty acids in the diet.

Chapter 3, Diets, Then and Now, Here and There gives the reader a historical overview of changes in dietary fat sources and usage over many lifetimes. Types of dietary fats have been changing in our food supply during the 20*th* Century. What do these changes mean? How do these changes affect our health? How do the changes affect the growth of infants and children for whom dietary fat is so important? How do the changes affect our choices of foods? There has not been very much agreement from decade to decade about what all these changes mean. Nonetheless, since these changes have been discussed periodically by clinicians and basic researchers in nutritional medicine, they need to be summarized and interpreted in order to present a valid historical perspective for the reader to evaluate.

In **Chapter 4, The Many Sources of Fats and Oils**, an overview of all the different types of food fats and oils usually found in the U.S. and Canadian food supply is presented. The reader will learn where the different fats and oils originated. Fats and oils play various roles in foods and food preparation, including the following: they provide palatability, flavor, aroma, and emulsification; they are the most efficient energy source; they are needed for plant membrane structure; and they serve as carriers for some vitamins. Some fats and oils are the best sources of essential fatty acids; some are almost devoid of essential fatty acids. Technical and historical information about the fats and oils is presented in this chapter.

Chapter 5, Labeling Fats and Oils for the Marketplace addresses the current regulations and practices. Whatever the in-vogue recommenda- tions may be, the balance of fatty acids in the diet can be determined by the consumer and evaluated by the professional if the amount of each fatty acid class is known either by appropriate labeling on the various food items or by available charts that list the amounts of fatty acid classes in each food. The extent to which mislabeling is a problem for the consumer and also for the professional who uses the label as a source of information for food composition tables or for dietary evaluation and recommendations is an issue that needs clarification. The extent to which the 1992 U.S. federal labeling law has exacerbated the mislabeling and misinformation that have been noted will be addressed; the potential effect of a proposed labeling regulation for the *trans* fatty acids will be discussed. These and other important aspects of food labeling in the United States compared to countries such as Canada and Great Britain are reviewed.

Chapter 6, An Overview of Dietary Fat Intake Recommendations provides an overview as indicated. In the United States, recommendations concerning fats and oils in the diet have come from federal government agencies such as the United States Department of Agriculture (USDA) and the Department of Health and Human Services (HHS), as well as from quasi-government agencies such as the National Research Council of the National Academy of Science (NAS-NRC). Within HHS, several agencies have been involved in recommendations about dietary fat. These include the National Heart, Lung and Blood Institute (NHLBI) of the National Institutes of Health (NIH), the Food and Drug Administration (FDA), and the Surgeon General's Office. Within USDA, the Human Nutrition Information Service (HNIS) has been responsible for the Dietary Guidelines.

The dietary advice from these agencies regarding the most appropriate balance of dietary fats has been evolving over the past several decades. For example, the recommendations in the 1970's were to consume twice the amount of polyunsaturates relative to saturates, i.e., a polyunsaturate-to-saturate (P/S) ratio of 2. By the late 1980's this ratio had been reversed, and the recommended P/S ratio became 0.7 to 1.0 depending on the agency to which you listened. Some of the recommended changes have been contradictory and have confused the public as well as the professional. The history of these changes as they pertain to dietary fat is reviewed, the latest recommendations from the Canadian government's Health and Welfare are also presented for comparison, and the role of the food industry in promoting these changes is documented.

Chapter 7, Small Summaries of Fat Facts will give some short sections on some of the critical topics.

Chapter 8, Frequently Asked Questions and Their Answers hopes to anticipate any burning queries the reader may have by the time this part of the book has been reached. This chapter is based on the many email, regular mail, and telephone requests for information received by the author over the years. This, plus the **General Glossary** (Appendix A), and the **Index** should be helpful to the reader.

The final sections of the book include the following: **Appendix A: General Glossary; Appendix B: Table of Acronyms; Appendix C: Fat Composition of Common Foods; Appendix D: Tables of Fatty Acid Sources and Nomenclature; Chapter Notes; Index;** and **About the Author**. The General Glossary includes technical information on many topics in lipids including some of the technicalities about the fatty acids not found in the narrative portions of this book. The Food Composition Tables include only those foods that are natural sources of fats and oils. Foods such as baked goods would not have a particular composition that could cover all of the products out in the market so they are not included. On the other hand, the composition of unprocessed fats and oils, meats, poultry, fish and seafood, eggs, and dairy products would be relatively unvarying and these are included. The final appendix includes several tables of technical information including nomenclature.

Chapter 1

Knowing the Basic Facts
About Fats

What Are Fats and Oils?

Fats and **oils** (technically called **lipids**) are basically made up of collections of molecules called **triglycerides**. If the collection is liquid at ambient temperature, it is called an oil; if it is solid, it is called a fat. The shorthand designation commonly used for triglycerides is **TG**.

A triglyceride is formed from three **fatty acids** attached to a **glycerol** molecule. The three fatty acids are held together through a special attachment to the glycerol and thus form a single molecular structure. Glycerol is the same molecule whether it is found in a plant or an animal. Basic fatty acids are also the same molecules regardless of whether they come from plants or animals (including people), although the proportions of each fatty acid on the triglyceride molecule will vary from plant to plant, from animal to animal, and from plant to animal.

What Are Bonds and Why Are They Important?

The shape of each triglyceride molecule will depend on the specific kinds of fatty acids found in the triglyceride. The shapes of the fatty acids are in turn related to the fact that fatty acids are formed from the elements carbon (**C**), hydrogen (**H**) and oxygen (**O**). Carbon is one of the few elements that will form chains or rings of atoms joined by chemical bonds in which one, two, or three pairs of electrons may be shared. If one pair of electrons is shared, the bond is called a *single bond* and is shown like this, **C-C**. If two pairs are shared, it is called a *double bond* and is shown as **C=C** in pictures of molecular structures. Likewise, the sharing of three pairs gives a *triple bond* and is shown as **C≡C**.

A bond in which more than one pair of electrons are shared is called an *unsaturated bond*, e.g., double carbon bonds, and since the unsaturated bonds are up for grabs, another element could come and "steal" one of those electrons and form a new bond. This makes unsaturated bonds relatively reactive and chemically unstable. If a fatty acid molecule has several unsaturated bonds it is called *polyunsaturated* and is generally very reactive chemically.

A carbon bond that shares only one pair of electrons is called a *saturated bond* (-C-C-), and generally in the case of fatty acids, the other electrons of the carbons are shared by hydrogen atoms when they are not shared by another carbon.

H H
-C-C-
H H

Figure 1.1 below gives a good presentation of the way carbons and hydrogens are bonded to each other. Each C in the carbon chain diagram represents a carbon with 3 hydrogens at the end of the chain and with 2 hydrogens in the middle of the chain if there are no double bonds, or one hydrogen for each carbon that has a double bond. In the diagrams without the C shown, the point is understood to represent the C and its appropriate number of hydrogens. (See next page)

What Are Fatty Acids?

A *fatty acid* is an organic molecule made of a chain of carbon atoms. These chains come in varying lengths (1 to 24 carbon atoms) with a carboxyl (acid) group (COOH) at the end. Fatty acids can join with other compounds such as glycerol, cholesterol, etc. Fatty acids are given different names depending on the length of the carbon chain and the degree and position of unsaturation of the chain. Remember, each carbon in the middle of the chain has room for two hydrogens and the carbon at the very end of the chain has room for three hydrogens.

H H
-C-C-H
H H

The delta (Δ) symbol is used in designating the carbon number where a double bond is located along the fatty acid chain. For example, Δ-9 means that the double bond is located at the ninth carbon from the carboxyl end of the molecule as below. (See also Figure 1.8.)

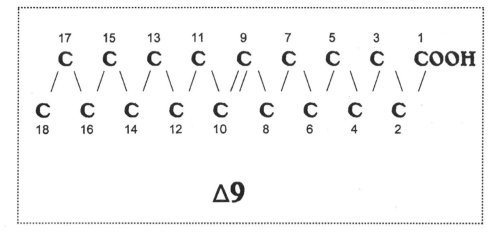

A fatty acid such as stearic acid (C18:0) can be shown like this:

H₃C-CH₂-CH₂-CH₂-CH₂-CH₂-CH₂-CH₂-CH₂-CH₂-CH₂-CH₂-CH₂-CH₂-CH₂-CH₂-CH₂-COOH

or like this:

H_3C-$(CH_2)_{16}$-COOH, Stearic acid, 18:0;

or it can be shown with or without the methyl (CH_3) end like this:

H₃C/\/\/\/\/\/\/\/\/COOH, Stearic Acid, 18:0

What About Saturated or Unsaturated or Isomers?

What is a *saturated fatty acid*? A fatty acid having no double bonds, i.e., having only single (-C-C-) bonds in the carbon chain, is a saturated fatty acid. If it is stearic acid, it is shown in abbreviated form as C18:0 where the zero indicates no double bond.

What is an *unsaturated fatty acid*? A fatty acid having at least one double (-C=C-) bond somewhere in the carbon chain is an unsaturated fatty acid. If only one bond is unsaturated it is called a *monounsaturated* fatty acid. Oleic acid is a monounsaturated fatty acid. A fatty acid having several double (-C=C-C-C=C-) bonds in the carbon chain is a *polyunsaturated fatty acid*. The essential fatty acids, linoleic acid and alpha-linolenic acid are polyunsaturated fatty acids. These bonds are shown in abbreviated labels as C18:1 (for one double bond), C18:2 (for two double bonds), etc.

What is an *isomer*? Single bonds can "wiggle" around so that the chain can "wag," but the double bonds cannot; they are held in a fixed position. The hydrogen atoms (**H**) attached to the carbon atoms (**C**) of the double bond, however, can be in one of two arrangements (isomers) relative to each other: both hydrogens can be on the same side of the bond (both on the head side or both on the feet side) or they can be opposite sides (head:foot). If they are both on the same side, they are called *cis* to each other. But if both hydrogens are on opposite sides, they are called *trans* to each other.

    H H
-C=C- *cis* unsaturated double bond

    H
-C=C- *trans* unsaturated double bond
      H

The bond geometry of several fatty acids is pictured in 2-dimensional drawings (2-D) in Figure 1.1. The top molecule is stearic acid, the middle molecule is oleic acid, and the lower molecule is the *trans* fatty acid elaidic acid.

The geometry of the glycerol molecule is shown below in a 2-D drawing, as a ball and stick 3-dimensional (3-D) molecule, and as a space-filling 3-D molecule.

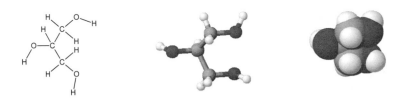

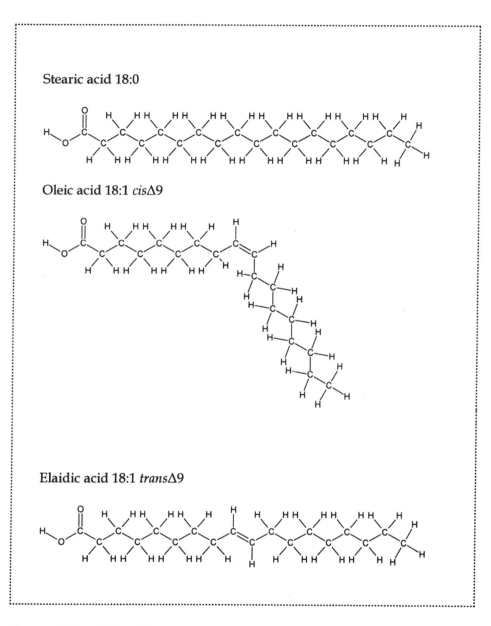

Figure 1.1 Basic Bond Geometry

Figure 1.2 gives a picture of a basic triglyceride. The fatty acids on this triglyceride are (clockwise starting at the upper right) palmitic acid (a saturated fatty acid), oleic acid (a monounsaturated fatty acid), and linoleic acid (a polyunsaturated fatty acid). These are very common fatty acids on typical triglycerides found in the original oils used in this country. There is almost always more palmitic acid than stearic acid in these oils and it is usually found attached to the position of the first carbon of the glycerol; linoleic acid is typically found attached to the second glycerol carbon and oleic acid and other fatty acids more often attached to the third carbon of the glycerol molecule.

If most of the fatty acids on the triglyceride are straight chains such as the saturated fatty acids or the *trans* **fatty acids**, the triglycerides can pack together into a crystalline structure that will form into a solid fat; if most of the fatty acids in the triglyceride molecule are curved chains as are the unsaturated fatty acids such as, oleic, linoleic, and linolenic acid, the triglycerides cannot pack together into crystals as readily and they will form into an oil instead.

Figure 1.3 pictures different triglycerides and how they fill space. From this we can imagine how they would pack together when they are in an oil or in a fat. The curved chains can not get as close together as the straight chains and they are the ones that form an oil instead of a crystalline solid.

These fatty acid structures, and those in later figures, are mostly shown as 3-dimensional space-filling models representative of a preferred conformation, usually thought of as the molecule at its lowest energy state. The structures have been drawn initially in 2-D, as shown in Figure 1.1, and then further developed with the 3-D optimization equations that are built into the chemical drawing software package, ACD/ChemSketch and ACD/3D Viewer (Version 4.0 for Microsoft Windows) from Advance Chemistry Development Inc, Toronto, Canada. A few of the structures are presented as 3-D stick models and they also have been drawn with the same computer program.

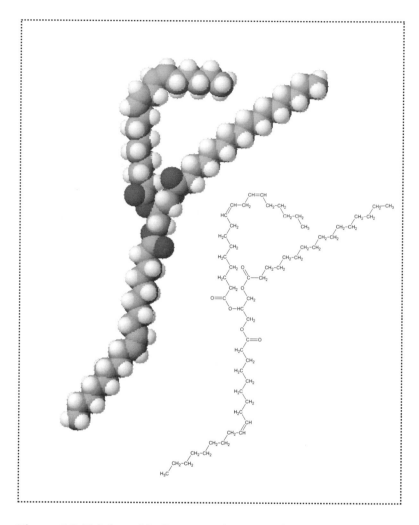

Figure 1.2 Triglyceride Structure in 2-D and 3-D

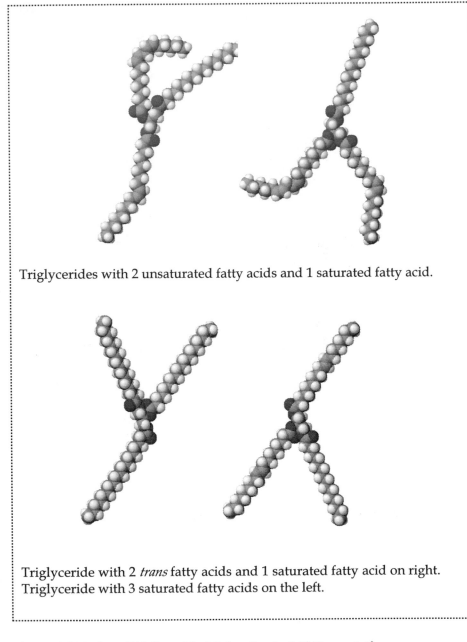

Triglycerides with 2 unsaturated fatty acids and 1 saturated fatty acid.

Triglyceride with 2 *trans* fatty acids and 1 saturated fatty acid on right. Triglyceride with 3 saturated fatty acids on the left.

Figure 1.3 Various Triglyceride Molecules in 3-D Presentation

How Many Triglycerides Are in a Common Measure?

The average triglyceride has a molecular weight of 865.9 grams/mole and a density of 0.91g/cc. You can use the molecular weight and Avogadro's number (6.022 x 10^{23} molecules/mole) to calculate the number of molecules in a given measure. If a tablespoon of oil has about 150 drops (this is the approximate number for a light oil), one drop will have approximately 63 quintillion (63 x 10^{18}) triglyceride molecules. You would need a really special electron microscope to see an individual triglyceride molecule.

Why Are the Oils Liquid and the Fats Solid?

Oils are liquid if they melt below ambient temperatures, and fats are solid if they do not melt at ambient temperatures. At the usual room temperatures in the United States, lamb tallow is one of the hardest fats, butter is a soft fat, chicken fat is almost liquid, lard can be a hard fat or a soft fat depending on what kind of a diet the animals ate, palm oil is a soft fat, and olive oil is a liquid. Canola, corn, cottonseed, peanut, safflower, soybean, or sunflower oils are very liquid *if* they have not been partially hydrogenated. Thus the natural fats range from very hard fats to very soft fats to viscous oils to liquid oils.

Whether these food lipids are called fats or oils sometimes depends on the ambient temperature where they originate. Palm oil and olive oils are fruit oils, and coconut oil is from a fruit, which is also a seed; they are liquids at the ambient temperature where they are produced. Palm kernel oil is a seed oil that is liquid in the tropics. Some of the oils like olive oil are very solid when they are stored in the refrigerator. Some like palm oil are separated into several semi-solid forms for use in foods. Figure 1.4 shows what these fats and oils look like at different temperatures. (See also Table 4.4 in Chapter 4 for melting temperatures of common fats and oils.)

The practice of calling animal fats "saturated" is not only misleading, it is just plain wrong. For example, beef fat is 54 percent **unsaturated**, lard is 60 percent **unsaturated**, and chicken fat is about 70 percent **unsaturated**. This makes these animal fats "less than half" saturated. Therefore, they really should be called unsaturated fats. In fact, none of the naturally occurring fats and oils is made up of *only* all saturated or all unsaturated fatty acids; rather they are mixtures of different amounts of various fatty acids. See Chapter 4 for a discussion of the physical characteristic of the individual fats and oils.

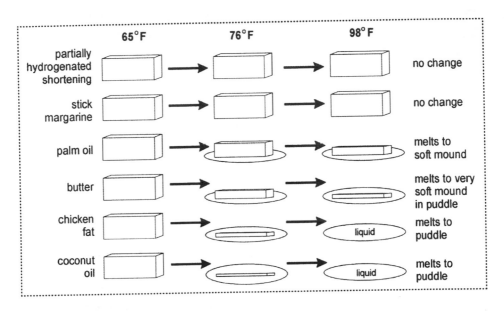

Figure 1.4 Melting Characteristics of Fats and Oils

Why are Animal Fats Called Saturated Fats?

These fats are called "saturated" because people have been misinformed and because they don't understand what the term saturated means when it is applied to edible fats and oils. When fats are totally "saturated," they are usually as hard as wax and they are not digested. When fats are almost totally unsaturated they are well digested, but they are very uncommon in the natural food supply. Totally unsaturated oils are nonexistent in the natural foods. (See Chapter 4)

How are Fats and Oils Processed?

Fats from animals are usually rendered, although they can be used in their unrendered form. The latter is the case when "suet" from beef or "fat back" from pork was used in cooking.

Typically, pork fat is wet rendered into lard and used as a bakery shortening. It is not normally deodorized because it does not have an objectionable odor or flavor. Sometimes it is partially hydrogenated to eliminate some of the unsaturated fatty acids.

Beef and lamb fat are dry rendered into tallow, for use as a frying fat. Because of its strong flavor, tallow is frequently deodorized unless the use requires the flavor to be retained. In the past, some tallows were used for french frying potatoes without deodorization. A traditional use of some of the fat from beef and lamb has been as finely chopped suet.

Poultry fat, especially chicken fat, is commonly rendered and used commercially in soups and in animal foods. A hundred years ago it was used for commercial baking.

Fats or oils from some seeds, such as sunflower, are extracted fresh from the seed by grinding of the seeds, followed by expeller pressing with or without a solvent such as hexane. Some seeds require precooking of the seeds before the grinding and the pressing. Rapeseed is such a seed.

Mechanical extraction is considered a safe method, but because the recovery of oil by this method is less than the industry desires, most oils are extracted using a solvent unless the oil is meant for a natural foods market. In this case, the oils are pressed from the seeds without the use of solvents, and without the increased yield. These oils are usually more costly in the marketplace.

The steps in commercial processing from the seed to the oil include crushing, extracting (by mechanical means or by use of solvents), degumming, neutralization, dewaxing, bleaching, filtration, and deodorization. Oils are frequently referred to as RBD, which stands for "refined, bleached, and deodorized." See also Chapter 4 and the Glossary.

Why Are Oils Partially Hydrogenated?

Most vegetable (primarily seed) oils cannot be used extensively for baking or deep fat frying unless they are changed from a liquid oil to a solid fat. You can cream a cup of fat into a cup of sugar and two cups of flour, and the resulting dough can be baked into a well-shaped cookie. If you try to substitute a cup of oil for the fat, you will be disappointed with the greasy flat "cookie." Foods that are fried in unrefined oil are also frequently greasy. The food industry knows that cookies and crackers, as well as cakes, pastries, and donuts have to be made with a fat at least as firm as a soft fat like lard or palm oil, so the industry changes the very liquid **oils**, such as soybean, corn, canola, cottonseed, and sometimes peanut oils and safflower oils, into **fats** by a process called

"partial hydrogenation."

These plastic, man-made fats are usually much firmer than the natural baking fats like lard and palm oil, and the baker can pack more of this fat into a product without producing a greasy feel. This is because these man-made fats have a wide range of high melting points for their individual triglyceride molecules, and even though they are very flexible, they hold their shape very well, and they don't melt at room temperature.

Oils such as soybean and canola that are going to be used by restaurants for deep frying do not need to be as solid as fats for baking, but they need to be stabilized by partial hydrogenation to prevent such undesirable problems as oxidation, polymerization, or heat damage. The result is what is called liquid shortening.

Some oils, such as cottonseed oil, have been traditionally used for frying potato chips and are not hydrogenated for this purpose. The limited amount of cottonseed oil available in the United States food supply precludes extensive usage.

Most oils cannot be substituted for butter as a spread, so they are partially hydrogenated to make solid spreads. You can churn cream for less than an hour and the result will be butter; but you could churn soybean oil or corn oil for years and you could not produce solid margarines, although you could produce something with the texture of mayonnaise if an emulsifier (e.g., cooked starch or egg) is added.

It is possible to make a margarine without partially hydrogenating the oil, and this has been done in Europe for a number of years using palm oil, palm kernel oil, or coconut oil because these oils have triglycerides that crystallize satisfactorily. There are also methods of making soft margarines out of other unhydrogenated oils, using a process called interesterification, and there has been at least one soft margarine marketed in Canada that was produced by this rather expensive process. The resulting product, however, is not very satisfactory to many people. There are also several spreads made with emulsifiers that use unhydrogenated liquid oils and a process similar to the one used for making mayonnaise. These spreads have not been widely available in the United States market until recently. There are more being sold in England and Canada at the present time than in the United States.

Just How Are Partially Hydrogenated Fats Different from the Original Oil?

Partial hydrogenation increases the degree of "saturation" of the fat by converting the polyunsaturated fatty acids into less unsaturated forms and differently unsaturated forms. In fact, a whole new class of fatty acids called *trans* fatty acids is formed. Sometimes these *trans* fatty acids have several unsaturated bonds in the *trans* configuration; sometimes the *trans* fatty acids have only one unsaturated bond in the *trans* configuration. But the *trans* fatty acids are mostly straight chains like the saturated fatty acids and they turn the formerly liquid oil into a solid "plastic" fat. If the new fat has *trans* fatty acids, there is proportionally less of the other fatty acids. Some of the partially hydrogenated fats in the United States have 50 percent or more of their fatty acids as *trans* fatty acids. Figure 1.5 shows how the process of partial hydrogenation changes the fatty acids in an oil that is intended for use in baked goods such as cookies, crackers, cakes, and pastries, as well as in snack chips.

Fats that have been partially hydrogenated have very, very long shelf life, unlike the original, highly unsaturated oils they were made from. The unsaturated oils can become rancid easily if they are not stored very carefully. The proneness to rancidity is due in part to the fact that some of the natural **antioxidants** usually found in the seed oils are lost when these seed oils are extracted with solvents, and since these oils are so highly unsaturated, they really need the antioxidant protection.

Some oils, like palm oil and olive oil when they are not extracted with solvents, contain high levels of many compounds that are natural antioxidants, and therefore they are well protected. Additionally, these two oils do not contain much of the highly unstable polyunsaturated fatty acids. This reactivity of the polyunsaturated fatty acids is the reason linseed oil makes a good drying oil for furniture. The gummy residue in salad bowls and frying pans is due to the polymers that are formed when the polyunsaturates are not adequately protected.

One of those common misstatements about hydrogenated fats and oils that we referred to in the introduction is the statement that hydrogenated soybean and cottonseed oils are not as highly saturated as palm, palm kernel, and coconut oil. However, these two oils (soybean and cottonseed) in their partially hydrogenated forms are often higher in long-chain "saturate-equivalents" (saturated fatty acids plus *trans* fatty acids, which are all 18 carbons long) after typical hydrogenation than are palm, palm kernel and coconut oils. Coconut and palm kernel oils have much lower levels of long-chain saturate-equivalents, since 65 percent of their fatty acids are medium-chain fatty acids. Palm oil is not usually partially hydrogenated and does not have any *trans* fatty acids.

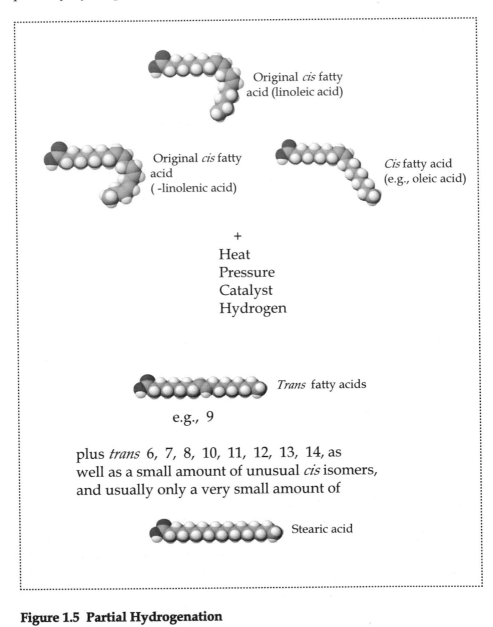

Original *cis* fatty acid (linoleic acid)

Original *cis* fatty acid (-linolenic acid)

Cis fatty acid (e.g., oleic acid)

+
Heat
Pressure
Catalyst
Hydrogen

Trans fatty acids

e.g., 9

plus *trans* 6, 7, 8, 10, 11, 12, 13, 14, as well as a small amount of unusual *cis* isomers, and usually only a very small amount of

Stearic acid

Figure 1.5 Partial Hydrogenation

Another common misstatement is that the only hydrogenation that increases saturates is hydrogenation of palm, palm kernel, coconut oil and animals fats. This is completely incorrect. Hydrogenating the so-called tropical oils hardly changes the levels of saturated fatty acids at all. Table D.1 in Appendix D gives the values for comparing the composition of different fats and oils.

As the reader will see later in this book, the natural long-chain saturated fatty acids and the *trans* fatty acids (long-chain saturate equivalents) produced by partial hydrogenation are equivalent in their physical properties in food manufacturing and food preparation. They act and react, however, very differently from each other in biological systems. Because of their equivalent physical properties, these fatty acids can be used interchangeably in many foods. Nonetheless, the differences in their actions in biological systems lends a critical spin to their unqualified acceptance or rejection.

What Is Meant by the Terms Saturated, Monounsaturated, Polyunsaturated, and *Trans*?

Fats are made up of several different classes of fatty acids. In naturally-occurring fats there are basically three major classes of fatty acids. One class of fatty acids, the saturated fatty acids, should really be divided into two or three separate subclasses, i.e., short-, medium- and long-chain. The second class is called monounsaturates. The third class is called polyunsaturates. There is also a fourth category of fatty acids, the *trans* fatty acids, which do not really belong with the naturally-occurring monounsaturates or polyunsaturates. Figure 1.6 presents the classification of fats in a chart that should make it easy for the reader to recognize the category to which the different fats belong.

In the fats and oils terminology, "unsaturated" equals "double bonds" and "saturated" equals "no double bonds." Another important aspect of the "double bonds" involves the geometry of those bonds. The naturally-occurring monounsaturated and polyunsaturated bonds are "*cis*" double bonds with the hydrogens that belong to the double bond on the same side of the molecule. The chemically-altered "monoun-saturated" and "polyunsaturated" bonds are "*trans*" double bonds with their hydrogens (for the double bonds) on opposite sides of the molecule. The former geometry (i.e., *cis*) introduces one or more permanent bends in the fatty acid molecule. The latter geometry (i.e., *trans*) straightens the fatty acid molecule.

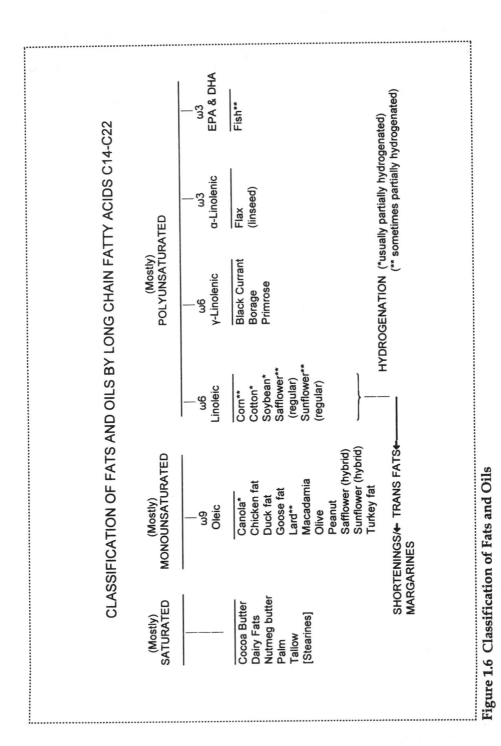

Figure 1.6 Classification of Fats and Oils

What is Meant by the Term Omega?

Fatty acids also are identified by the "families" to which they belong. Families differ from classes, and the term "families" uses the word "omega" for its descriptor. The Greek symbol "ω" is omega, and it will sometimes be used. Figures 1.7 through 1.10 give examples of these various families and will list the fatty acids that are formed from the first fatty acid in the family to the last most common fatty acid in the family. You will notice that the title of each of the figures refers to an n-9, n-7, n-6, and n-3, and then tells you in the table that the n-9 is also called the omega-9 or ω-9. This is because technically, these families are designated by the "n-" in the nomenclature (naming and numbering) in the newer chemical literature. The older literature used "omega" and now much of the popular literature is using omega. So, if you see the term n-3 in an article or book about fats and oils, realize that what is meant is omega-3.

As noted above, fatty acids are molecules with a carbon chain, and they have two ends. One end has a methyl group, and the other end has a carboxyl group. The term "omega" refers to the methyl end of a fatty acid. Thus "omega oxidation" refers to the oxidation of a fatty acid that starts at the methyl end of a fatty acid. The other end of the fatty acid is the carboxyl end, and oxidation from that end is called "beta(β)-oxidation" because the oxidation begins with the second (beta) carbon of the fatty acid chain.

Omega is also used to designate unsaturated fatty acid families. Saturated fatty acid families do not have an omega designation. Omega-3 refers to the family of fatty acids in which the first *cis* double bond (unsaturation) closest to the methyl end is in the 3rd position. Omega-6 refers to the family of fatty acids where the first *cis* double bond closest to the methyl end is in the 6th position. Omega-9 refers to the first *cis* double bond appearing in the 9th position.

There are numerous omega-3 fatty acids with varying numbers of *cis* double bonds ranging from three to six depending on how long they are. The basic omega-3 fatty acid has 3 double bonds, it is 18 carbons long, it is called alpha-linolenic acid, and it is an **"essential"** fatty acid, i.e., it cannot be produced in the human body but must be provided in the diet.

There are numerous omega-6 fatty acids with varying numbers of *cis* double bonds ranging from two to six depending on how long they are. The omega-6 fatty acid with 2 double bonds is 18 carbons long, is called linoleic acid, and is an essential fatty acid.

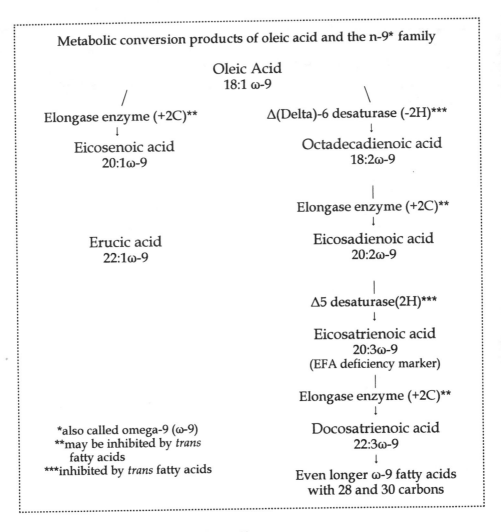

Metabolic conversion products of oleic acid and the n-9* family

Oleic Acid
18:1 ω-9

Elongase enzyme (+2C)**

Eicosenoic acid
20:1ω-9

Δ(Delta)-6 desaturase (-2H)***

Octadecadienoic acid
18:2ω-9

Elongase enzyme (+2C)**

Eicosadienoic acid
20:2ω-9

Erucic acid
22:1ω-9

Δ5 desaturase(2H)***

Eicosatrienoic acid
20:3ω-9
(EFA deficiency marker)

Elongase enzyme (+2C)**

*also called omega-9 (ω-9)
**may be inhibited by *trans*
   fatty acids
***inhibited by *trans* fatty acids

Docosatrienoic acid
22:3ω-9

Even longer ω-9 fatty acids
with 28 and 30 carbons

Figure 1.7 Omega-9 Fatty Acid Family

The omega-9 fatty acid is not essential because the body can make it. Oleic acid is an omega-9 fatty acid. Palmitoleic acid, a 16 carbon monounsaturated fatty acid, is an omega-7 fatty acid. In the omega-9 family, oleic acid is either elongated or desaturated as a first step. When it is desaturated, it gains a double bond and is then elongated to make a 20 carbon fatty acid with 2 double bonds, which is then desaturated again to form eicosatrienoic acid. This 20 carbon fatty acid with 3 double bonds is called the Mead acid (or Mead's acid), and it was named after James Mead, a lipids researcher at the University of California at Los Angeles (UCLA), who first identified it. When its level is increased in the body, it is a marker of essential fatty acid deficiency. Some people have mistakenly considered it a sign that the body can make its own essential fatty acids. The Mead acid, however, is not an essential fatty acid. In fact, it is an example of the need for the essential fatty acids because eicosatrienoic acid does not convert into the prostaglandins that the body needs. See section on Essential Fatty Acids.

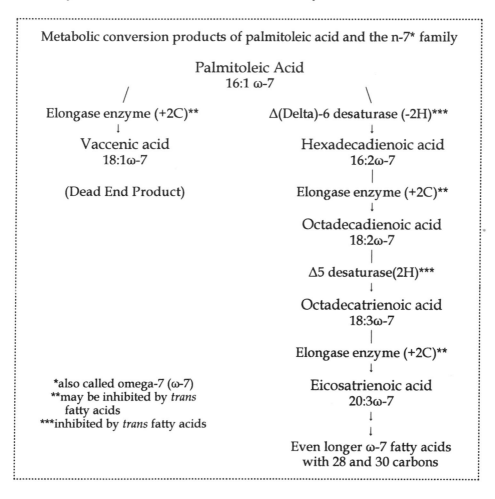

Figure 1.8 Omega-7 Fatty Acid Family

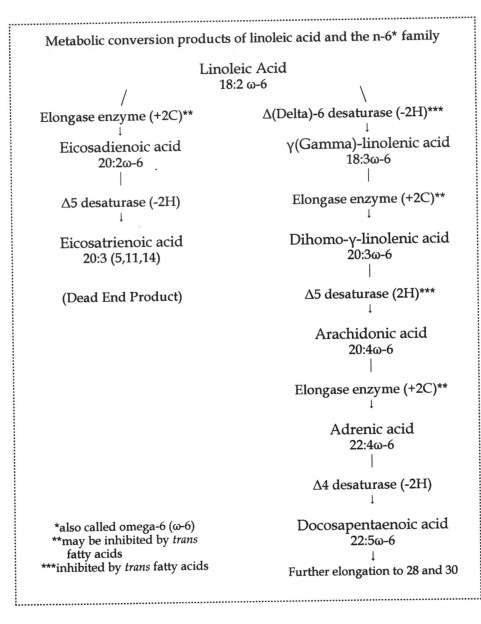

Metabolic conversion products of linoleic acid and the n-6* family

Linoleic Acid
18:2 ω-6

Elongase enzyme (+2C)**   Δ(Delta)-6 desaturase (-2H)***

Eicosadienoic acid   γ(Gamma)-linolenic acid
20:2ω-6   18:3ω-6

Δ5 desaturase (-2H)   Elongase enzyme (+2C)**

Eicosatrienoic acid   Dihomo-γ-linolenic acid
20:3 (5,11,14)   20:3ω-6

(Dead End Product)   Δ5 desaturase (2H)***

                                           Arachidonic acid
                                           20:4ω-6

                                           Elongase enzyme (+2C)**

                                           Adrenic acid
                                           22:4ω-6

                                           Δ4 desaturase (-2H)

*also called omega-6 (ω-6)   Docosapentaenoic acid
**may be inhibited by *trans*   22:5ω-6
    fatty acids
***inhibited by *trans* fatty acids   Further elongation to 28 and 30

Figure 1.9 Omega-6 Fatty Acid Family

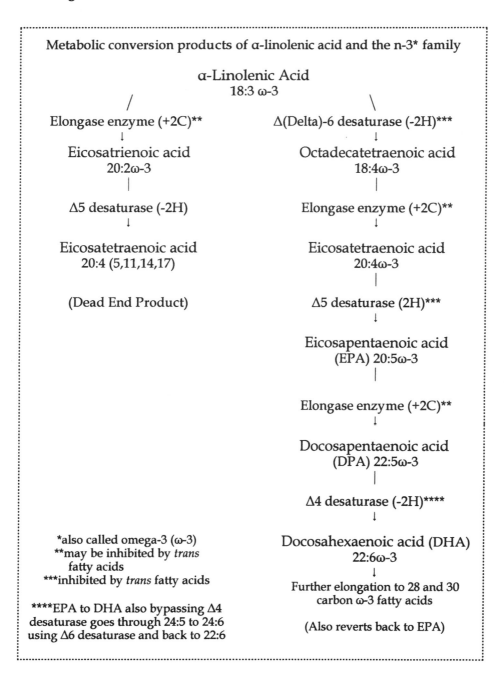

Metabolic conversion products of α-linolenic acid and the n-3* family

α-Linolenic Acid
18:3 ω-3

Elongase enzyme (+2C)**   Δ(Delta)-6 desaturase (-2H)***

Eicosatrienoic acid   Octadecatetraenoic acid
20:2ω-3   18:4ω-3

Δ5 desaturase (-2H)   Elongase enzyme (+2C)**

Eicosatetraenoic acid   Eicosatetraenoic acid
20:4 (5,11,14,17)   20:4ω-3

(Dead End Product)   Δ5 desaturase (2H)***

                                 Eicosapentaenoic acid
                                 (EPA) 20:5ω-3

                                 Elongase enzyme (+2C)**

                                 Docosapentaenoic acid
                                 (DPA) 22:5ω-3

                                 Δ4 desaturase (-2H)****

*also called omega-3 (ω-3)   Docosahexaenoic acid (DHA)
**may be inhibited by *trans*   22:6ω-3
  fatty acids
***inhibited by *trans* fatty acids   Further elongation to 28 and 30
                                 carbon ω-3 fatty acids
****EPA to DHA also bypassing Δ4
desaturase goes through 24:5 to 24:6   (Also reverts back to EPA)
using Δ6 desaturase and back to 22:6

Figure 1.10 Omega-3 Fatty Acid Family

Saturated Fatty Acids

The **saturated** fatty acids are not all the same. They come in different lengths. The shorter ones, with chain lengths from three to twelve carbons, of the type found in butter, coconut oil, and palm kernel oil, have much lower melting points than the more common longer chain saturated fatty acids. Most texts refer to them as short-chain if they are less than 8 or 10 carbons long, and medium-chain if they are 10 to 12 carbons long. Some lipids researchers consider the 14 carbon fatty acid, myristic acid, a medium-chain fatty acid and some researchers consider it a long-chain fatty acid.

When these **shorter-chain saturated fatty acids** are used by the body for energy, they do not produce as many calories as the longer chain fatty acids. That is why there are fewer kilocalories in a pound of butter than in a pound of margarine made with seed oils. Not a lot less -- only 8 kilocalories per pound to be exact -- but most people have been wrongly led to believe that butter has more calories than regular margarine. A pound of coconut oil or palm kernel oil has 100 kilocalories less than a pound of soybean oil.

The short-chain saturated fatty acids are **propanoic acid** (3 carbons), **butyric acid** (4 carbons), and **caproic acid** (6 carbons).

Medium-chain saturated fatty acids are found in several different foods. In the form of medium chain triglyceride oils (called MCT oils), they are used in special medical formulas for people who need the energy from fat, but who cannot absorb the longer chain fatty acids.

The complete set of medium-chain fatty acids, which are not found in commercially available MCT oils, are especially important in infant formulas where they duplicate the medium-chain saturated fatty acids found in human milk; especially the 12 carbon saturated fatty acid, lauric acid, that functions as a special antimicrobial (antiviral, antibacterial, and antiprotozoal) fatty acid in human milk. Until just recently, the only practical commercial source of these medium-chain saturated fatty acids was coconut oil and palm kernel oil. Recently, the U.S. domestic oil industry developed a genetically-engineered canola oil called "laurate canola," which is a source of some of the medium-chain fatty acids. (See Chapter 4 for information on the individual fats and oils.)

The medium-chain saturated fatty acids are **caprylic acid** (8 carbons), **capric acid** (10 carbons), and **lauric acid** (12 carbons). (Some fats and oils experts also consider myristic acid (14 carbons) a medium-chain saturated fatty acid, but it is generally included with long-chain saturated fatty acids in tables.) (See the General Glossary for details of these fatty acids.)

These short- and medium-chain saturated fatty acids are not deposited to any extent in the adipose tissue. They are also not usually found on the chylomicrons unless they are consumed in relatively large amounts. (Chylomicrons are the special carriers in the blood that take the fat that people absorb through the lymph system and the blood stream to the liver, the adipose, and other tissues. See Chapter 2)

The **longer-chain saturated fatty acids**, range from 14 to 24 carbons. Palmitic acid with 16 carbons and stearic acid with 18 carbons are the most common of the saturated fatty acids in food. Humans and other animals make palmitic acid and stearic acid out of carbohydrates and protein, and these two saturated fatty acids are changed into both 16 and 18 carbon monounsaturated fatty acids to maintain desirable physiological balances. The palmitic acid that man eats can end up as oleic acid because the liver and other tissues add two more carbons and turn palmitic acid into stearic acid, which in turn can become oleic acid through a special function called desaturation that puts a double bond into the molecule, causing it to bend. Palmitic acid is the major fatty acid in normal lung surfactant. The very long-chain saturated fatty acids (20 to 24 carbons) are membrane fatty acids found especially in the brain.

The long-chain saturated fatty acids are **myristic acid** (14 carbons), **palmitic acid** (16 carbons), **stearic acid** (18 carbons), **arachidic acid** (20 carbons), **behenic acid** (22 carbons), and **lignoceric acid** (24 carbons). (See the General Glossary for details of these fatty acids)

Figure 1.11 shows a series of common saturated fatty acids typical of the kind found in both food and the body tissues. These include capric acid (10 carbons with no double bonds, i.e., C10:0), lauric acid (C12:0), myristic acid (C14:0), palmitic acid (C16:0), stearic acid (C18:0), arachidic acid (C20:0), and behenic acid (C22:0).

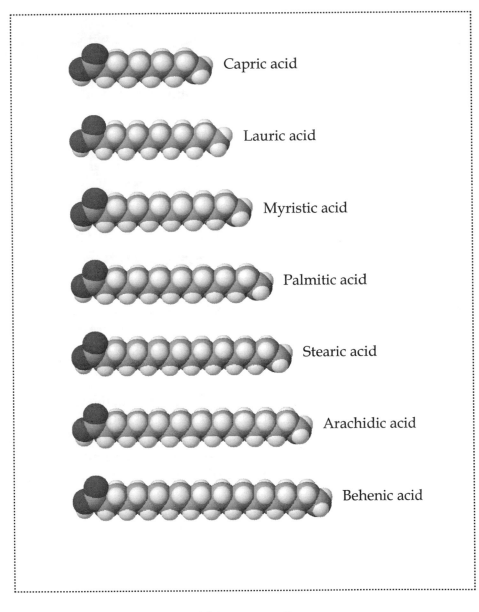

Capric acid

Lauric acid

Myristic acid

Palmitic acid

Stearic acid

Arachidic acid

Behenic acid

Figure 1.11 Common Fatty Acid Structures: Saturates

Unsaturated Fatty Acids

Figure 1.12 is shown on two pages and pictures a series of common unsaturated fatty acids. These fatty acids all have one or more *cis* double bonds and they include monounsaturated fatty acids palmitoleic acid (C16:1) and oleic acid (C18:1), followed by the polyunsaturated fatty acids linoleic acid (C18:2), γ-linolenic acid (C18:3), α-linolenic acid (C18:3), arachidonic acid (C20:4), eicosapentaenoic acid (C20:5), and docosahexaenoic acid (C22:6). Docosahexaenoic acid is shown in two views; the second view is a spiral view where the methyl end (tail) is tucked behind the carboxyl group.

Examples of fatty acids with one double bond, two double bonds, three double bonds, four double bonds, five double bonds, and six double bonds are shown below in the 2-D form.

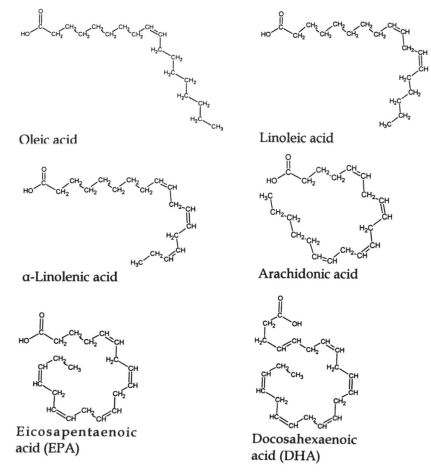

Oleic acid

Linoleic acid

α-Linolenic acid

Arachidonic acid

Eicosapentaenoic acid (EPA)

Docosahexaenoic acid (DHA)

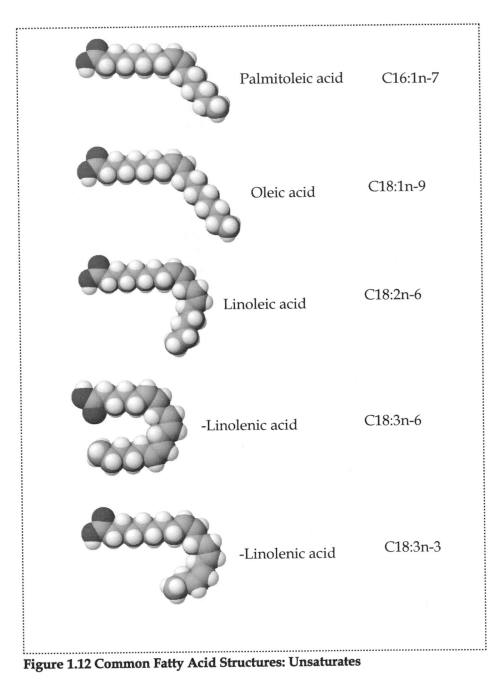

Palmitoleic acid   C16:1n-7

Oleic acid   C18:1n-9

Linoleic acid   C18:2n-6

-Linolenic acid   C18:3n-6

-Linolenic acid   C18:3n-3

Figure 1.12 Common Fatty Acid Structures: Unsaturates

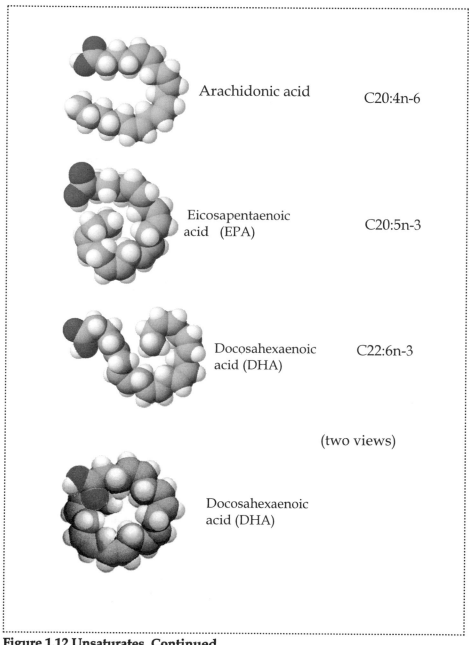

Arachidonic acid C20:4n-6

Eicosapentaenoic acid (EPA) C20:5n-3

Docosahexaenoic acid (DHA) C22:6n-3

(two views)

Docosahexaenoic acid (DHA)

Figure 1.12 Unsaturates Continued

Monounsaturated Fatty Acids

The **monounsaturated** fatty acids are found in 14, 16, 18, 20 , 22 and 24 carbon lengths, but by far the most common is the 18 carbon monoun-saturate, oleic acid. The best known source of oleic acid in oils has been olive oil, although there are oils from foods such as avocado and nuts such as hazelnut (filbert) that have inherently higher levels of oleic acid than olive oil (See Chapter 4). More recently, the low-erucic acid rapeseed oil known as canola oil has become a popular source of oleic acid. New high-oleic varieties of safflower oil and sunflower oil are starting to come onto the scene. A new variety of palm oil also has been grown that produces a high-oleic oil. Many animal fats such as lard and tallow are high in oleic acid. See Figure 1.13 for a list of high-oleic acid fats and oils.

It should be noted that the fatty acid oleic acid is the same oleic acid whether it comes from olive oil (or any other plant oil) or dairy fat (or any other animal fat). The same holds true for any of the saturated fatty acids or polyunsaturated fatty acids. The saturated fatty acid palmitic acid is the same saturated fatty acid whether it is found in soybean or canola oil or in palm oil or in any animal fat.

The 16 carbon monounsaturate, palmitoleic acid, is formed when an unsaturated bond is placed in palmitic acid, or by taking away 2 carbons from oleic acid. The former is made by a mechanism called desaturation, and the latter by a mechanism called "chain-shortening". Palmitoleic acid is found in all animal and fish fats, especially chicken fats, and is an identifying marker of an animal fat. Vegetable oils usually contain less than 1 percent palmitoleic, but pork fat (lard) usually has 3-4 percent and chicken fat has 6-8 percent. One exception in the vegetable fats is macadamia nuts with approximately 20 percent palmitoleic acid. Palmitoleic acid is one of the fatty acids that the body uses as an antimicrobial fatty acid. The pathways showing the elongated fatty acids in the omega-9 and omega-7 families (which start with monounsaturated fatty acids) are depicted in Figures 1.7 and 1.8 above.

```
┌────────────────────────────────────────────────────────────────────────┐
  Fats and Oils Whose Major Fatty Acid is Oleic Acid

                    (% of total fatty acids)

  Animal Fats                       Vegetable Oils
  Beef tallow (48)                  Canola, rapeseed (56)*
  Butter (29)                       Olive (78)
  Chicken (36)                      Palm olein (43)
  Egg (50)                          Peanut (45)*
  Human milk (36)                   Safflower, high oleic (74)*
  Lard (44)                         Sunflower, high oleic (81)*


  * Only if unhydrogenated
└────────────────────────────────────────────────────────────────────────┘
```

Figure 1.13 High-Oleic Fats and Oils

Rapeseed and mustard oils are known as common sources of the 22 carbon monounsaturate, erucic acid. Fish oils are also sources of the 20 carbon monounsaturates gadoleic and gondoic acids, and the 22 carbon monounsatuate cetoleic acid. The fish oils that are partially hydrogenated are also sources of 20 and 22 carbon monounsaturated fatty acids, which are not the same as the original gadoleic acid or erucic acid (see section on *trans* fatty acids.)

The dominant naturally occurring monounsaturated fatty acids are **myristoleic** acid (14 carbons), **palmitoleic acid** (16 carbons), **oleic acid and vaccenic acid** (18 carbons), **gadoleic acid** and **gondoic acid** (20 carbons), **cetoleic acid** (22 carbons), **erucic acid** (22 carbons), and **nervonic acid** (24 carbons). (See General Glossary for details of these fatty acids)

Polyunsaturated Fatty Acids

The **polyunsaturated** fatty acids are usually found in 18, 20, and 22 carbon lengths. The best known are the "omega-6" fatty acids, linoleic, gamma[γ]-linolenic, and arachidonic acids, and the "omega-3" fatty acids, alpha[α]-linolenic, eicosapentaenoic (EPA) and docosahexaenoic (DHA) acids. As noted above, they are called omega-6 and omega-3 to designate the position of the first double bond relative to the omega end of the fatty acid as opposed to the carboxyl end of the fatty acid. These fatty acid families are shown in Figures 1.9 and 1.10.

Linoleic acid is commonly known as "the essential fatty acid." It is 18 carbons long and has 2 double bonds. Arachidonic acid is 20 carbons long and has 4 double bonds. Arachidonic acid is not technically considered essential because the properly functioning body can supposedly make all the arachidonic acid it needs out of linoleic acid. Linoleic acid cannot be made by animals and must be supplied by foods on a regular basis. All unhydrogenated seed oils are good sources of linoleic acid. Arachidonic acid is found in animal fats, especially pork. (Some text books have erroneously said that arachidonic acid is found in peanut oil. It is not. What is actually found in peanut oil is a 20 carbon saturated fatty acid sometimes called *arachidic* acid.)

The other known essential fatty acid is α-linolenic acid. This fatty acid is the precursor to the 20 and 22 carbon "omega-3" fatty acids popularly called EPA and DHA. The best known most concentrated sources of α-linolenic acid are unhydrogenated flax oil (65 percent), unhydrogenated and unrefined canola oil (10-15 percent) or unhydrogenated and unrefined soybean (6 to 10 percent) oils, but many green leaves that are commonly eaten are adequate sources of this fatty acid. Lesser known oils such as perilla oil and hemp oil also contain about 60 percent α-linolenic acid. Corn oil and cottonseed oil have very little α-linolenic acid. Unhydrogenated fish oils are the best sources of EPA (up to 18 percent) and DHA (up to 13 percent), although small amounts are found in some animal fats and some egg yolks.

The essential fatty acids are precursors for the special hormone-like substances known as eicosanoids such as prostaglandins. Prostaglandins are potent regulators of metabolism both in health and disease. (See **Chapter 2** for discussion of essential fatty acids and prostaglandins.)

The polyunsaturated fatty acids are: **linoleic acid** (18 carbons), **gamma-linolenic acid** (18 carbons), **alpha-linolenic acid** (18 carbons), **dihomo-gamma-linolenic acid** (20 carbons), **arachidonic acid** (20 carbons), **eicosapentaenoic acid** (20 carbons), **docosapentaenoic acid** (22 carbons), **clupanodonic acid** (22 carbons), and **docosahexaenoic acid** (22 carbons). (See **General Glossary** for details of these fatty acids)

Trans Fatty Acids

The *trans* **fatty acids** are found in very minor amounts (usually less than 2 percent but sometimes up to 5 percent of the total fat) in all of the ruminant fats (antelope, buffalo, cow, deer, goat, sheep), but they are found in major amounts (as much as 50 to 60 percent or more of the total fat) in the partially hydrogenated vegetable oils. These fatty acids are usually 18 carbons long.

Actually the kinds of *trans* fatty acids found in ruminant fats differ considerably from those found in partially hydrogenated vegetable oils because of the average placement of the *trans* double bonds. The major *trans* fatty acids in ruminant fats have the double bond in the Δ-11 position. This 18 carbon fatty acid has been given the name of *trans*-vaccenic acid and it is a precursor to conjugated linoleic acid (CLA), which is reported to be anticarcinogenic (Chin et al 1992). (See section on **conjugated linoleic acid** below.)

The major *trans* fatty acids in the partially hydrogenated vegetable fats have their double bonds in the delta(Δ)-8,-9,-10,-11, and -12 positions. The *trans* Δ-9 position has been identified as a health problem fatty acid by much research. The common name given this 18 carbon *trans* fatty acid is elaidic acid. Health questions about the *trans* Δ-10 and *trans* Δ-12 have also been raised. The combined *trans* Δ-9,-10, and -12 usually make up half or more of the total *trans* in partially hydrogenated vegetable oils. These same *trans* usually make up about one fifth of the total *trans* in ruminant fats.

Figure 1.14 pictures the typical *trans* fatty acid structures, and these are all 18 carbons long with the *trans* double bond in different places as indicated. There are some *trans* fatty acids with more than one *trans* bond, and they are also usually 18 carbons long. They have not been pictured in this figure. Generally there are not nearly as many of these *trans* fatty acids in fats like the margarines and shortenings. They are, however, sometimes found in partially hydrogenated oils in amounts of several percent of the total fatty acids.

The *trans* fatty acids found in hydrogenated fish oils are 14, 16, 18, 20 and 22 carbons long with varying numbers of *trans* double bonds all along the fatty acid chains. There are many more different kinds of *trans* fatty acids in partially hydrogenated fish oils than in any other partially hydrogenated fat.

Although *trans* fatty acids are unsaturated fatty acids by chemical definition, they cannot be legally designated monounsaturates or poly-unsaturates for the purpose of food labeling in the United States, in Canada, or in Great Britain (U.K.). In the United States, authorities in the F.D.A. had early on recognized that the *trans* polyunsaturated fatty acids were *not* biologically equivalent to the *cis* polyunsaturated fatty acids, and that they could not function as essential fatty acids. (Recall that essential fatty acids are used in the body to form important hormone-like regulators of metabolism called *prostaglandins*. For complete discussion see section on prostaglandins in Chapter 2).

Prior to the new labeling law in the United States, the *trans* fatty acids could not have been legally included in the fat labeled as polyunsaturates, and no provision existed at that time for determining that the monounsaturates could not be *trans*. (See Chapter 5 for more discussion on labeling issues.)

Originally the U.K. had issued regulations to add the *trans* fatty acids to the saturates for labeling purposes since it had been decided (by the COMA committee of the Ministry of Health) that the function of the *trans* fatty acids was the same as that of the saturated fatty acids. Then, in January 1988, the *trans* fatty acids were put into their own separate category for labeling purposes. Since the research published from 1990 and afterward clearly showed that the *trans* fatty acids do behave differently than saturated fatty acids, the move to place them in their own category was fortuitous.

In Canada the *trans* fatty acids are considered the equivalent of saturated fatty acids for the purposes of determining the balance of essential fatty acids needed in special formula diets. Some fats and oils researchers in Canada and the United States had gone on record to state that *trans* fatty acids are the equivalent of saturated fatty acids. Some representatives of the edible oil industry do not want the *trans* fatty acids to be identified; they would like to pretend that the *trans* fatty acids are like oleic acid even though all the properly conducted research studies show that *trans* fatty acids are unlike oleic acid in every function. Some members of the edible oil industry prefer to compare the *trans* fatty acids only to stearic acid when confronted with the statement that the *trans* behave "like saturates." The *trans* fatty acids do **not** behave like saturated fatty acids in biological systems although they do behave like numerous saturated fatty acids in food preparation. (See Chapter 2 for discussion of differences between saturated fatty acids and *trans* fatty acids in biological systems.)

The *trans* fatty acids from commercial partial hydrogenation that have been added to our diets in ever increasing amounts during the latter part of the 20th Century have been aptly termed by some as "molecular misfits." (See Chapter V, Labeling Fats and Oils for the Marketplace.)

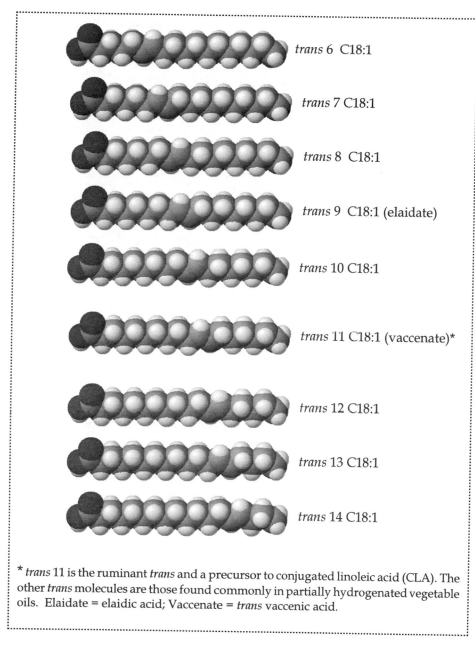

trans 6 C18:1

trans 7 C18:1

trans 8 C18:1

trans 9 C18:1 (elaidate)

trans 10 C18:1

trans 11 C18:1 (vaccenate)*

trans 12 C18:1

trans 13 C18:1

trans 14 C18:1

* *trans* 11 is the ruminant *trans* and a precursor to conjugated linoleic acid (CLA). The other *trans* molecules are those found commonly in partially hydrogenated vegetable oils. Elaidate = elaidic acid; Vaccenate = *trans* vaccenic acid.

Figure 1.14 Common *trans* Fatty Acid Structures

Why Do We Need to Know about the *Trans* Fatty Acids?

When people eat fats containing *trans* fatty acids, these fatty acids are deposited in varying amounts in some of the tissues, and they have an effect on the way the organs in the body function. For some people, eating margarines with high *trans* levels raises their serum cholesterol levels 20 mg percent (mg/dl) (e.g., from 220 mg percent to 240 mg percent) more than does a margarine with a lower *trans* level.

Feeding partially hydrogenated fats to pigs causes the serum HDL cholesterol (the so-called good cholesterol) to be decreased in a dose-response manner. These *trans* fatty acids also make pig's platelets more "sticky." Since pigs are considered an ideal animal model for studying dietary effects of importance to human health, these findings have important implications for humans.

Feeding *trans* fatty acids from partially hydrogenated vegetable oils to adult humans lowers HDL cholesterol and raises lipoprotein [a]. Feeding human infants with milk containing *trans* fatty acids that came in through the mother's diet causes a significant decrease in visual acuity.

See the next section for more details on the effects of *trans* fatty acids in the diet.

What Do Research Studies Say about the *Trans* Fatty Acids?

Several research studies have been conducted with humans to measure the effect of *trans* fatty acids on serum cholesterol, which also included HDL cholesterol. The first study was published in August 1990 in *The New England Journal of Medicine* and the Dutch researchers reported that feeding *trans* fatty acids did lower HDL cholesterol in humans in addition to raising LDL cholesterol and total serum cholesterol. The same kind of study was completed in 1992 by the human nutrition laboratory of USDA. In this industry-sponsored feeding study using lower levels of *trans* fatty acids, the same results, i.e., lowering of HDL cholesterol, were reported. Further research in this government laboratory has shown (in 1998) that the lowering of the HDL cholesterol is statistically significant, and therefore very troublesome. Another kind of study from a government laboratory in the U.K. reported that *trans* fatty acids caused blood platelet adhesiveness (stickiness).

Each time another study is reported, we see that the results are the same. The HDL cholesterol is significantly decreased, the LDL cholesterol is increased, and the more recent studies have shown that the heart disease marker called Lipoprotein [a] (Lp[a]) is increased, especially in people who already have high levels of this lipoprotein. Interestingly enough, saturated fatty acids lower Lp[a], so an adequate amount of saturated fatty acids in the diet is a good thing to have.

When monkeys are fed *trans-* containing margarine in their diets, their red blood cells do not bind insulin as well as when they are not fed the *trans* fatty acids. Research has shown that consuming *trans* fatty acids raises the blood sugar levels and causes people to weigh several kilograms more that people consuming the same amount of fat that is not hydrogenated. This means that people who have a tendency to develop diabetes will be made more likely to respond poorly to *trans* fatty acids in their diets and be pushed in the direction of developing diabetes.

When lactating animals are fed fats containing *trans* fatty acids, they produce milk that has significantly lower cream volume and consequently has lower nutrient density. There is some evidence that the same thing happens to human mothers. When the researchers have examined the fat in milk that mothers are producing, they have found up to 17 percent of the fatty acids as *trans* fatty acids. That is very high, but when they measured the levels in mothers who were not eating foods with *trans* fatty acids, the levels were so low that they found less than 1 percent. Further, when researchers examined the visual acuity of the babies who received *trans* fatty acids from their mother's milk, the higher levels of *trans* fatty acids were noted to produce significantly lower visual acuity scores at 14 months.

Many of the reproductive functions are changed in animals or people fed *trans* fatty acids relative to those who are not fed *trans* fatty acids. For example, male animals have much lower levels of testosterone in their blood when they are fed *trans* fatty acids and they produce significantly more abnormal spermatozoa. Female animals showed altered gestation patterns when they were fed *trans* fatty acids.

How important these changes in reproduction are for humans is not really known because *none* of the studies that have been done to compare the kinds of fats people eat with their health status have ever addressed this particular issue. However, several recent studies in Europe showed that low birth weight infants had more *trans* fatty acids in their cord blood because their mothers were consuming *trans* fatty acids in foods. The same researchers reported that the critical very long-chain omega-3 polyunsaturated fatty acids were lost from the important membranes in the brain when there was evidence that the mothers consumed *trans* fatty acids.

Large United States government studies such as the big National Health and Nutrition Examination Survey (NHANES), the USDA Food Consumption Survey, or the Lipid Research Clinics did not include any *trans* fatty acid data in their data banks. For that matter none of these big surveys had really accurate data for any of the fatty acid classes, including saturated, monounsaturated, or polyunsaturated fatty acids.

As should be apparent to everyone, *if you do not have the trans fatty acid numbers accounted for in the data bases, the other fatty acid numbers are all wrong for all of the foods that contain fats and oils that are partially hydrogenated.* This statement is true for a lot of foods because approximately 70 percent of all the vegetable oils used in foods such as crackers, cookies, pastries, cakes, snack chips, imitation cheese, candies, or fried foods are partially hydrogenated. This means that we really don't know what kind of fatty acid patterns people are consuming, so we certainly don't know whether the people with certain adverse health patterns consume more or less of any given class of fatty acids than those people without the adverse health patterns.

All the rhetoric not-with-standing, we really do not know if, as adults, eating 50 percent of our fat as saturated fatty acids (this is the percentage that is found in human milk) causes any health problem or relieves any health problem *because we have never measured the dietary intake of the different fatty acid classes accurately!* However, when we have looked at what the fats were in our diets from the historical perspective, we don't find any problems with the natural fats that have been around for eons, and these diets were high in natural saturated fatty acids, and the only *trans* fatty acids in the diets were the small amount present in the ruminant fats. (See Chapter 3 for a discussion about this issue.)

But How Much *Trans* Do We Really Eat?

More than you realize. Over the years between the late 1970s and the late 1990s, when foods have been analyzed for *trans* fatty acid content, they have been found to have similar levels because the partial hydrogenation process was relatively consistent in its formation of *trans* fatty acids for different uses.

For example, one large order of french fried potatoes deep fried in partially hydrogenated soybean oil has 8-9 grams of *trans*. One tablespoon of a very popular margarine has 4.6 grams of *trans*, although there are some margarines that have been made with either low levels of *trans* or no *trans* fatty acids.

All the commercial shortenings made with partially hydrogenated soybean oil have 25-50 percent of the fat as *trans* fatty acids. Commercial shortenings made with partially hydrogenated canola oils have the same or even higher levels of *trans* fatty acids. This means that the fat ingredient in all those cookies, crackers, donuts, cakes, breadings, frostings, puddings, is between one-quarter and one-half *trans* fatty acids.

Typical snack chips can have as much as 6 grams of *trans* fatty acids in a 42 gram package, an 85 gram snack package of soft batch cookies is 7 grams of *trans* fatty acids, and a 78 gram snack pack of chocolate chip cookies had 11.5 grams *trans* fatty acids, and the snack pack of a popular brand of pecan cookies had 10 grams of *trans* fatty acids.

Two ounces of imitation cheese (American sliced) was found to have as much as 8 grams of *trans* fatty acids because this type of food is also made with partially hydrogenated soybean oil. By contrast, two ounces of natural cheese (American sliced) has less than half a gram of *trans* fatty acids.

Specialty breads such as croissants are traditionally made with butter and have less than half a gram of *trans* fatty acids for a typical 57 gram croissant, which has 12 grams of fat. Because these specialty rolls have become very popular, they are frequently made with partially hydrogenated vegetable oils. Croissants from nationwide popular donut companies have more fat in each croissant (17 grams) and approximately a third of the fat is *trans* fatty acids, so we find that this type of croissant has between 5 and 6 grams of *trans* fatty acids each. (Also see Chapter 3.)

Odd-Chain and Branch-Chain Fatty Acids

The **odd-chain** fatty acids are found in ruminant fats, especially in milk fats, in low levels. They are produced by microbial synthesis in the rumen. They are also found in very small amounts in human milk lipids and in certain animal and fish tissues.

The **branch-chain** fatty acids are minor components of animal fats, marine oils, and microbial lipids. The ones that have an even number of carbons are called iso acids, and the ones that have an odd number of carbons and are called anteiso acids. One fairly well known branch chain fatty acid is phytanic acid, which has 20 carbons and four branches; this fatty acid is involved in one of the lipid storage diseases called Refsum's disease (See **Chapter 2** and the **General Glossary**).

What is Conjugated Linoleic Acid?

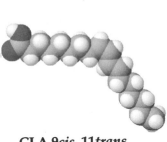

CLA 9*cis*, 11*trans*

Conjugated linoleic acid (CLA) is a unique fatty acid found almost exclusively in ruminant animal and dairy fats. This fatty acid has only been recognized for some two decades. It was first reported by the Australian lipid biochemist Peter Parodi, whose research with composition of dairy fats is well known. Since Dr. Parodi was the person to discover this fatty acid, he had the traditional privilege of giving this fatty acid its trivial name. He selected the name alpha-rumenic acid, because the origin is the rumen. In the future CLA will probably be referred to as alpha-rumenic acid in texts but the abbreviation CLA will probably be around for awhile.

A decade after Parodi's discovery, a group at the University of Wisconsin, headed by biochemist Michael Pariza did the major research identifying the anticarcinogenic properties of CLA. More recently, the Wisconsin group has done research that suggests that CLA may have properties that tend to normalize body fat deposition. In chickens, CLA prevents eggs from hatching.

Conjugated linoleic acid is formed in the rumen of ruminant animals. So when a university biochemist wrote in a nutrition article about CLA on his internet site "Nutritional Basics" that individuals should consume linoleic acid and have their bodies make the CLA, it was somewhat amusing but also disconcerting to see such a mistake. Making your own CLA would be possible only if humans were herbivores and chewed their cud. Human beings do a number of odd things, but chewing the cud like a sheep, goat, or cow is not one of them. Nonetheless, we can make CLA from the *trans*-vaccenic acid that comes to us from milk fat, because that fatty acid with its Δ-11 *trans* fatty acid (*trans* vaccenic acid) can be desaturated by the same desaturase system in our bodies that makes oleic acid out of stearic acid.

What About Olestra and the Other Fat Replacers?

The low-fat, no-fat craze of recent years has led companies to make numerous fat replacers. There are several categories of fat replacers, which include carbohydrate-based products, protein-based products such as microparticulated proteins, and those fat-based products referred to as lipid analogues.

A commercial example of the carbohydrate-based products is Oatrim. Others include cellulose in the form of a gel, dextrins, various fibers, hydrocolloids (gums), inulin, maltodextrins, polydextrose, polyols and various starches. These carbohydrate-based fat substitutes have the ability to make baked goods moist because they hang on to water.

An example of a protein-based product is Simplesse, which is made of a micro-particulated egg-white protein; modified whey proteins are also used. Reduced-fat (margarine-like) table spreads are formulated with the addition of both hydrocolloids (carbohydrate-based) and microparticulated proteins.

Examples of lipid analogues include structured triglycerides, which utilize interesterified fatty acids such as Caprenin and Salatrim and sucrose polyesters such as olestra (Olean).

The fat replacer olestra is a sucrose polyester, in other words, a molecule of sucrose with a bunch of fatty acids (six, seven or eight) esterified to the OH positions on the sucrose molecule. Because the body does not have the enzymes to hydrolyze the total olestra molecule to release the fatty acids, the product does not provide calories. Since olestra behaves like shortening in deep fat frying in the manufacture of snack chips, it has become popular with some of the snack chip companies and is being marketed in the United States. Because it acts like mineral oil or like resins such as cholestyramine, and because any fat soluble nutrients will adsorb onto it, the fat soluble nutrients can be lost to the individual. Thus, the consumption of olestra has the potential for causing nutrient deficiency problems, especially in growing children or in individuals with disorders such as macular degeneration who need those lipid-soluble nutrients found in foods being eaten along with the olestra-containing snacks. Figure 1.15 shows a triglyceride molecule and a sucrose polyester molecule.

The structured triglyceride Caprenin, which is made from caprylic acid, capric acid, and behenic acid, has been touted as low calorie because the very long-chain behenic acid was only partially digested and absorbed in some people. (See the General Glossary for detailed discussion of the individual fatty acids.)

A GRAS petition was filed by Procter & Gamble, which holds the patent for Caprenin, with the F.D.A. for the use of Caprenin in confectionary products. One of the candy makers made a reduced calorie form of one of its major candy bars using Caprenin, but reportedly did not order the second load of the so-called "reduced calorie tailored fat." The structured lipid Salatrim (also called Benefat™) is composed of a long-chain fatty acid and two very short-chain fatty acids. This man-made fat is used for confections and baked goods as well as dairy products and is reported to have almost half fewer calories than regular fat.

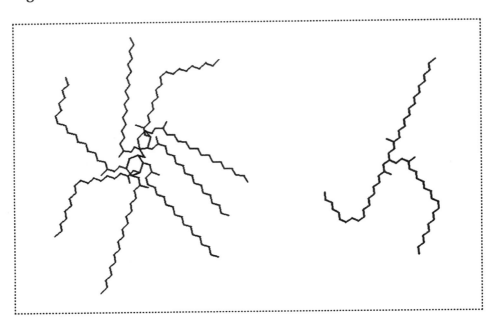

Figure 1.15 Sucrose Polyester Molecule and Triglyceride Molecule

What about Cholesterol?

Cholesterol is a high molecular weight alcohol (not to be confused with the common alcohol, ethanol). That means that it is a large alcohol molecule relative to other alcohol molecules. Glycerol is the alcohol molecule that holds the fatty acids together in triglycerides. Glycerol has 3 carbons, 3 oxygens and 8 hydrogens. Ethanol has 2 carbons and 6 hydrogens, but only one oxygen. Cholesterol is an alcohol molecule with 27 carbons, one oxygen and 46 hydrogens. Technically, it is a sterol, and cholesterol is the animal sterol.

There are also plant sterols. Plant sterols are very similar in their structure to cholesterol but they are not identical. Sitosterol is one of the many plant sterols; it also has 27 carbons and one oxygen, but it has 50 hydrogens (4 more than cholesterol). In fact, all plant sterols have more hydrogens than cholesterol. The difference between animal and plant sterols can be seen in Figure 1.16.

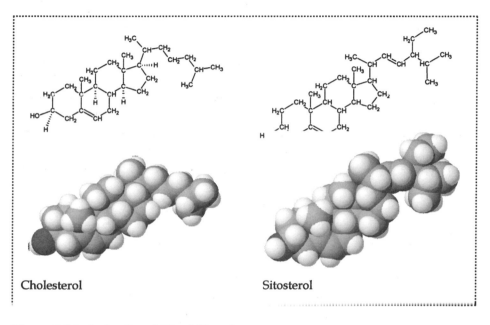

Cholesterol   Sitosterol

Figure 1.16 Animal and Plant Sterols

Cholesterol and plant sterols are referred to as "fatty substances" because they are soluble in fats and oils and fats and oils solvents, but they are not the same as fatty acids or triglycerides and they play completely different roles in animal and plant physiology.   One important difference between cholesterol and regular triglycerides in fats and oils is that only the triglycerides supply calories. Cholesterol is not used by the body for energy. Also, the amounts that are eaten are quite different. Cholesterol comes in milligram amounts in the foods where it is present, but triglycerides are found in gram amounts (a gram is equal to a thousand milligrams). For example, 3 ounces of fish such as salmon would have from about 3 to 10 grams of fat and about 30 to 70 milligrams of cholesterol.

Both cholesterol and plant sterols are important parts of the membrane systems in cells (animal cells or plant cells). Cholesterol is essential to life. Without cholesterol the body could not function.

Cholesterol is the basic building block for many important hormones and other constituents, but it is never used by the body for energy. Cholesterol is found only in animal tissues (e.g., meat, poultry, fish, insects), where it is a component of the membranes. That is why there is more cholesterol in the lean tissue than there is in the adipose tissue. Cholesterol is a major component of egg yolk where it is essential for the development of the chick. The cholesterol in the milk fat is part of the milk fat globule membrane.

Cholesterol has been reported in trace amounts in vegetable oils. Originally it was thought that the cholesterol was probably in the oils because of contamination of the original seeds or grains by cholesterol from insects since cholesterol is soluble in fats and oils and in the solvents used for extracting the fats and oils. Recent research suggests that all plants make trace amounts of cholesterol in addition to making their own particular plant sterols. The amounts are too small to end up on food labels.

It is not possible for humans to eat enough cholesterol-containing foods every day to supply the amount that a human needs. To make up for the difference between what is consumed in the diet and what is needed by our bodies to function properly, our livers and other organs have very active cholesterol synthesis capability (i.e., the capability of manufacturing cholesterol from basic raw material such as carbohydrate, protein, and fat). When there is some cholesterol in the diet, our own synthesis declines, and when there is no cholesterol in our diets (as would be the case with strict vegetarians), the body's cholesterol synthesis is very active.

See Chapter 2 for additional discussion of the role of cholesterol in physiology and the role of lipoproteins in the transport of cholesterol and other lipid substances. (Also see General Glossary)

Chapter 2

Lets Get Physical With Fats

The Digestion, Absorption, and Metabolism of Carbohydrates and Proteins as Related to Fats, Oils, and Cholesterol

Although we usually think of our digestive tract as being inside of our bodies, from the standpoint of that part of the body that has the liver, heart, lungs, kidneys and the blood vessels and lymph system, the digestive tract is still "outside" the most inner part of our bodies. Foods and parts of food that don't make it into the most inner parts do not really become part of us. They may act as surface irritants or stimuli or food for the intestinal microflora.

It is only those parts of food that are transported across the wall of the intestine that are truly being digested. In brief, the food and drink that we consume travels through the digestive tract, which is represented by the mouth, the esophagus, the stomach, the small (upper) intestine with three parts known as the duodenum, the jejunum, and the ileum, and the large (lower) intestine known as the colon with the final section known as the rectum. Swallowed food moves through the esophagus, into the stomach where it is churned, partially processed, and prepared for the further processing it receives as it proceeds along the rest of the intestine.

Diagrams and cartoons of the digestive and metabolic pathways are presented here in Figures 2.1, 2.2, 2.3, and 2.4 for you to refer to as you read this next chapter.

What Do Carbohydrates and Proteins Have to Do With Fat?

In order to fully understand fat digestion, it is necessary to know something about the digestion and metabolism of **carbohydrates**.

Digestion of carbohydrates starts in the mouth and continues in earnest in the small intestine. If the carbohydrate is the type that is called "complex" -- the kind that is made up of large (multiple) units -- then it needs to be broken into smaller (single) units for the final stages of absorption into the **portal blood** and transport thereafter to the liver.

The smaller carbohydrate units are sugars like glucose, fructose, and galactose. These sugars are ultimately broken apart in the cells into even smaller units, unless they are to be used for building complex tissue molecules such as glycolipids. When the sugar molecules are broken apart, energy molecules (called **ATP**) are formed. Since only so many of these energy molecules can be formed at any one time (either for immediate use by the cells or for short-term storage), and since only so much of these sugar units can be stored as glycogen (no more than 1 to 1.5 grams total), something has to be done with the extra carbohydrate units that are rapidly being absorbed and transported to the liver, and that something is that these smallest units are put together in a special way to make fatty acids (see "The Digestive Pathway" pictures).

The more carbohydrate you eat the more fat your liver and adipose tissue makes from any excess carbohydrate. Thus the end product of much of the carbohydrate that is eaten is **fat**, and this fat is stored either for the short term or for the long term, depending on the energy requirements of the body.

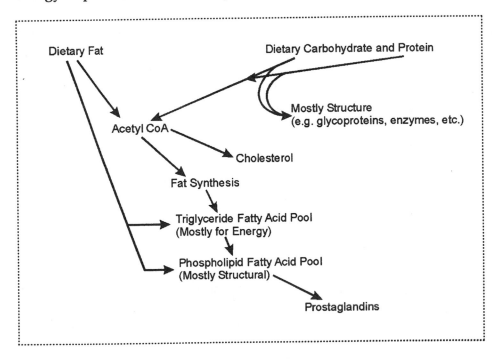

Figure 2.1 Outline of Digestive and Metabolic Pathways

Mouth
chewing and mixing
salivary enzymes split starch

Esophagus
food slides down
no enzyme function

Stomach
food churned into chyle
cells produce hydrochloric acid
pepsin starts to digest proteins
gastric lipase may work
carbohydrates hydrolyzed by acid

Upper (Small) Intestine
bile acids from gallbladder
enzymes from pancreas
  amylases, lipases, trypsin
  and other proteases
Duodenum, Jejunum, Ileum
absorb digested nutrients

Large Intestine
Colon
conserves water and minerals
passes undigested waste

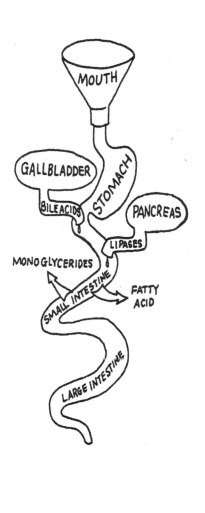

Figure 2.2 Digestive Pathways -- Where Things Happen

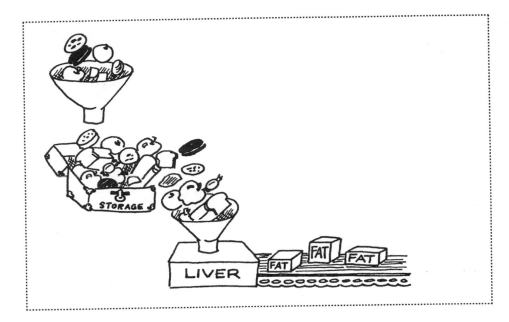

Figure 2.3 Metabolic Pathway Cartoon for Fat Synthesis

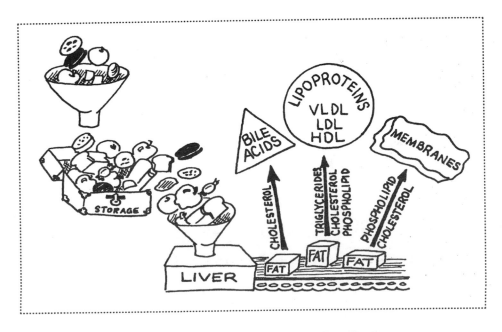

Figure 2.4 Metabolic Pathway Cartoon for Lipid Synthesis

Although nature has seen to it that simple carbohydrate is digested fairly rapidly, quite the opposite is true for fat; in other words, fat is much more *slowly* digested than carbohydrate. This is the natural appropriate process.

Protein is not usually considered along with carbohydrate and fat as a source of energy, and when the protein that is eaten is just the right amount to supply the body with the necessary amino acids for tissue building and repair there is no extra for energy use. In most diets today, however, there is an excess of protein and that protein must be dealt with by the body.

The way the normal body deals with excess amino acids is to remove the nitrogen from each amino acid molecule to form a fragment that is going to be further processed. (The nitrogen is put into a form that is secreted by the normal kidneys. Diseased kidneys cannot handle extra nitrogen, and this is the reason low-protein diets are advocated for some people.)

The fragments from the amino acids are then sent to be used for making glycogen if the body needs glycogen and doesn't have readily available glucose, or they are sent into the part of the body's organs where fatty acids are made. So the excess protein very readily can end up as fat. The fat is *de novo* fat, i.e., fat newly made by the body, so it is saturated fat.

How Does the Digestion and Absorption of Fat Happen?

When fat is eaten, it must first be digested before it can be absorbed through the intestinal wall. Most of the digestion of fat occurs in the upper part of the small intestine and is accomplished by special digestive enzymes called **lipases**. The lipases act on fat (triglycerides) that has been emulsified with the aid of **bile acids** (see discussion about cholesterol and emulsification below). The lipases work by breaking the emulsified fat into smaller units. Some of the fat that is "digested" is broken down into individual fatty acids and glycerol, some is broken down into the special intermediate molecules called monoglycerides, which are made of glycerol with one remaining fatty acid still attached. These monoglycerides are absorbed as monoglycerides, and some of them have very special functions.

By the time some of these fatty acids and monoglycerides and glycerol have traveled through the intestinal cell to the lymph stream, they are repackaged into triglycerides. The fat molecules that have long-chain fatty acids are ultimately put onto carriers in the lymph system called **chylomicrons**, which are manufactured in the intestinal cells for the purpose of transporting these exogenous fat molecules. The short-chain and most of the medium-chain fatty acid molecules go into the portal blood and are transported to the liver in much the same way that the carbohydrate goes to the liver. These short-chain and medium-chain fatty acid molecules also supply energy more rapidly like carbohydrates.

The triglycerides that are put onto the chylomicrons for the final journey go to the liver or to other tissues. Once those triglycerides (and their fatty acids) enter the cells, they are again broken apart into increasingly smaller units until they are formed into the final energy molecule called ATP. This process, which produces energy, is called oxidation, either beta-oxidation or omega-oxidation (See Chapter 1 and the General Glossary for additional discussion of oxidation). Sometimes the oxidation takes place in the peroxisomes but usually it takes place in the mitochondria. If the cells don't need the energy molecule at the moment, the small units that have been formed are shunted into the synthesis of fatty acids, and then as triglycerides, they are stored in adipose tissue.

The slow digestion of fat allows for the gradual release of energy so that there is no need for the liver and adipose tissue to synthesize fat. This slow digestion of fat also helps the body to absorb more of the nutrients that are along with the fat. Excess fat intake, however, results in storage of that excess ingested fat in the adipose cells all over the body. Of course, if there is an adequate intake of the natural fats found in whole foods most people will have good satiety and then they are less likely to overeat.

What About Cholesterol?

Cholesterol is not "digested" in the sense that the term is usually meant. In other words, there is no breaking of larger particles into smaller particles such as happens with fat being broken apart into fatty acids as noted above, or with carbohydrate digestion, or when protein is "digested" to its component amino acids. The amount of cholesterol that is absorbed by the intestinal cells varies, but generally it amounts to much less than half (50 percent) of the amount consumed (except in the special case of infants where most of what is consumed is absorbed -- see below for details). The statement "even if you didn't eat any cholesterol, your liver would manufacture enough for your body's needs" has been made so frequently it is often believed. But in fact, there is evidence that for some people cholesterol is an absolute dietary essential because their own synthesis is not adequate. Research at the University of California, Berkeley (Singer, M. 1995), has shown that the cholesterol in eggs is helpful to older people whose memory is declining. The evidence is clear that for most people the more that dietary cholesterol is ingested, the less it is synthesized by their body tissues.

All cholesterol is made from the basic molecule called acetyl CoA. Acetyl CoA is the product made from the metabolism of carbohydrate, from the metabolism of extra protein, and from the metabolism of fat. The synthesis of cholesterol is increased more from consumption of polyunsaturated fatty acids than from the consumption of saturated fatty acids. The effect of natural fatty acids on serum cholesterol levels is dependent on the original serum cholesterol levels: high serum cholesterol *decreases* with consumption of most fatty acids, including all saturates; low serum cholesterol *increases* with many of the fatty acids, including saturates, monounsaturates and sometimes the polyunsaturates.

Infants need cholesterol for proper brain development. Large amounts of cholesterol are supplied to the infant in human milk. Also the mammary gland secretes a special enzyme into the human milk that ensures that almost all of the cholesterol will be absorbed by the infant. Whole cows milk also supplies about the same amount of cholesterol, but infants fed most infant formulas get either very small amounts of cholesterol or no cholesterol. (The scientists in the companies that manufacture infant formulas generally know that infants need to consume adequate amounts of cholesterol, but they have let the anti-cholesterol propaganda control the composition of their products to the detriment of the growing infant.)

Cholesterol may be needed to form properly the part of the brain that allows the eyes to develop normally. Research has recently identified the cyclopian eye as the result of inadequate cholesterol in certain tissues. (Strauss 1998)

Cholesterol is used by the body as a raw material for the healing process. This is the reason the injured areas in the arteries (as in atherosclerosis) or the lungs (as in tuberculosis) have cholesterol along with several other components (such as calcium and collagen) in the "scar" tissue that is formed to heal the "wound." Research in Germany has identified the likely mechanism whereby the body delivers cholesterol to the cells of the body involved in tissue repair. (Pfohl et al

1999) In addition to being the body's basic repair substance, cholesterol has important structural and other basic functions (see section on physiology of cholesterol below).

The Physiology of Fats and Cholesterol

It has not been generally recognized by most people that fat plays such a very important role in maintaining the structure of all the cells in our bodies. Our bodies are made up of many billions of cells. These cells come in many different shapes and sizes and are joined together in many different amounts to form many different organs, including the blood vessels, the liver, the kidneys, the lungs, the heart, and the brain.

Within the cells of the various organs (the liver, the lungs, the heart, the pancreas, etc.), there are many different subcellular parts called **organelles**. These organelles have specialized functions just like different departments or machinery in a factory. If the departments are not complete, or if the machinery is not working efficiently, quality goods cannot be produced.

Fats and Lipids in Cell Membranes

A common factor in the makeup of all the cells is the presence of structures called **membranes**. Each cell (as shown in Figure 2.5) has many membranes surrounding or separating the different parts of the cell. In a cell that divides and multiplies, there is a central part called a **nucleus**, which is surrounded by the nuclear membrane.

The "machines" in the cell that clean up unwanted material are called **lysosomes**. Different types of cells have differing numbers of lysosomes, some of which have different functions. All of the lysosomes are surrounded by the lysosomal membranes. All the different compartments in each cell are separated from each other by membranes, e.g., plasma membranes, microsomal membranes, mitochondrial membranes.

The structure of each of the individual membranes is similar enough to allow for the use of a general description. All membranes are made primarily of special lipid molecules such as **phospholipids** and **cholesterol**, special **glycolipids** and **glycoproteins**, and various kinds of **protein** molecules called extrinsic or intrinsic proteins. (The protein molecules sitting on the exterior part of the membrane are called extrinsic and protein molecules sitting within the membrane are called intrinsic.)

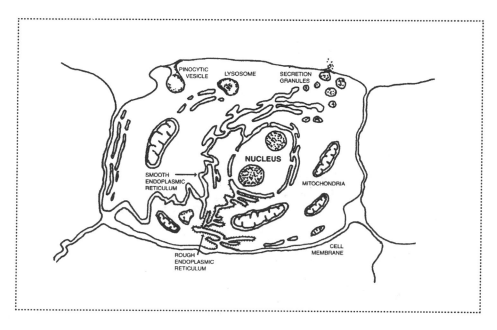

Figure 2.5 Typical Cell

These membranes have a "generic" name. They are called lipid bilayers because they are made of lipid (fat) and they have two layers (see Figure 2.6).

Different membranes have different amounts of lipid, and most of the lipids are phospholipids. For example, the lipid part of the membranes in the mitochondria is 90% phospholipid, but the lipid part of the plasma membranes are only 50% phospholipid. The phospholipid and cholesterol molecules provide flexible structure to the membrane.

Membrane Fatty Acids and Phospholipids

As we learned in **Chapter 1**, fatty acids come in different lengths and different shapes. In biological membranes the fatty acids are found mostly in the phospholipid molecules: two fatty acids for each phospholipid molecule. Remember, in triglycerides, fatty acids come in sets of three, and they are attached to glycerol.

The phospholipids are also formed with the glycerol backbone, but the third component of the phospholipid molecule is one of several vitamin-like metabolites. Different phospholipid molecules usually have

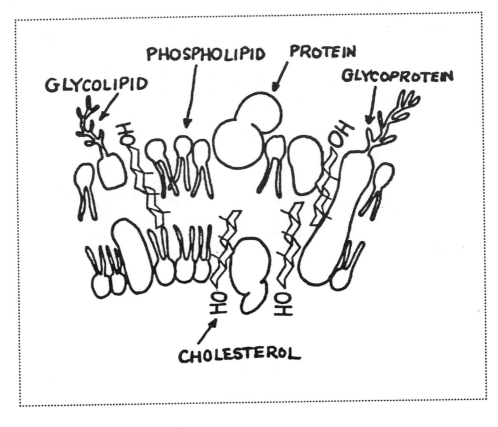

Figure 2.6 Lipid Bilayer Cartoon

their own assortment of fatty acids, but a large portion of these fatty acids are very long (20 and 22 and even 24 and more carbons long) and when they are very unsaturated (4, 5, and 6 double bonds), they may be used by the various organs for forming prostaglandins.

You may recognize the name of one of the common egg or plant phospholipids called lecithin (phosphatidylcholine). The other common phospholipids include phosphatidylethanolamine, phosphatidylserine, phosphatidylinositol, sphingomyelin, and cardiolipin. Phosphatidylserine has recently been reported to be needed to maintain appropriate age-related cognitive function. Sphingomyelin and its metabolites help suppress tumors.

The fatty acids found on the different phospholipids are different in different tissues. For example, in the red cell membrane, the most common fatty acids on phosphatidylcholine are palmitic acid (31.2 percent) and linoleic acid (22.8 percent). The fatty acids most often found on phosphatidylserine are stearic acid (37.5 percent) and arachidonic acid (24.2 percent). These two phospholipids as well as the phosphatidylcholine with two palmitic acids known as the lung surfactant are all shown in Figure 2.7.

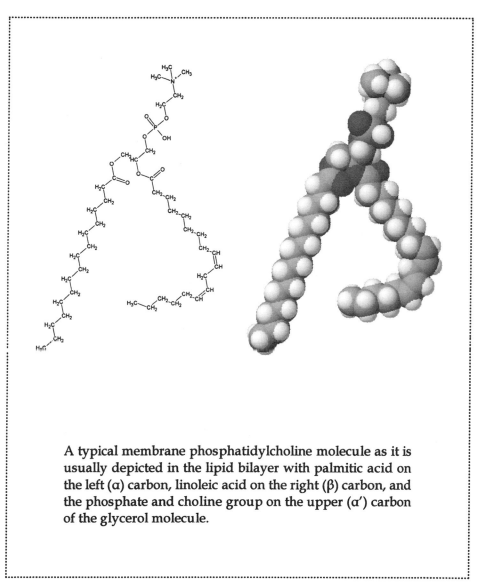

A typical membrane phosphatidylcholine molecule as it is usually depicted in the lipid bilayer with palmitic acid on the left (α) carbon, linoleic acid on the right (β) carbon, and the phosphate and choline group on the upper (α') carbon of the glycerol molecule.

Figure 2.7 Phospholipid Molecules

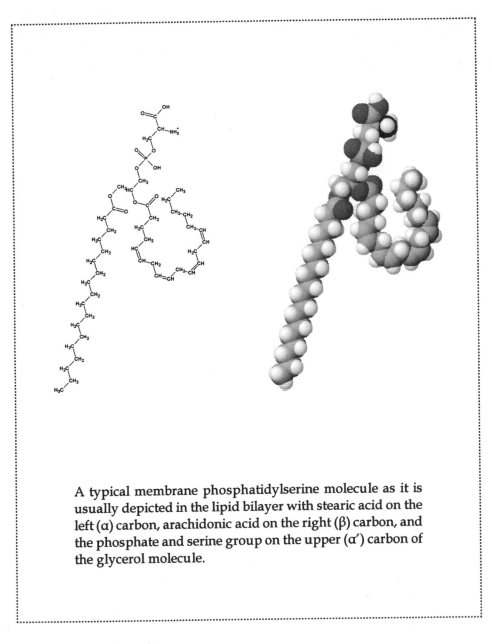

A typical membrane phosphatidylserine molecule as it is usually depicted in the lipid bilayer with stearic acid on the left (α) carbon, arachidonic acid on the right (β) carbon, and the phosphate and serine group on the upper (α') carbon of the glycerol molecule.

Figure 2.7 Continued

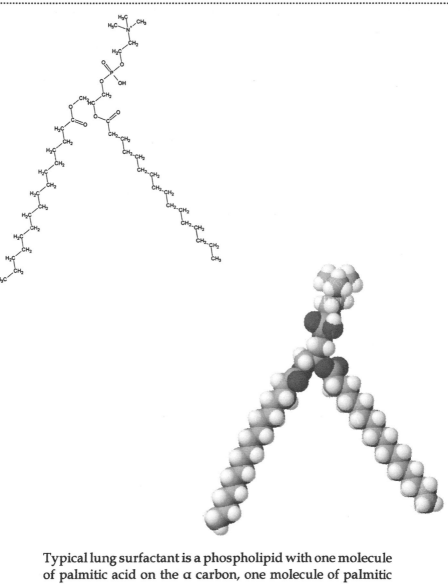

Typical lung surfactant is a phospholipid with one molecule of palmitic acid on the α carbon, one molecule of palmitic acid on the β carbon, and the phosphate and choline group on the α' carbon of the glycerol molecule. It is called dipalmitoyl phosphatidylcholine.

Figure 2.7 Continued

In the white matter of the human brain, which is largely myelin, 87 percent of the phospholipids such as phosphatidyl-choline and 82 percent of the phosphatidylserine have been shown to be only saturated fatty acids and monounsaturated fatty acids. In the phosphatidylcholine, the combination is palmitic acid and oleic acid; in the phosphatidylserine, the usual combination is stearic acid and oleic acid. In the phospholipid called phosphatidylethanolamine, more than half of the fatty acids are saturated and the rest are polyunsaturated. Very long-chain saturated fatty acids with 22 and 24 carbons are important parts of the myelin fatty acids.

As noted above, the body needs saturated fatty acids for at least half, and sometimes much more, of the fatty acid part of the phospholipids that form the membranes of the cells. For those who don't understand why the human body makes saturated fatty acids -- it is because the saturated fatty acids are required by the body, and for some people, the fats in the diet are either too polyunsaturated or too low.

Membrane and Tissue Cholesterol

One of the more important components of cell membranes is cholesterol. In addition to an antioxidant role, cholesterol molecules give the proper amount of rigidity to the membranes. In other words, cholesterol helps a membrane keep its proper shape. The cholesterol molecules are also critical components of some of the cell receptors. Receptors are mostly protein molecules that bind specific chemicals to enhance their uptake into the cell. One such receptor is the glutamate receptor.

How much cholesterol a membrane has depends on how unsaturated the fatty acids of the phospholipids are; the more unsaturated they are, the more cholesterol is needed to provide the membrane with just the right amount of stiffness or flexibility.

Cholesterol in the skin is used as the substrate for the production of the precursor of vitamin D (provitamin D_3); the cholesterol is in a form called 7-dehydrocholesterol. Cholesterol is also a component of the scar tissue formed during the healing process.

Fat as An Enzyme Regulator

Enzymes are the basic machinery in cells that are responsible for putting things together or taking things apart. Some enzymes are on the inside of the cell membrane, some are on the outside of the cell membrane, and some stretch all the way across the membrane so that they are in touch with both the internal portion of the cell and an external part. Enzymes are protein molecules that are referred to as *"biocatalysts"* because they catalyze reactions that otherwise would not occur at the typical temperatures and pressures found in the cell.

The way the enzymes function is often related to the kinds of lipids (e.g., fatty acids) surrounding them in the membrane. For example the part of the enzyme called the active site might be hidden and unavailable if the membrane fatty acids were of one type, but exposed and available if they were of another type. Just how flexible (fluid) the membranes are is dependent on both the fatty acids of the membrane phospholipids and the cholesterol molecules; together they essentially make up the lipid portion of the membranes. So, when we think of enzymes that are working well, we should probably think of them in terms of them as being "well-oiled machinery."

Essential Fatty Acids

There are two absolutely essential fatty acids, i.e., linoleic acid and alpha-linolenic acid; and there are several other conditionally essential fatty acids. An essential fatty acid cannot be made in the human body and must be provided in the diet.

Chemically, essential fatty acids are carboxylic acids with hydrocarbon chains 18 carbons in length, with an appropriate number of attached hydrogens and oxygens that are arranged, at the molecular level, in a specific shape and have certain temperature-related characteristics. Fatty acids range from 3 to 24 carbons in length; the major essential fatty acids are both 18 carbons long.

The conditionally essential fatty acids include gamma-linolenic acid (GLA), arachidonic acid (AA), eicosapentaenoic acid (EPA), and docosahexaenoic acid (DHA). All four of these fatty acids *can* be made by cells in the body, but there are a number of interfering food substances or illnesses or genetic inadequacies that make these latter fatty acids become dietary essentials for some people. These conditionally essential fatty acids are 18, 20, and 22 carbons long.

Essential fatty acids are needed by each animal the, human included, for proper nutrition and health. The essential fatty acid status of individuals, however, cannot always be predicted with ease, in part because the range of levels of *trans* fatty acids in peoples' diets has complicated the situation.

Because the *trans* fatty acid isomers, in amounts frequently consumed in the U.S., can greatly interfere with normal fatty acid storage and metabolism, it is desirable to evaluate the dietary intake of *trans* fatty acids by individuals. This has not always been easy due to a lack of adequate listing of *trans* fatty acid content of foods. As noted below, there are ways of estimating the levels of *trans* fatty acids in many foods, and the removal of all processed foods from the diet, although not always easy, is a possible approach to removing them that can be recommended.

The minimum amount of the essential fatty acid linoleic acid thought to be required in the diet is 2-3% of calories; the minimum amount of the essential fatty acid alpha-linolenic acid currently thought to be required in the diet is approximately 0.5-1.5% of calories. (See Chapter 3 for sources and amounts of essential fatty acids.)

The essential fatty acids are precursor molecules to one or another of eicosanoids such as the prostaglandins (PGs). Prostaglandins are locally produced hormones that control different physiological functions; they are arranged in several different series, e.g., E, F, I. The conditionally essential fatty acids are those fatty acids formed from the essential fatty acids that are the immediate precursors to the prostaglandins, or a precursor to the immediate precursor (e.g., gamma-linolenic acid becomes PGE_1; arachidonic acid becomes PGE_2, PGI_2, $PGF_{2\alpha}$, or assorted other prostaglandin-like substances; eicosapentaenoic acid becomes PGE_3 or PGI_3 or one of several other prostaglandin-like substances).

The essential fatty acids and their elongated forms are part of the structural matrix of the cell membranes along with many other fatty acids.

Fatty Acids as Hormone Regulators

There are special hormone-like substances that the body cannot get along without. They are made from the elongated forms of the essential fatty acids. These elongated forms are, for example, gamma-linolenic acid, dihomo-gamma-linolenic acid, and arachidonic acid made from linoleic acid, and eicosapentaenoic acid made from alpha-linolenic acid.

These hormone-like substances are called eicosanoids because they are 20 carbons long, or prostaglandins because they were originally found in the prostate gland, or leukotrienes because of their original identification in leukocytes (white blood cells). They are thought to be formed in the cells' membranes, and they are very potent and important in their actions. For example, they regulate substances that act as the cells' messengers for doing things like opening and closing different channels to let substances in and out of the cell.

There has been a lot of misinformation in the popular literature about the function of the prostaglandins that the body makes out of arachidonic acid. Some writers have suggested that all the prosta-glandins that are made from arachidonic acid are "bad," but this is not true, and this kind of misinformation has resulted from not understanding the multiple actions of the prostaglandins. Some prostaglandins, such as thromboxanes (TXA_2) promote aggregation of, for example, blood platelets, while other prostaglandins such as prostacyclins (PGI_2) have the opposite effect. When they are working properly in the same tissue, they provide the fine tuning necessary for proper maintenance of physiological equilibrium (i.e., homeostasis) in the body.

See Figure 2.8 for the prostaglandin pathways and the General Glossary for more detailed description of the individual eicosanoids and their precursors.

See also the discussion of Essential Fatty Acids in Chapter 1 and Chapter 3 as well as the General Glossary.

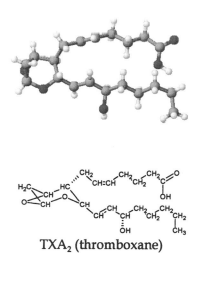

TXA$_2$ (thromboxane)

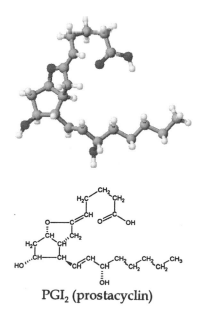

PGI$_2$ (prostacyclin)

Arachidonic acid   **Dihomo-γ-linolenic acid**
(AA) 20:4ω6   **DGLA 20:3ω6**
↓   ↓

Prostaglandins   *Prostaglandin*
PGE_2 PGE_1
PGI_2
$PGF_{2d\alpha}$ ------------------

or   **Eicosapentaenoic acid (EPA)**
                                        20:5ω3
Thromboxanes   ↓
TXA_2 *Prostaglandins*
                                        PGE_3
or PGI_3

Leukotrienes   *or*
5-HPETE
5-HETE   *Thromboxanes*
LTA_4 TXA_3
LTB_4
LTC_4 *or*

or   *Leukotrienes*
                                        LTB_5
Lipoxins LTC, D, E_5
12-HPETE
12-HETE

Figure 2.8 Prostaglandin Pathways

Cholesterol as Hormone Precursor

The body uses cholesterol as the raw material from which it makes all sorts of hormones. The best known is perhaps vitamin D, the so-called sunshine vitamin. Vitamin D starts out as cholesterol and undergoes several changes, first in the skin, then in the liver, and lastly in the kidneys, before it is finally in the form that is active in regulating calcium metabolism and calcium absorption.

Equally as important, if not more so, are all of the steroid hormones (better known as the sex hormones), which are made out of cholesterol. (See Figure 2.9) When blood cholesterol has been measured in people who are under stress, the levels of cholesterol are always increased, and this is because the adrenal hormones used by the body for response to stress are made from cholesterol.

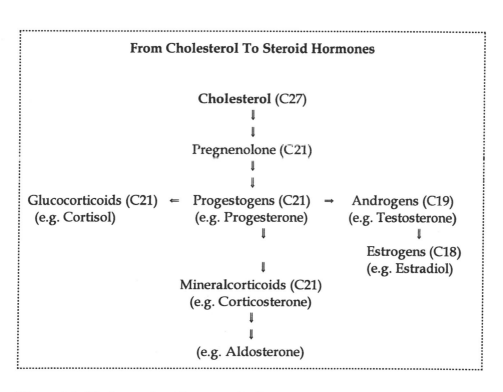

Figure 2.9 Cholesterol to Hormone Pathways

Lipoproteins

Fat, cholesterol, and other fat-soluble molecules are not water-soluble so they need special carriers that allow them to be transported through the body in the bloodstream because the bloodstream is a water-based fluid. The lipoproteins act as the carriers because they have a water-soluble exterior and a fat-soluble core (interior).

There are a number of classes of lipoproteins, and they are categorized on the basis of their density. Figure 2.10 presents a chemical content description of the common lipoproteins and their density characteristics. The commonly measured and/or evaluated serum lipoproteins include chylomicrons, very low-density lipoproteins (VLDL), low-density lipoprotein(LDL), intermediate density lipoproteins (IDL), and high-density lipoproteins (HDL). Attention has also been given to lipoprotein [a], so-called "lipoprotein little a" (see General Glossary for more details on the individual lipoproteins).

	Lipoprotein Classes				
	Chylo-microns	VLDL	IDL	LDL	HDL
Total protein %	1.5-2.5	5-10	15-20	20-25	40-55
Total lipid%	97-99	90-95	80-85	75-80	50-55
Phospholipids %	7-9	15-20	22	15-20	20-35
Cholesterol					
Esterified %	3-5	10-15	22	35-40	12
Unesterified %	1-3	5-10	8	7-10	3-4
Triglycerides %	84-89	50-65	30	7-10	3
Density (g/ml)	<0.95	0.95-1.006	1.006-1.019	1.019-1.063	1.063-1.210
Particle diameter (Å)	10^3-10^4	250-750	250	200-280	50-130

Figure 2.10 Characteristics of Lipoproteins

Fat for Emulsification

Special kinds of fats (lipids) called bile acids are needed for the emulsification of food fats and oils. The bile acids (also called bile salts) are made from cholesterol in the liver, they are stored in the gallbladder, and they are used by the body to aid in the digestion and absorption of fats and oils and the absorption of fat-soluble vitamins such as vitamins A, D, E, and K.

Other kinds of fat that the body uses for emulsification include the monoglycerides and the diglycerides formed from phospholipids or triglycerides. There are many activities in the cells that use the mono-glycerides and the diglycerides as intermediates in physiologically important reactions.

Phospholipids such as lecithin act as emulsifiers. Lecithin is a major lipid component in egg yolk. Most commercial lecithin today is extracted from soybeans during oil processing.

Fat as Carriers of Fat-soluble Vitamins and Other Fat-soluble Nutrients

A most important role played by fat involves transport of some of the vitamins and fat soluble phytochemicals such as carotenoids. Without enough fat in our foods, the fat soluble vitamins such as **Vitamins A, D, E and K** are not efficiently absorbed. In fact, a low-fat diet can very easily become a vitamin-deficient diet, in part because these vitamins are only found in the fatty (or oily) part of food. Since it is now recognized that the fat soluble vitamins play important roles as antioxidants, a situation that encourages their loss would be undesirable.

Vitamin A is a very important fat soluble vitamin. It is critical for many functions, including successful reproduction, normal cell division, vision (especially night vision), function of the immune system, bone remodeling, the formation of enamel on teeth during their development in childhood, and skin health. It is referred to an anti-infective vitamin in the *Merck Index*.

Vitamin A was first recognized in butter and egg yolk when these foods were found to correct an experimental deficiency in laboratory animals. True vitamin A occurs only in foods of animal origin and requires fat for absorption. The best sources are liver and other meats, cod liver oil, egg yolks, butter and cheese from grass-fed cows, and fortified dairy products. Green and yellow fruits and vegetables contain β-carotene, some of which is converted to vitamin A in well-fed healthy adults whose diets include adequate animal fats.

Vitamin D is both a fat soluble vitamin and a hormone. Vitamin D can be made in the body through a series of steps starting in the skin when it is exposed to adequate sunlight. The form of vitamin D made in the skin from cholesterol (see discussion above on tissue cholesterol) is further changed to another form in the liver and then to the final active form in the kidney.

Natural vitamin D is not widely available in food and is mainly found in egg yolks, cod liver oil, pork liver sausage and other liver, fatty fish, butter, fortified milk, and other fortified foods. Milk is usually fortified with vitamin D_3, known as cholecalciferol, and other foods such as margarine are usually fortified with ergocalciferol, the irradiated yeast (plant) form known also as vitamin D_2. Some questions have been raised about the safety of large amounts of D_2.

Vitamin E is a fat soluble vitamin that was first identified in the early 1920s by researchers studying experimental diets being given to rats. One of the diets did not support reproduction in these rats. At the time the missing substance was not known as other vitamins were ruled out. The newly recognized necessary nutrient was called vitamin E, and it was found in many natural foods but not in the synthetic diet mixes. Because it was necessary for supporting reproduction, it was given the technical name tocopherol from the Greek words descriptive of something supporting childbirth together with the suffix "ol" that described the chemical as an alcohol. During the next half a century, vitamin E was further identified as an important antioxidant. By the end of the 1990s, vitamin E was recognized as important for maintaining cardiovascular health.

Sources of vitamin E include unrefined vegetable oils, green leafy vegetables, wheat germ, whole-grain products, liver, egg yolks, nuts, and seeds. Vitamin E supplements are sold as both the natural *d*-alpha and mixed tocopherols and the synthetic *d,l*-alpha tocopherols. The latter are not the same as the natural vitamin E, and final determination of effectiveness has not been made.

Vitamin K is a fat soluble vitamin necessary for proper blood clotting, and it too was discovered when certain experimental diets caused hemorrhages in the experimental animals. Vitamin K also is now known to play a role in maintaining adequate bone density; it helps the bone protein matrix pick up and keep adequate calcium.

Some of the bacteria in the intestine manufacture vitamin K, which provides a complementary source. Food sources of vitamin K, however, turn out to be very important, and they include liver, leafy green vegetables, cabbage-type vegetables, dulse, and green tea leaves.

Phytochemicals such as carotenoids, including α-carotene, β-carotene, lutein, lycopene, and zeaxanthin, are important fat-soluble nutrients, which are vitamin-like plant substances. These phytonutrients are involved in numerous tissue functions playing major roles as antioxidants, and in the case of lutein and zeaxanthin, they are antioxidants that serve as light-absorbing pigments in the retina and are protective of the macula. Lutein and zeaxanthin are found in egg yolks. Tomatoes are a source of lycopene and zeaxanthin.

Biotonutrients such as carnitine, coenzyme Q10, inositol, and lipoic acid, are important fat-soluble nutrients, which are vitamin-like substances from both animal and plant sources.

Fat as a Factor for Satiety

As discussed above in the section on digestion, fat is digested slowly. This means there is a slow release of the fat molecules from the food, with a slower emptying of both the stomach and the upper part of the small intestine than there would be if no fat was present in the food. As a result of the presence of fat in the small intestine, special hormones are produced that prevent the hunger contractions. This role of delaying the onset of hunger is thought to be helpful for dieters; thus, a careful balance of fat in the diet becomes critical for someone trying to lose weight. Too much fat in the diet and the loss of weight is thwarted; too little and the hunger pangs play havoc with good intentions and usually lead to overeating carbohydrates.

Fat as Protective Padding and Covering

It is important to realize that *obesity* is the excess storage of *unnecessary* depot fat. That is quite distinct from the appropriate storage of an adequate amount of depot fat.

Because of the unusual emphasis today on fat, some people hold the misconception that all fat storage in the body is unnecessary. This is unfortunate because the normal amount of depot fat varies from one person to another, and preoccupation with those fat deposits that are genetically determined can only be counterproductive. The person who has lost a major portion of fat padding due to illness may have great difficulty sitting or lying on hard surfaces. The internal organs are supported and cushioned by the internal fat padding. A normal amount of fat under the surface of the outer skin keeps that organ from sagging and wrinkling by providing necessary support for the tissues. The fat layer also prevents undo dehydration of the skin. (See discussion on obesity)

Fat For Energy Storage

The role of fat in energy storage has been frequently misunderstood; in all probability because some of us tend to store too much fat in places where we think it doesn't look so good when we see ourselves in the mirror. But are we being reasonable?

Each pound of fat supplies us with approximately 4000 kilocalories of reserve energy. That is the way nature intended it to be. This means that a slender person who weighs 150 pounds will be carrying about 25 to 35 pounds of fat as energy reserve. If that reserve was in the form of carbohydrate it would have to weigh 50 to 70 pounds to give the same amount of energy, and the person would weigh about 175 to 185 pounds. In addition to being heavier, relative to the amount of energy that can be produced, stored carbohydrate is bulky whereas stored fat is compact. (See below)

How Much Fat Reserve Do We Need Stored in Our Bodies?

Probably more then most people realize.

Let's consider, for example a case of a slender person who weighs 150 pounds. If we are talking about a male, then close to 20 percent of that weight would be fat, i.e., 30 pounds. Normal slender females usually maintain closer to 25 percent of their weight as fat; i.e., 37.5 pounds for someone weighing 150 pounds. This is a minimum amount of energy reserve nature intended to have stored in our bodies as fat. And these amounts of energy reserves, which were needed early in man's evolution, provided just enough for surviving during times of short -term famine or illness.

If carbohydrate was stored in the body for spare energy, it would weigh more than twice the amount that fat does for the same amount of energy that is provided, and it would be very bulky. That 150 pound male would weigh a bulky 180 pounds because he would have to carry about 60 pounds of carbohydrate to provide the spare energy. The 150 pound female would weigh a bulky 187½ pounds for the same amount of spare energy stores.

People who have too much fat, or those people who are afraid of gaining too much fat, probably have a difficult time believing that they are better off carrying their necessary energy reserves as fat in the form of triglyceride rather than as bulky carbohydrate such as glycogen.

Protein also weighs more than twice as much as fat does for the same energy potential. Also, when protein is "burned" for energy there is extra nitrogen that the kidneys have to process and eliminate. By comparison, fat burns as a pretty clean "fuel"; it goes to carbon dioxide and water.

Health Issues and Fats and Oils

In this section we will touch briefly on some of the "popular" disease states that are considered as having a connection to dietary fats. These currently include various forms of vascular disease (both cardiovascular and cerebrovascular), several cancers, diabetes, obesity, immune dysfunction, and mental illness (schizophrenia and depression). There are also a number of genetic disorders, which involve lipids, and a few of these are tied to dietary fats. See for example Refsum's disease, sphingolipids, leukodystrophies in the **Glossary**.

It is not the intention of this section to provide a comprehensive, therapeutic listing of all the causes and treatments of these disorders. Rather it is the intent to provide some insight into some of those research reports about the effects of fats and oils as they pertain to these disease states; especially those diseases and their "fat connection" that have had wide coverage by the media. The reader may wish to discuss this with his or her health care professional.

What the reader should know, is that there is an important question of how valid is the current diet and heart disease research debate. Today, in the food/nutrition/health research market, any researcher who finds results that are contrary to the current, government supported consensus, has a most tricky task. The researcher has to publish everything very carefully in a manner that supports the current consensus in such a way that he/she will continue to receive funding and at the same time report the findings the way they came out.

Some people are very clever at this kind of doublespeak. They repeat the going hypothesis, as if it was valid and written-in-stone, early in the introduction section of their scientific or clinical paper; they then give the actual findings in the tables without discussing any results that are disparate from the hypothesis, and sometimes without certain averages or baseline numbers that would give away the inconsistency at a glance; then they discuss the meaning of the going hypothesis in the discussion section of the paper, the summary section, and/or the abstract; and after this has been published, they apply for the next grant from the appropriate industry or government agency.

The next thing that happens is that the news media journalists pick up the information from these convoluted reports, usually because someone has put out a press release about what is to appear in a "prestigious" scientific or medical journal, and these journalists who are not trained in scientific method fill the television, magazines, books, and newspapers with continued validation of garbage.

One of the best recent articles exposing this type of situation is by Uffe Ravnskov, M.D., Ph.D. from Lund, Sweden, which appeared in the *International Journal of Epidemiology*.

Atherosclerosis (or coronary heart disease) and a causative relationship between dietary fats, oils, and cholesterol has been the object of much research and conjecture for more than four decades. The popular consensus during this time has been: 1) that the consumption of natural saturated fats and oils was causing heart disease; 2) that the consumption of polyunsaturated oils would cure and prevent heart disease; and, further, 3) that the consumption of cholesterol-containing foods was also a causative factor.

The popular literature of epidemiological studies usually attributes an increased risk of coronary heart disease (CHD) to elevated levels of serum cholesterol, which in turn are thought to derive from a dietary intake of saturated fats and cholesterol. But, saturated fats may be considered a major culprit for CHD only if the links between serum cholesterol and CHD, and between saturated fat and serum cholesterol, are each firmly established. Decades of large-scale tests and conclusions therefrom have purported to establish the first link. This relationship has reached the level of dogma. Through the years metabolic ward studies on humans and various animal studies have claimed that dietary saturated fats increase serum cholesterol levels, thereby supposedly establishing the second link. But the scientific basis for both of these relationships has now been challenged as resulting from large-scale misinterpretation and misrepresentation of the data (Smith 1991, Enig 1993, Mann 1993, Ravnskov 1995, 1998).

As regards the currently popular concept that saturated fat in the diet is the major culprit, the lipid biochemist Professor Michael Gurr (1996) wrote knowledgeably on the subject. He noted in his conclusion

> "...that whatever causes CHD [coronary heart disease], it is not primarily a high intake of SFA [saturated fatty acids]. By the same token, major changes in SFA consumption are unlikely to lead to major benefits from CHD reduction."

Prominent researchers have periodically provided examples of contradictions to the hypothesis blaming saturated fat for CHD. In 1990, an editorial by Harvard University's Professor Walter Willett acknowledged that even though

"The focus of dietary recommendations is usually a reduction of saturated fat intake, no relation between saturated fat intake and risk of CHD was observed in the most informative prospective study to date." (Willett 1990)

Then in 1995, Dr. Willett's group published one of their studies examining "...the association between fat intake and the incidence of coronary heart disease in men of middle age and older." One of their stated conclusions was that

"[t]hese data do not support the strong association between intake of saturated fat and risk of coronary heart disease suggested by international comparisons." (Ascherio et al 1995)

Research published from Willett's group or in collaboration with his group in 1997 reported either a nonsignificant association between CHD events and saturated fat intake (Hu et al 1997) or no association (Pietinen et al 1997).

Even Dr. William P. Castelli, the director of the famous Framingham study, the results of which have been interpreted by many in ways so as to link saturated fats to CHD, declared for the record in a 1992 editorial that

"...in Framingham, Mass, the more saturated fat one ate, the more cholesterol one ate, the *more calories one ate*, the lower the person's serum cholesterol...the opposite of what the equations provided by Hegsted et al (1965) and Keys et al (1957) would predict..."

Castelli, who usually supports the hypothesis, further admitted that

"...In Framingham, for example, we found that the people who ate the most cholesterol, ate the most saturated fat, ate the most calories,, weighed the least, and were the most physically active." (Castelli 1992)

Coronary heart disease is recognized by many researchers as having multiple causes of both known and unknown origin, e.g., cigarette smoking, genetics. Environmental and dietary causes have been under investigation for many decades. Some of the environmental and common dietary theories, which are alternatives to the saturated fat hypothesis, are outlined in Figure 2.11.

What causes heart disease? Alternative dietary and environmental theories proposed to explain the CHD epidemic

Price	Deficiency of fat soluble vitamins
Yudkin, Ahrens	Refined carbohydrates
Kummerow, Mann, Willett	*Trans* fatty acids from hydrogenated fats
Hodgson	Excess omega-6 from refined vegetable oils
Addis	Oxidized cholesterol and oxidized fats
Shute	Vitamin E deficiency
Pauling	Vitamin C deficiency
McCully	Deficiency of folic acid, B6 and B12
Annand	Heated milk protein
Anderson	Magnesium deficiency
Huttunen	Selenium deficiency
Ellis	Microbial agents (viruses, bacteria)
Benditt	Monoclonal tumor theory
de Bruin	Thyroid deficiency
LaCroix	Coffee consumption
Morris	Lack of exercise
Stern	Exposure to carbon monoxide
Smith	Changes & fashions in reporting cause of death

Figure 2.11   Alternative Causes of CHD

Some of the theories involving fats and oils for which there is currently substantial proof include: 1) regular intake of *trans* fatty acids from partially hydrogenated vegetable oils; 2) excess intake of omega-6 fatty acids from refined vegetable oils; 3) consumption of oxidized cholesterol and oxidized fats; and 4) a deficiency of fat soluble vitamins. Various vitamin deficiencies such as those of vitamin E, vitamin C, folic acid, vitamin B6 and vitamin B12 as well as deficiencies of magnesium and selenium have also been causally linked to CHD.

Professor Fred Kummerow, who did the earliest research on the *trans* fatty acids in the United States, and his colleagues have just reported on new research (Kummerow et al 1999) that has identified a mechanism for an adverse effect of *trans* fatty acid intake in the presence of magnesium deficiency on a known cardiovascular risk factor. This research showed that there was a significant increase of calcium influx into human arterial endothelial cells when there was a combination of *trans* fatty acid intake and deficient magnesium status. These are common dietary problems in the United States. Stearic acid, a common saturated fatty acid, and oleic acid, the common monounsaturated fatty acid, did not show the same undesirable effect.

Everyone who is truly interested in understanding the politics of fats and oils and cholesterol should find a copy of *The Cholesterol Controversy* by Edward R. Pinckney, M.D. and Cathey Pinckney and read it from cover to cover. This small volume was published in 1973 by Sherbourne Press, Inc. of Los Angeles (ISBN number is 0-8202-0155-3). The book contains a very good documentation of early fats and oils industry skulduggery, of the exchanges of industry lawyers and other personnel with Food and Drug Administration personnel, and some of the game-playing of the committee hearings on diet and disease chaired by Senator George McGovern. Dr. and Mrs. Pinckney were helpful to the late Russell Smith, Ph.D. who authored several massively documented exposes in the 1990s of the cholesterol issues. A smaller version of some of Dr. Smith's work titled *The Cholesterol Conspiracy* was published in 1991 by Warren H. Green, Inc. (ISBN 0-87527-476-5)

Another source of critical and objective information about cholesterol, fats, and coronary heart disease can be found in the writings of George V. Mann, Sc.D., M.D., especially the 1993 proceedings of the Veritas Society "Coronary Heart Disease: The Dietary Sense and Nonsense" edited by Dr. Mann and published by Janus Press (ISBN 1-85756-972-8).

And for those who have access to the internet, there is a superb web site with essays and references on the topic written by Uffe Ravnskov, M.D., Ph.D. (http://home2.swipnet.se/~w-25775/ is the web address). Dr. Ravnskov, who is a clinician and researcher in Lund, Sweden, has written a book *The Cholesterol Myth* and the English translation may be available by the time you are reading this book. Look for it.

Cerebrovascular disease has also been touted to be the result of too much "saturated" fat in the diet. Nonetheless, in the late 1990s, the research has been showing that those with higher intakes of polyunsaturated fats have been more likely to have strokes, and the more saturated fats are protective. The research has also reported that older individuals with serum cholesterol below 200 mg percent are at greater risk for stroke.

Cancer is another disease that has been tied periodically to dietary fats and oils. (See the discussion on animal fats and cancer below)

An example of alleged health hazards concluded from incorrect data is provided by the following example. In 1975, Kenneth Carroll, Ph.D., a Canadian biochemist active in cancer research, presented a graph of the positive relationship between breast cancer and dietary fat intake across the world. There were major problems with the supporting data because some numbers represented actual intake data and most represented disappearance data (i.e., the food available in a given country to be consumed as opposed to what is actually consumed). For example, Puerto Rico was shown as having less than 80 grams of total dietary fat intake using published intake data whereas the disappearance data for Puerto Rico was 121 grams of total dietary fat at that time. Other countries such as the U.S., which had a value greater than 145 grams of total dietary fat, represented disappearance data. You cannot put such disparate numbers together into a graphical comparison. A further major complication relates to the fact that this is a gender-related cancer and the fat disappearance/intake data being used was across genders.

Dr. Carroll was probably best known for his animal research, and that research clearly showed that the more polyunsaturated the fats were in the diets, the more they were cancer promoting; and that the more saturated the fats were, the more they were cancer reducing. In these studies by Carroll, the most cancer reducing fat was coconut oil. The conclusions from these studies are usually given an edible oil industry spin so that the problems with the polyunsaturates are pretty much ignored, and the safer more saturated fats come out as the problem.

The frequent contention that various cancers such as colon cancer are related to animal fat intake, which is usually translated as saturated fat intake, is based on acceptance of misinformation that began nearly four decades ago. See section below on **Animal Fats and Health Issues: What is the True Story?**

Diabetes has two forms: one that requires an outside source of insulin because the beta cells in the pancreas do not produce insulin, and one where the body produces insulin but the body does not utilize the insulin.

The first form is called insulin-dependent diabetes mellitus (IDDM), type I diabetes, or insulin-requiring diabetes, and it usually develops in childhood. Currently, the exogenous insulin has be given by some form of injection. Lack of insulin causes a loss of fat tissue triglycerides along with very high blood glucose levels because insulin is required for maintaining adequate fat stores.

The second form of diabetes is called non insulin-dependent diabetes mellitus (NIDDM), type 2 diabetes, or maturity onset diabetes, and it usually develops in overweight adults. In this form of diabetes, the body produces adequate or even excessive insulin, but insulin receptors on cells do not function appropriately.

Many clinicians believe that diabetes is made worse by "saturated fats." This consensus appears to be based on the prevailing attitude about causes of heart disease. Research has shown that dietary *trans* fatty acids have adverse effects in diabetes, including interference with insulin binding. There is no proven mechanism for any adverse effect from consumption of saturated fatty acids.

People who have poor control of their diabetes are very susceptible to the potentially damaging effects of oxidized lipids. When polyunsaturated fats and oils are not carefully protected, the levels of oxidized lipids is increased. Diabetics should avoid oxidized fats and oils.

Obesity is a major health problem, the cause of which is currently under intense investigation. Although obesity is an abnormal accumulation of fat cells and triglycerides, the exact reasons for this accumulation, beyond what is caused by the simple consumption of excess calories, are not known with any certainty. There have been reports in the scientific literature that individuals who consume diets high in partially hydrogenated fats tend to weigh more for the same caloric intake. It has been noted that saturated fatty acids in the adipose and in other cell membranes pack more densely than the unsaturated fatty acids. Thus, obesity, as it is related to size as opposed to weight, may reflect different tissue compartments and storage. There is anecdotal evidence that people with a large dietary intake of highly processed foods tend to accumulate excess adipose tissue.

If you look at the research data related to fat cells in normal and obese individuals, you find that those who are of normal weight with normal size fat cells (0.66 µg lipid per cell) and a normal number of fat cells (26±6.8 × 10⁹) carry about 37.8 pounds of fat. Someone with what is called juvenile-onset obesity has larger size fat cells (0.9µg lipid per cell), many more fat cells (85±6.9 × 10⁹), and carries about 168.3 pounds of fat. When someone develops adult-onset obesity, their fat cells become quite large (0.98 µg lipid per cell), they have many more fat cells (i.e., 62±4.2 × 10⁹) than the normal weight person (although less than the juvenile-onset obese person), and they carry about 133.7 pounds of fat. If the adult-onset obese person loses weight, the amount of fat that is carried is 61.4 pounds even though their fat cell size (0.45 µg lipid per cell) is smaller than the normal weight individual because the number of fat cells is still the same (i.e., 62 × 10⁹). Since the body does not like to have empty fat cells, the reduced formerly adult-onset obese person understandably has difficulty remaining reduced. (data from Linder 1985)

Immune dysfunction has been recognized as related to an inappropriate balance of fatty acids. Lipids are considered important nutrients in the regulation of immune function (Meydani 1991). Diets high in omega-6 fatty acids, and diets high in partially hydrogenated vegetable fats have been reported to adversely alter immune function. On the other hand, diets high in coconut oil or fish oil have been reported to improve immune response by decreasing pro-inflammatory cytokines (Sadeghi et al 1999).

Mental illness has recently been connected to inadequate omega-3 fatty acid consumption or to inappropriate processing of alpha-linolenic acid to the longer-chain omega-3 fatty acids such as docosahexaenoic acid and eicosapentaenoic acid. Research is being conducted at the National Institute on Alcohol Abuse and Alcoholism of the National Institutes of Health in Bethesda, Maryland.

Problems such as attention deficit disorders (ADD) and attention deficit hyperactivity disorders (ADHD) have been studied in relationship to essential fatty acid deficiency and adverse effects of the partially hydrogenated vegetable fats and oils.

Other ailments such as **cystic fibrosis** are being studied for a newly discovered connection to the longer-chain omega-3 fatty acid docosahexaenoic acid.

Animal Fats and Health Issues: What is the True Story?

In 1965, Ernst Wynder, M.D. of the American Health Foundation gave a talk at a meeting. During the talk he presented a slide, which he said showed that animal fat and colon cancer were positively correlated across many countries. Unfortunately, the data on the slide represented mostly processed vegetable fat for the many countries. The numbers were remote from the amount of animal fat in these countries, both in amounts and proportions. About 89 percent of the number for the U.S. represents processed vegetable fats.

Then in 1973, Haenszel and other statisticians and clinicians from Hawaii and the National Institutes of Health analyzed the colon cancer and diet relationship among Japanese Hawaiian patients. They actually found that the highest risk relationship came from macaroni, green peas, green beans, and soy, yet the conclusions drawn from this research was that beef was related to colon cancer, and that it fit the hypothesis of Wynder.

By 1975, Peter Greenwald, Ph.D. from New York State Cancer Institutes, who later became a high-level bureaucrat at the National Cancer Institute, surmised that one group of people who were noted for their high rates of colon cancer must be consumers of a lot of beef and that this fit the Haenszel findings. Gradually the antibeef agenda gathered momentum and eventually became accepted by the media who pushed it and by the unfortunate consumer who swallowed this big fraud, hook, line, and sinker.

In 1979, cancer researchers Saxon Graham and Curtis Mettlin wrote a review and commentary on "Diet and Colon Cancer" for the American Journal of Epidemiology. They wrote:

> "We first encountered the animal fats hypothesis with colon cancer etiology about 1965 at a symposium chaired by Ernst Wynder...Prior to this...[Wynder] had found no differences of note. At the symposium, Dr. Wynder presented the data shown in figure 1. Note that he found the mortality from colon cancer in countries increases as the *per capita* amount of animal fats ingested in those countries increases. This graph and others like it have many times subsequently been shown as being fundamental in support of the meat and fat hypothesis."

As noted above, these were not animal fat data. And now, more than three (3) decades after the initial fraudulent report, the anti-animal fat hypothesis continues to lead the nutrition agenda. It was a false issue then, and it remains a false issue today.

Health Concerns Related to Consumption of Partially Hydrogenated Vegetable Fats and Oils

It is evident from published studies of the *trans* fatty acids that a number of earlier researchers had questioned the biological safety of the *trans* fatty acids viz a viz their relationship to both cancer and heart disease. In fact, Ancel Keys had originally claimed that the partially hydrogenated vegetable oils with their *trans* fatty acids were the culprits in heart disease. This was in 1958, and the edible oil industry was very swift in their squelching of that information; they shifted the emphasis to "saturated" fat and started the unwarranted attack on meat and dairy fats. It has taken 30 years for research to get back on track. Now research is being reported on adverse effects from *trans* related to heart disease, diabetes, cancer, low birth weight, obesity, and immune dysfunction.

Because *trans* fatty acids disrupt cellular function, they affect many enzymes such as the delta-6 desaturase and consequently interfere with the necessary conversions of both the omega 6 and the omega-3 essential fatty acids to their elongated forms and consequently escalate the adverse effects of essential fatty acid deficiency (this latter effect was shown especially by the work of Dr. Holman and his colleagues at the Hormel Institute at the University of Minnesota).

Some adverse effects of consuming *trans* fatty acids reported in humans and animals are the following:

• Lowers the "good" HDL cholesterol in a dose response manner (the higher the *trans* level in the diet, the lower the HDL cholesterol in the serum);

• Raises the LDL cholesterol in a dose response manner;

• Raises the atherogenic lipoprotein (a) (Lp(a)) in humans (whereas saturated fatty acids lower Lp(a));

• Raises total serum cholesterol levels 20-30mg%;

• Lowers the amount of cream (volume) in milk from lactating females in all species studied, including humans, thus lowering the overall quality available to the infant;

• Causes a dose response decrease in visual acuity in infants who

are fed human milk with increasing levels of *trans* fatty acids, which extends to 14 months of age;
- Correlates to low birth weight in human infants;
- Increases blood insulin levels in humans in response to glucose load, increasing risk for diabetes;
- Affects immune response by lowering efficiency of B cell response and increasing proliferation of T cells;
- Decreases levels of testosterone in male animals, increases level of abnormal sperm, and interferes with gestation in females;
- Decreases the response of the red blood cell to insulin, thus having a potentially undesirable effect in diabetics;
- Inhibits the function of membrane-related enzymes such as the delta-6 desaturase, resulting in decreased conversion of, e.g., linoleic acid to arachidonic acid;
- Causes adverse alterations in the activities of the important enzyme system that metabolizes chemical carcinogens and drugs (medications), i.e., the mixed function oxidase cytochromes P-448/450;
- Causes alterations in physiological properties of biological membranes including measurements of membrane transport and membrane fluidity;
- Causes alterations in adipose cell size, cell number, lipid class, and fatty acid composition;
- Adversely interacts with conversion of plant omega-3 fatty acids to elongated omega-3 tissue fatty acids;
- Escalates adverse effects of essential fatty acid deficiency;
- Increases peroxisomal activity (potentiates free-radical formation);
- Precipitates childhood asthma

Two of the early researchers into the *trans* problems, Professor Fred Kummerow and Dr. George Mann, have continued their research and writing. A recent published paper (Nelson 1998) from a USDA researcher states:

> "Because *trans* fatty acids have no known health benefits and strong presumptive evidence suggests that they contribute markedly to the risk of developing CHD [coronary heart disease], the results published to date suggest that it would be prudent to lower the intake of *trans* fatty acids in the U.S. diet."

Some "Surprising" Health Effects of Selected Fats and Oils

Milk fat intake has recently been studied in 70 year old males. The research showed that the milk fat was inversely associated with a large number of cardiovascular risk factors. In other words, the milk fat was good. The researchers were surprised at their findings because they had believed the propaganda that saturated fat was bad. (Smedman et al 1999)

Coconut oil and **fish oil** decrease pro-inflammatory cytokines (TNF-α, IL-1β, IL-6) relative to omega-6 oils. Research suggests that these oils might be useful as therapies in acute and chronic inflammatory disease. The enhanced production of IL-10 by coconut oil shows an additional anti-inflammatory effect (Sadeghi et al 1999). Coconut milk (which contains the coconut fat) and fish (which contain fish oil) have been combined in many traditional diets in tropical countries for thousands of years.

Gamma-linolenic acid (GLA) from sources such as borage oil, and **eicosapentaenoic acid** (EPA) and **docosahexaenoic acid** (DHA) from sources such as fish oil can enhance the effectiveness of radiation treatment against malignant cells and are protective of normal cells (Hopewell et al 1993, Devi and Das 1994, Vartak et al 1997, Vartak et al 1998).

❦❦❦❦❦

What (Fats) Fatty Acids Found in Foods Are Natural to the Human Body?

Saturated fatty acids
**	palmitic acid
**	stearic acid
**	myristic acid
***	lauric acid

Monounsaturated fatty acids
**	palmitoleic acid
**	oleic acid

Polyunsaturated fatty acids
*	linoleic acid
*	linolenic acid - α
**	linolenic acid - γ
**	arachidonic acid
**	eicosapentaenoic acid
**	docosahexaenoic acid

* these fatty acids are used and needed by the body, but they are not made by the body; they are called essential fatty acids

** these fatty acids are used and needed by the body and they are made by the body

*** this fatty acid is made by certain parts of the body such as the lactating mammary gland, but it must come from the diet so it is a conditionally essential fatty acid

What Fatty Acids Found in Foods Are Not Natural to the Human Body?

almost all of the *trans* fatty acids

ଟ୍ଟଟ୍ଟଟ

Chapter 3

Diets, Then and Now, Here and There

What Fats Are In, What Fats Are Out

There was a time when a cookbook or a treatise on cookery discussed the use of different fats based on the qualities those fats bestowed to the foods they were part of. The special flavor imparted to a sauce by olive oil, the superior flavor and texture imparted to a crust or pudding by beef tallow (suet) or lard, the subtle flavor of Chinese foods fried in peanut oil, and the distinctive flavoring of coconut oil in Polynesian cooking were all important to the cook. That emphasis is almost completely gone today. No longer is the cook encouraged to salvage the fat that cooks out of the meat by turning it into gravy to top the potatoes or the rice or the homemade biscuit (and chances are the biscuit is no longer homemade).

Any discussion about fats today, in cookbooks or in magazines devoted to food and cookery, is likely to be negative about fat and additionally to reflect the "anti" saturated-fat propaganda, which started about forty years ago in the United States and spread to most of the world where the United States has influenced the food, nutrition, and biomedical communities. As a result, nearly every article about fats and oils in the diet begins with a faulty premise. That faulty premise is that cholesterol and the saturated fats are the culprits for the myriad of chronic ailments that afflict modern populations. This premise was basically invented in the late 1950s for the purpose of protecting the margarine and shortening industry from the challenges that were newly emerging from some of the scientific critics of hydrogenation who saw this as the cause of the epidemic of heart attacks. This chain of events has been reviewed by Hastert in a 1983 article on hydrogenation.

The resulting misinformation that was generated has virtually removed the safe and important natural fats from the diets of many people and has replaced these desirable fats with various partially hydrogenated fats and oils, or with a myriad of nonfood stabilizers, extenders, and emulsifiers in the low-fat and no-fat versions of traditional foods.

This unfortunate action has had a particularly devastating effect on the coconut oil industry. Coconut oil is one of the most saturated of the natural fats, one of the oldest in use, and one of the most desirable of the natural fats to have at least small amounts of in the diets of people.

Thus, we have ended up with a situation where the fats that have been used for centuries are out, and the fabricated fats that should be out are in. The emphasis is on low fat, but most of the foods that are being marketed today are filled with fat. Usually this fat is a partially hydrogenated fat that has such a high melting point it is not always noticed by the consumer when the food containing it is eaten.

Fats and oils in the U.S. food supply can come from several sources. They are either added fats such as table spreads, shortenings, and salad and cooking oils, or they come from the fat component of the meat and dairy products, from nuts and seeds, or from vegetables and fruit tissues. Added fats in the form of oils, shortenings, spreads (butter and margarine), salad dressing, etc. are listed in government documents such as those published by USDA and/or the Commerce Department as "table and cooking fats," etc. As shown in Figure 3.1, there have been major changes in the source oils for these products during the last hundred years.

```
                              1890 vs 1990

        FATS AND OILS IN THE U.S. FOOD SUPPLY

        1890                        1990

        LARD                        SOYBEAN OIL (70%
        TALLOW (SUET)                 PARTIALLY HYDROGENATED)
        CHICKEN FAT                 RAPESEED OIL
        BUTTER FAT                    CANOLA OIL (USUALLY
        OLIVE OIL                     PARTIALLY HYDROGENATED)
        PALM OIL                    COTTONSEED OIL
        COCONUT OIL                 PEANUT OIL
        PEANUT OIL                  CORN OIL
        COTTONSEED OIL              PALM OIL
                                    COCONUT OIL


     (IN DESCENDING ORDER OF MARKET SHARE)
```

Figure 3.1 Source of Fats and Oils in the United States 1890 vs1990

Fat in Human Diets in Antiquity

When we think about changing the fat in our diets or recommending new diets for purposes of improving health, we need to consider what the fats in past diets of many people have been. We also must consider the present diets of various groups of people around the world for whom the specter of heart disease, diabetes, or cancer in middle age is *not* a problem.

What was the fat content of a diet prior to 1920 before the incidence of coronary heart disease supposedly started to increase dramatically? What about the diet and its fat content in the 1800's? What was and is the fat content of the low-risk cultures?

Comparison of the diets of healthy groups of people shows a wide range of dietary intake of carbohydrate and fat. As an example, fat intake in healthy groups can vary from 10 percent of the calories (desert nomads) to 50 percent or more of the calories (e.g., Greenland Eskimos). Desert nomads consume less fat than Mediterranean people who consume less fat than northern European people, who in turn consume less fat than Eskimos. These varying amounts of dietary fat intakes may reflect the different energy needs due to diverse climates as well as the available fats in the different parts of the world. What is clear is that coronary heart disease incidence does not parallel dietary intake of fat for these groups since the nomads and the Eskimos both have the lowest *incidence* of heart disease.

The fats that humans have consumed for millennia, such as the fats that they added to mixed dishes, were almost always more saturated than they were unsaturated. It was the easily extractable fat or oil, the fat that came from the animal, or in the case of areas such as the tropics, it was the oil that came from the coconut or the palm fruit that was used in cooking. Sometimes it was one of the very stable oils like olive oil (or sesame paste) that had a lot of built-in antioxidant and wasn't too polyunsaturated.

People didn't really have the ability to extract oil from vegetables like corn, or from many seeds, as they do today. However, they got their essential polyunsaturated fatty acids from many of these plants when they were included in the foods they were eating. People used the intact leaf, root, nut, grain, or seed, along with all the plant's inherent antioxidants, in the stews or in the porridges that most people ate. This was the way the polyunsaturates were historically consumed. The polyunsaturated fatty acids didn't have to be hydrogenated to keep them from going rancid because they were consumed in a protected whole-food state. (As we learned in Chapter 1, the process of hydrogenation effectively destroys the part of the polyunsaturates that is the aspect of their essentiality.)

People on low fat diets historically consumed adequate amounts of essential fatty acids from such foods as grains, vegetables, and nuts; they made their own saturated fat (*de novo*) for use in their membranes, for the necessary support adipose, and for energy storage. Those people with higher fat intakes in their diets still had about the same amount of essential fatty acids, and ultimately the same amount of saturated fat for the specialized storage or as the energy source.

Regardless of whether they ate it or their bodies made it, the fat in the adipose tissues of our ancestors was relatively saturated, and therefore the fatty acid supply to the metabolic tissues was predictably saturated. Today with the high levels of partially hydrogenated vegetable and marine oils in the diets of many people, everyone's tissues and organs are faced with a new situation, and many researchers have concluded that the presence of the *trans* fatty acids in the diet is causing shifts in favor of chronic disease.

Today, we hear talk about diets such as the Mediterranean diet or the French diet or the Chinese diet. When it comes to the fat in those diets, most of the information being given out is not accurate. Surprisingly enough, the diets of these groups are rather predictably saturated in and of themselves, or they are saturated fat-producing diets when they are low fat diets. These diets are reviewed below.

How Much Fat Do We Really Eat in the United States?

What about eating patterns in the United States? There are many different ways of eating, and no one way is necessarily the "right" way.

It is a commonly held belief today that we have had a large increase in our dietary fat intake during this century. What we have had is a large increase in our intake of fats from vegetable sources (along with a substantial decrease in our intake of fats from animal sources). At the same time the amount of fat in our diets as a percent of calories has not changed that radically.

Figure 3.2 and Figure 3.3 graphically depict the changes in fat sources over the 20th Century beginning in 1910 when the United States Department of Agriculture records were first kept. Table 3.1 gives the USDA values for changes in fat intake (availability) from the 1930/1935 period to 1985. These data show that the major change in fat intake, during this period when there was beginning evidence of increased disease in our population, is a 127 percent increase in polyunsaturated fat

---

Table 3.1   Dietary Fat Intake Data 1930 to 1985

1930-1935
Saturated fat	59 grams = 48 percent
Monounsaturated fat	50 grams = 40 percent
Polyunsaturated fat	<u>15 grams</u> = 12 percent
	124 grams

1985
Saturated fat	62 grams = 38 percent
Monounsaturated fat	68 grams = 41 percent
Polyunsaturated fat	<u>34 grams</u> = 21 percent
	164 grams

Changes from 1930/35 to 1985

Saturated fat	+ 3 grams (5 percent increase)
Monounsaturated fat	+18 grams (36 percent increase)
Polyunsaturated fat	+19 grams (127 percent increase)

(Change as percentage)

Saturated fat	↓ 21 percent
Monounsaturated fat	↑ 2.5 percent
Polyunsaturated fat	↑ 75 percent

Much of the "polyunsaturated fat" and the "monounsaturated fat" has been partially hydrogenated.

Data from: DHHS Publication No.(PH)89-1255

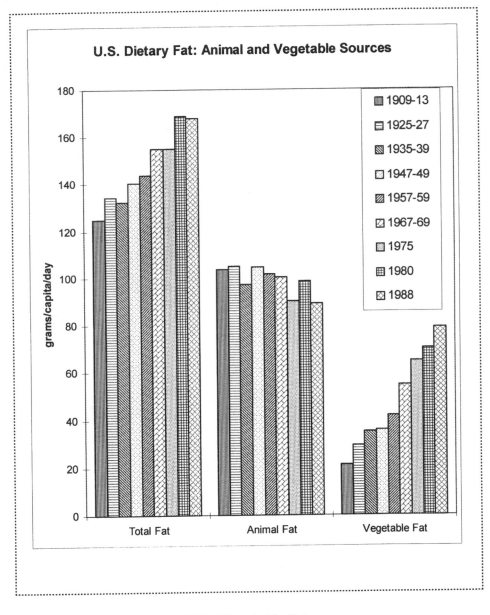

Figure 3.2 Total Fat, Animal Fat, Vegetable Fat

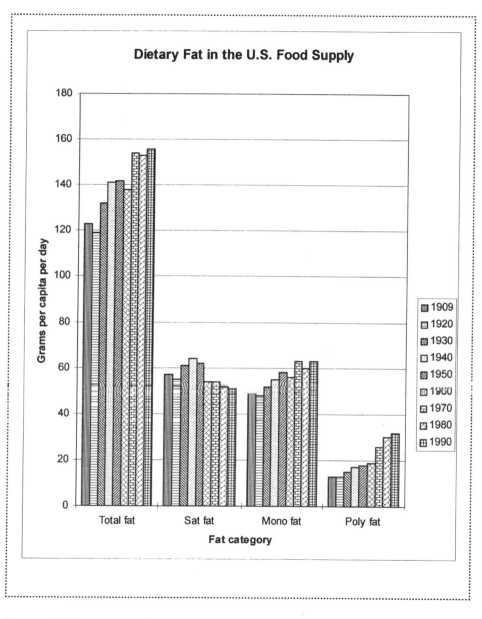

Figure 3.3 Categories of Dietary Fats 1909-1990

Food Fat Production and Eating Habits in Late 1800s

In the late 1800s, commercial shortenings advertised to the housewife were fats such as cotolene (a blend of cottonseed oil and beef tallow), refined leaf lard, or coconut butter (oil).   These commercially available fats, as well as fat rendered from beef, poultry, chicken, and pork in the home, were used for frying and as shortening in baking.   Figures 3.4 and 3.5 are typical advertisements for fats and oils sold to the housewife.

Butter and cream were valued for table use as well as for cooking and baking. In addition to cottonseed oil and coconut oil, olive oil and poppyseed oil were listed as principal vegetable oils.

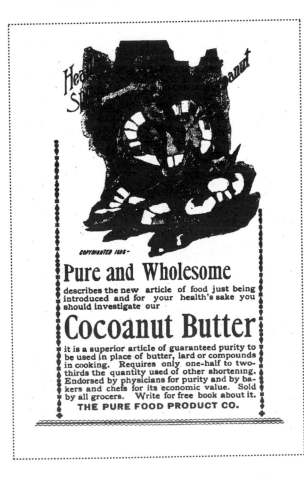

Figure 3.4 Coconut Oil Advertisement 1896

Fat in Diets in the 1890s and Early 1900s

Fat in the diets of Americans has always ranged from 30 percent to 43 percent of the calories depending on which survey you look at, and even in the 1890s the amount of fat in diets seems to have been this amount. A typical diet in the 1890s contained more fat than most people realize. Meals were larger, but people were also more physically active so they needed more food.

Averaging close to 3000 kilocalories for a day, the fat, which was mostly the more saturated fats, made up 36 percent of those calories.

The article on diets in the 1911 *Encyclopaedia Britannica* included information on many dietary surveys. There were 339 diet surveys to be exact of which 238 were done in the U.S. The highest level of fat intake reported was for American lumbermen at 43.6 percent of kilocalories, closely followed by Danish physicians at 42.9 percent of calories . Except for inmates in "insane hospitals" in the U.S., who averaged 29.9 percent of their kilocalories as fat, the average American family/adult ranged from 32.4 percent to 36.5 percent of kilocalories as fat.

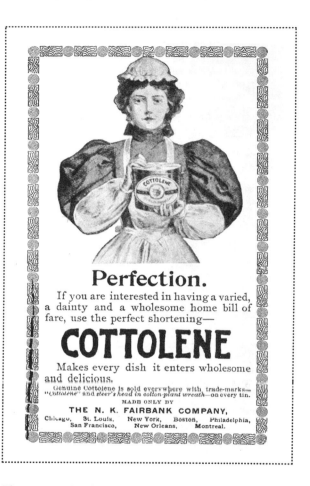

Figure 3.5 Cooking Fat Advertisement, 1896

Fat in the Diets in the 1930s, 1940s, 1950s, 1960s...

The "recommended" diets (e.g., General Foods) in the 1930s contained even more fat (40 percent of kilocalories). The sets of therapeutic diets recommended in the 1930s, which were deliberately high in protein or high in fat, contained, respectively, 46 percent and 61 percent of kilocalories as fat, while recommended diets made deliberately high in carbohydrates contained 29 percent of kilocalories as fat. It is quite apparent from these documents that, historically, diets in the U.S. have not been as low in fat as is currently touted as desirable.

An adequate daily diet for an average adult in the 1930s was listed in an authoritative text (Chapter 9 in Proudfit) as including 77 grams of dairy fat in the 114 grams of total fat. The dairy fat included 19 grams from whole milk, 22 grams from cream, and 36 grams from butter. This type of diet would have provided 2.5 grams of the antimicrobial(e.g., antibacterial, antiviral) fatty acids (e.g., lauric acid) and other desirable components such as sphingolipids and CLA.

In the preface to The Yearbook of Agriculture 1966 (also known as House Document No. 89 of the 89th Congress, 2nd Session) *Protecting Our Food*, the editor reminds us that the purpose of the yearbook is to "inform all Americans about the great scientific achievements that assure us a safe and plentiful supply of food." Causes of food deterioration were reviewed.

The discussion of fats and oils was particularly illuminating. The reader in 1966 learned that "[f]ats and oils in foods may be particularly subject to [rancidity] oxidation," especially during storage with resultant "off-flavors and odors that characterize rancidity." The foods that can be affected in this manner include high fat foods such as "cooking oils, meats, dairy products, eggs, fish, and nuts" as well as foods like bakery products, which usually contain added fat. Even vegetables with small amounts of fat could develop serious flavor problems if the fat became oxidized.

The reader at that time further learned that "[f]ats are composed of molecules of glycerin [glycerol] linked to fatty acids." These fatty acids "may be saturated or unsaturated, terms which refer to the ability of fatty acids to combine with other substances such as oxygen." "Saturated fatty acids are rather stable chemically and account for much of the firmness of fats at room temperatures."

"The unsaturated fatty acids ... are softer -- some even liquid at room temperature -- and are much less stable. Hence, these are most subject to attack by oxygen."

"But the attack on fats by oxygen can be prevented by antioxidants. These antioxidants are present naturally in most vegetable oils, but those classes of antioxidants and synergists (which potentiate antioxidants) were generally lost in the refining process...because of our desire for ...vegetable oils that are clear and sparkling..."

There was at this time no mention of saturated fatty acids in unfavorable terms, and the problems with the unsaturated fatty acids were clearly recognized by the writers.

Perhaps it is more meaningful for us to think about the changes over time for the amounts of fat in our diets that come from refined and/or partially hydrogenated vegetable fats/oils. It is clear that there has been a large increase in this kind of fat in most diets in the U.S. and Canada.

The "Industrial Revolution" for Fats and Oils Began in 1910

Hydrogenation of vegetable oils was introduced into the U.S. in 1910, and Crisco went on sale in 1911. Just as the earlier cottonseed/tallow blends had been intended as replacement competition to lard, this new vegetable shortening was also marketed as a replacement for lard.

In the 1930s, published texts on nutrition and dietetics included corn oil and peanut oil in lists of vegetable oils, and also referred to the commercial hydrogenation of cottonseed oil and its sale in the form of a solid fat.

Up until shortly before World War II, the margarines (which had originally started as blends of animal fats for a cheap butter substitute) were largely (90 percent) made of coconut oil, animal tallow, or lard; very little hydrogenation was required or used. By the 1940s, domestic vegetable oils made up 90 percent of the fat in margarines and hydrogenation was both required and used.

Prior to World War II, and depending on where one lived in Europe, much of the added fat or oil in the diet, other than the animal, poultry, and dairy fats, came either from small presses such as those used for flaxseed oil in Eastern Europe, the larger presses used for olive oil in the Mediterranean area, or from the hydrogenation plants in countries such as Holland or Denmark. These hydrogenation plants were closed down during the war, and the native populace consumed whatever animal and dairy fats were available. Even though the war led to marked restrictions in food and the fat rations were limited, there were available fats from animal and dairy sources.

Role of Edible Oil Industry in Promoting Consumption of *Trans* Fatty Acids

Beginning in the 1950s, the food industry capitalized on its ability to turn the domestically produced seed oils, which were plentiful, but not sufficiently marketable as liquid oils, into solid fats for the budding fast food industry and for the expanding baking and snack food industry.

In the late 1950s, an American researcher, Ancel Keys, announced that the CHD epidemic was being caused by the hydrogenated vegetable fats; previously this same person had introduced the idea that saturated fat was the culprit. The edible oil industry quickly responded to this perceived threat to their products by mounting a public relations campaign to promote the belief that it was only the saturated fatty acid component in the hydrogenated oils that was causing the problem. The industry then announced that it would be changing to partially hydrogenated fats and that this change would solve the problem. In actual fact, there was little change then because the oils were already being partially hydrogenated and so the levels of saturates remained similar, as did the levels of *trans*. From that time on, the edible fats and oils industry promoted the twin ideas that saturates (namely animal and dairy fats) were troublesome, and polyunsaturates (mainly corn oil and later soybean oil) were health-giving.

In 1965 the American Heart Association (AHA) changed its Diet/Heart statement by (i) deleting the recommendation to decrease the intake of hydrogenated fats and by (ii) removing a negative reference to the *trans* fatty acids. The revised statement encouraged the consumption of partially hydrogenated fats (Committee Print, Dietary Goals for the United States, 2nd Edition, U.S. Government Printing Office, Washington DC 1977). In the 1970s and the 1980s, the AHA continued to promote the partially hydrogenated fats as long as they contained twice as much polyunsaturates as saturates.

At the very times that U.S. government-sponsored research results, such as those of the National Heart Lung and Blood Institute's Lipid Research Clinic (LRC) trials, lent additional credence to the anti-saturated fat view, it became clear to some that the prevailing interpretations of these research results were fatally flawed: *The measurements of dietary fat intake did not acknowledge the existence of trans fatty acids and consequently were inaccurate.* The interpretations of the results of these LRC trials, however, were the basis for the 1984 National Institutes of Health Cholesterol Consensus Conference, which in turn gave rise to the National Cholesterol Education Program (NCEP). The NCEP program encouraged consumption of margarine and partially hydrogenated vegetable fats.

Perhaps one of the most remarkable aspects of the saturated fat issue is that the *trans* fatty acids were kept out of both government and private food composition data bases for several decades! *Trans* fatty acids were treated as a nonissue by most technical and government information sources and the media for several decades, though that situation has now changed. The Harvard University School of Public Health has established a data base that includes the *trans* fatty acids for a large number of foods; at least one of the commercial food analysis programs has begun the inclusion of *trans* fatty acids in its data base; in recent years, copies of the U.S. Department of Agriculture provisional table of *trans* fatty acids in foods have surfaced, although the table is not yet in final official form. As noted in Chapter 5, the FDA has announced at the end of 1999 that it will be putting out regulations for labeling the *trans* fatty acids, so there will have to be more complete information available within a matter of years.

By the mid-1980s, major changes were made in the food supply that were damaging to the image and markets of the naturally saturated fats. Some groups in the edible oil industry (e.g., soybean producers) and some of the consumer activist groups (e.g., Center for Science in the Public Interest (CSPI)) further eroded the status of saturated fats when they sponsored the antisaturated fat, antitropical oils campaign in the mid-to late-1980s. (See Chapter 5 for discussion of the involvement of CSPI.) The activism of these groups resulted in wholesale economic boycotting of the so-called saturated fats, especially the palmitic-rich tallows and palm oil and the lauric-rich oils; this activism resulted in their ultimate removal from very many foods. As a result, the partially hydrogenated vegetable oils replaced the naturally saturated fats and, there were major increases in the levels of unnatural *trans* fatty acids in popular food items in the U.S. and Canada, especially restaurant foods, bakery goods, snack chips, and other widely consumed processed foods.

Trans Fatty Acids in U.S. Foods and Elsewhere

Individual meals in fast food restaurants now provide many more times more *trans* fatty acids than they did a decade ago; for example, a meal of the "identical" foods showed 19.2 g *trans* fatty acids in 1992 versus 2.4 g *trans* fatty acids in 1982. This increase is largely due to the campaign waged by CSPI against the naturally saturated fats and oils.

How much fat and *trans* fat is in some of the most popular foods? Chicken nuggets and potato fries are very popular foods with many Americans, and especially with children. Chicken nuggets are reported by Davineni (1997) to be about 33 percent fat on average (range of 21 to 35 percent), and potato fried about 26 percent on average (13.5 to 28 percent range). An order of 6 chicken nuggets weighs between 100 and 130 grams according to restaurant and U.S. Department of Agriculture Handbook 8 guides; this means that the samples from typical fast food restaurants analyzed by Davineni would provide from 33 to 43 grams of fat, which is higher than the restaurants or USDA admit. With this much fat, of which about 35 to 42 percent could be *trans*, a serving of chicken nuggets could provide 12 to 18 grams of *trans*. A large order of potato fries is 122 grams, which would provide 13 to 28 grams of fat (also somewhat more than the above guides admitted), and 5 to 12 grams of *trans*. See Table 3.2 on the next page for published values of *trans* fatty acids in diets in various countries in addition to the United States.

One recent fad in some of the newer and more upscale restaurants has been the replacement of butter for spreading on bread with a plate or bowl of olive oil (sometimes flavored, but usually plain olive oil) for dipping bread. What is somewhat amusing and ironical is the fact that butter is only 80 percent fat while olive oil is 100 percent fat. When a piece of bread that has been saturated with olive oil is eaten, the amount of fat being consumed is easily 2 to 3 times the amount of a thin spreading of butter.

Table 3.2 Dietary Exposure to *Trans* Fatty Acids

Published Estimates of *Trans* Fatty Acid Availability[1,2] and Consumption[3] in Various Countries

		Grams/person/day	Percent of Total Fat	Reference
Canada	Average	9.1	9.5	Brisson (1981)
	Maximum	17.5	18.2	Brisson (1981)
England	Average	12.0	10.8	Gurr (1983)
	Maximum	27.0	24.3	British Nutrition Foundation (1987)
Germany	Range	4.5-6.5	NA	Heckers (1979)
Holland	Average	17.0	12.6	Brussaard (1986)
Scotland	Range[3]	0.4-47.6	0.3-11.6	Bolton-Smith et al (1995)
Sweden	Average[3]	5.0	5.0	Akesson et al (1981)
United States	Average[1]	12.1	7.8	Enig et al (1978)
	Average[1]	11.4	7.3	Applewhite (1979)
Adult ♀	Average	9.7	11.8	Craig-Schmidt et al (1984)
	Maximum	13.7	17.1	
Adolescent ♀	Average	3.1	6.5	Van den Reek et al (1986)
	Range	0.4-8.0	1.8-17.2	
	Average[1]	13.3	8.0	Enig et al (1990)
Adults 20-65 yrs	Range	1.6-38.7	5-15	
Teenage ♀	Average[2]	14.9	8.0	Enig et al (1991)
	Average[3]	>30.0	>26.0	Enig (1993)

[1] Available for total population, estimated from government fats and oils availability data and known *trans* fatty acids levels in foods;
[2] Available for selected age groups, estimated from government fats and oils availability data and known *trans* fatty acids levels in foods;
[3] Consumption based on food records and analytical data.

What Are Healthy Fats and Oils?

Healthy fats and oils are the ones that don't oxidize readily, or that are usually consumed before they can oxidize. Those fats and oils that are oxidized are either: (1) not available for use as energy or for structural purposes because they are either in a polymerized unusable form; or (2) they contain toxic components.

Naturally occurring fats and oils that have been consumed for thousands of years are invariably found to be the more saturated animal and plant fats. The more readily oxidizable oils historically have usually been consumed in their original packaging. In other words, they have been consumed as the seeds and plants before they have been extracted and had a chance to form oxidized products.

Fats and oils to be avoided, in addition to partially hydrogenated vegetable fats, include any rancid or overheated fats and oils that contain breakdown products such as oxidized fatty acids, oxidized sterols, peroxides, acrolein, hydrocarbons, and aromatic compounds. These types of abused fats and oils are not safe. They range from immediately toxic to chronically toxic. Free radicals are derived from, e.g., decomposition of unsaturated fatty acids, especially polyunsaturated fatty acids. Ozone-induced reactive free radicals can interact with sulfhydryl groups in proteins as well as with unsaturated fatty acids and are very destructive of membranes.

Oils, especially the "polyunsaturated" oils, that have been thought to be good, because they decrease serum cholesterol levels, actually have been shown to increase cholesterol in tissues; the reason being that the polyunsaturated fatty acids are deposited into the membranes and the body needs to put more cholesterol into these membranes to stabilize them and to maintain the melting point (fluidity) characteristics of the membrane.

The effect of fatty acids on serum cholesterol levels is dependent on the original serum cholesterol levels: high serum cholesterol decreases with most fatty acids, including all saturates; low serum cholesterol increases with many of the fatty acids, including saturates, monounsaturates, and sometimes the polyunsaturates.

What Balance of Fats Do We Need?

The important thing to understand is that all fats are basically mixtures of saturated, monounsaturated, and polyunsaturated fatty acids in different proportions. There isn't any real evidence that everyone needs to consume exactly the same balance of fatty acids, except that we do know that people need to take in at least 2 to 3 percent of their calories as fat in the form of omega-6 fatty acids and at least 1 to 1.5 percent of their calories as fat in the form of omega-3 fatty acids. This means that small people on fewer calories need fewer grams of essential fatty acids than larger or more active people who consume more calories. It also means that since people are being advised to consume about 30 percent of their calories as fat, the nonessential fatty acid portion is about 25.5 percent of their energy (kilocalories).

Some people have selected a type of diet that provides the correct amount of essential fatty acids from natural foods. Most people, however, consume many processed foods for which there is no certainty of essential fatty acids being left in the foods. This is especially true if the foods contain partially hydrogenated vegetable oils. In such case, some individuals may wish to add natural oils to their diets as a source of essential fatty acids.

Tables 3.3 and 3.4 give examples of measures of different oils that could be used to supply appropriate amounts of omega-3 fatty acids in the daily diet. Tables 3.5 and 3.6 give examples of measure of different oils that could be used to supply appropriate amounts of omega-6 fatty acids in a daily diet.

Contrary to prevailing propaganda, fats and oils are very important components of diet. The consumption of naturally-occurring, unprocessed or minimally processed fats and oils plays a role in maintaining good health. In addition to the well-recognized need for unprocessed omega-3 and omega-6 fatty acids, there is strong evidence that some of the medium-chain saturated fatty acids such as lauric acid are essential since they are needed for maintaining the natural ability of the individual to fight potentially harmful microorganisms. In addition to antimicrobial fatty acids such as lauric acid found principally in coconut oil and palm kernel oil, fatty acids such as the anticarcinogen conjugated linoleic acid (CLA) and immune-supporting fats, such as glycosphingolipids, are found in dairy and animal fats.

The bottom line is to consume as many whole foods and whole food mixtures as possible. Since we live in a society where other people prepare most of the foods many of us eat, it is important to look for those foods that are the least processed and, when it comes to fats and oils, the least likely to go rancid.

Table 3.3 The Essential Fatty Acid (EFA) α-Linolenic Acid (Omega-3) (ω-3)

How much ω-3 fat do we need? Enough to supply 1-1.5% of energy (kcal)

For 2000 kcal diet (20-30 kcal as ω-3 fat), we need 2.2 - 3.3 grams of ω-3 fat

To get 3.5 grams of the ω-3 EFA α-linolenic acid a day from added oils, you need to consume one of the following:

Flaxseed oil	~1.5 tsp	(~53% 18:3 ω-3)*
Canola oil	~1.5 TBS	(~15% 18:3 ω-3)*
Walnut oil	~2.0 TBS	(~12% 18:3 ω-3)*
Soybean oil	~3.0 TBS	(~7% 18:3 ω-3)*

tsp ≡ teaspoon, TBS ≡ tablespoon
*Only if unrefined

Table 3.4 The Fish Oil Omega-3 (ω-3) EPA and DHA
EPA ≡ eicosapentaenoic acid, DHA ≡ docosahexaenoic acid

How much is needed?

Connor & Connor (1997) suggest 2 to 3 g fish oil per day for individuals who do not eat fish for primary prevention of heart disease; more for treatment of existing disease.

(Capsules are ~ 0.2-0.5 g (200-500 mg) EPA per capsule)

Fish ranges from less than 0.5 grams of total omega-3 per 100 gram (3.5 oz) serving (e.g., cod, flounder, haddock, halibut); ~1 to 1.5 grams (e.g, anchovy, mullet, salmon); ~1.5 to 2.0 (e.g., herring, lake trout); and 2 to 3.3 grams (e.g., herring, mackerel, sardines) per 100 gram (3.5 oz) serving of the fish.

> **Table 3.5 The Essential Fatty Acid (EFA) Linoleic Acid (Omega-6) (ω-6)**
>
> How much ω-6 fat do we need? Enough to supply 2-3% of energy (kcal)
>
> For 2000 kcal diet (40-60 kcal as ω-6 fat, we need 4.4 - 6.7 grams of ω-6 fat
>
> To get 7 grams of the ω-6 EFA linoleic acid a day from added oils, you need to consume from one of the following:
>
> | | | |
> |---|---|---|
> | Sunflower oil | ~2.0 tsp | (~68% 18:2 ω-6) |
> | Evening Primrose oil | ~2.0 tsp | (~69% 18:2 ω-6) |
> | Corn oil | ~1.0 TBS | (~57% 18:2 ω-6) |
> | Borage oil | ~2.0 TBS | (~23% 18:2 ω-6) |
> | Flaxseed oil | ~2.0 TBS | (~17% 18:2 ω-6) |
> | Canola oil | ~2.5 TBS | (~19% 18:2 ω-6) |
> | Olive oil | ~5.0 TBS | (~10% 18:2 ω-6) |

There is nothing wrong with consuming your essential fatty acids from extracted oils (e.g., from the bottle instead of in the seed) as long as those oils are safely extracted and carefully stored, but a good balance needs to be maintained with sources of the more saturated fats such as the animal tallows and/or dairy fats for those who are not vegetarians, or the more saturated fats such as palm or coconut oils for those who are vegetarians. For those who like to use the "whole food" for their omega-3 fatty acids, 2 TBS of freshly ground flaxseed (which can be added to cereal or juice) would supply the same amount of alpha-linolenic acid as would ½ tsp of flaxseed oil (Table 3.2).

Note: Research has shown that saturated fat in the diet is needed by the body to enable it to adequately convert the essential omega-3 fatty acid (α-linolenic acid) to the elongated omega-3 fatty acids EPA and DHA. These latter fatty acids are necessary for prostaglandin formation and visual function, respectively. (Gerster 1998)

Table 3.6 Conditionally Essential Gamma Linolenic Acid (GLA) (ω-6)

How much is needed?

Some researchers have suggested 70-240 mg a day

This is the equivalent of

~1 capsule of Borage oil
~1-6 capsules of Evening Primrose oil
~1-2 capsules of Black Currant oil

Dietary Fat and Pregnancy and Lactation

Pregnant and lactating women have numerous requirement for additional nutrients during the period of pregnancy and while they are nursing their infant(s). In addition to the obvious need for additional energy from fats and carbohydrates, as well as the need for adequate protein, vitamins and minerals, there is a requirement for additional special fats and oils. This is because there is the need to include more adequate omega-3 and omega-6 essential fatty acid sources.

The whole diet should include about 3 to 5 percent of the energy (calories) as omega-6 fatty acids and half as much as omega-3 fatty acids. (See section above on dietary fat balance) To achieve easily adequate omega-6 and omega-3 essential fatty acid status means using only unhydrogenated fats and oils for preparation of foods. It also means including all the natural fats that come with the natural foods, because the best way to avoid the unnatural *trans* fatty acids is to consume adequate fat from natural sources.

Research carried out in Europe (Koletzko 1991) shows that the *trans* fatty acids have an undesirable effect on the birth weight of the infant. Dr. Koletzko (1992) in Germany has identified the partially hydrogenated vegetable fats and oils as a factor in low birth weight infants, and also in interference with proper levels of the elongated omega-3 fats (called DHA) in the brains of infants.

Research reported in the late 1990s from Canada has shown that the *trans* fatty acids consumed by the lactating mother go directly into her milk at levels up to 18 percent of the total milk fat, and the *trans* fatty acids in human milk were found to correlate significantly with decreased visual acuity in the infants. This shows quite clearly that *trans* fatty acid-containing products should be avoided by lactating women.

Dietary Fat and Growth

A normal diet in infancy is relatively high in fat. Human milk provides about 50 percent of its calories as fat. This way the protein is spared and utilized for growth. Carbohydrates are also spared for some quick energy, for maintaining glucose levels, and for membrane formation.

The sugar found in human milk, as well as in milk from the cow, goat, and sheep, is called lactose. Lactose is made up of two single sugars called glucose and galactose; they are joined together in much the same way that glucose and fructose are joined together to form sucrose, the common table sugar. Galactose is used by the body for building important membranes in the brain, for example. The body has limited ability to convert glucose to galactose, but can convert galactose to glucose unless there is a genetic lack of the enzyme that accomplishes this latter conversion.

Human milk fat has a unique fatty acid composition. It is approximately 45 to 50 percent saturated, about 35 percent monounsaturated, and 15 to 20 percent polyunsaturated. Of the saturated fatty acids made in the mammary gland, up to 18 percent can be the antimicrobial fatty acids lauric acid and capric acid. These antimicrobial fatty acids give the infant fed good quality human milk protection against lipid-coated viruses, bacteria, and protozoa.

In the United States, and to an extent in Canada, many pediatricians have mistakenly believed that they should recommend low fat diets to children. Several prominent pediatricians (Drs. Fima Lifshitz, Robert Olson, and Stanley Zlotkin), on the other hand, have recognized that children given low fat diets or low saturated fat diets develop many growth and health problems. Children need to eat foods that will give them only natural fats, and they need to have enough of their caloric intake as fat so that they grow properly, don't become ill, and are happy and active.

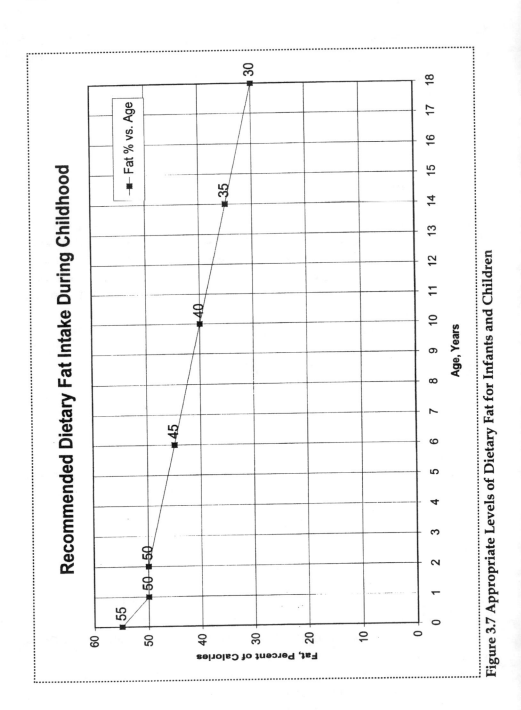

Figure 3.7 Appropriate Levels of Dietary Fat for Infants and Children

Recommendations for the amount of fat in a child's diet have been made by various groups and agencies. The US and Canadian government agencies and pediatric groups have recommended a **gradual decrease** in dietary fat intake. The appropriate levels of dietary fat between birth and two years of age are recognized as being approximately 50 to 55 percent of calories; the recommended level of dietary fat for adults is 30 percent of calories. If you wish to follow these recommended guidelines to lower fat content of a child's diet, do so gradually, to reach 30 percent of calories at the end of growth, which is approximately 18 years of age. Figure 3.7 gives a graphic picture that enables you to determine the appropriate amount at any given age.

During the first year of life, an infant who receives good nutrition, with adequate energy and adequate electrolytes such as chloride, will make a lot of fat for brain structure. What is made is a lot of saturated fatty acids, especially extra-long-chain saturated fatty acids, for building myelin for the brain.

Research in the late 1990s has shown that oils such as canola oil are not appropriate for growing animals and likely not appropriate for growing children. The use of canola oil is not allowed in infant formula in the U.S. or Canada.

A Dozen Important Dietary Does and Don'ts

❦ **Do consume optimal amounts** of fat-soluble vitamins A, D, E, and K and fat-soluble phytonutrients and biotonutrients (pages 71 to 73).

❦ **Do eat at least one egg a day if you are not allergic to them;** more than one is likely to be better for some people. If you are feeding children, be sure that they eat a minimum of one whole egg a day. (Fish eggs can take the place of poultry eggs for some purposes.)

❦ **Do consume optimal amounts of omega-3 fatty acids.** Use the information on page 106 in this chapter to determine how much you need and the composition information in Chapter 4 and Appendix 3 to identify appropriate sources.

❦ **Do limit excess omega-6 fatty acids in your diet.** Use the information on page 107 in this chapter to determine how much you need and the composition information in Chapter 4 and Appendix 3 for the numerous sources.

❦   **Do include sources of lauric acid in your diet.** Lauric acid is a healthy functional saturate and is found in lauric oils, so anything made with coconut oil or products made with desiccated or whole coconut (macaroons and coconut milk) are good sources. Full fat dairy products also supply small amounts. See page 115 and composition information in Chapter 4 and Appendix 3.

❦   **Do remember that full fat milk and dairy products are healthful foods** and should be eaten, particularly by children. Imitation dairy foods should be avoided. They usually are missing the important natural fats and often are sources of problematic *trans* fatty acids and other antinutrients.

❦   **Do include some fats in your diet from natural meats, fish, eggs, and/or dairy products.** They are necessary as sources for true vitamin A, vitamin D, and assure intake of vitamin B12.

❦   *Don't fear cholesterol.*   Cholesterol is the body's repair substance. It is needed for proper brain function and proper hormone balance.

❦   *Don't fear saturated fats.* Saturated fatty acids are the body's natural fats, which are used for appropriately functioning cell membranes and for critical energy in important organs such as the heart and other muscles.

❦   *Don't use only one fat or oil exclusively.* Fats and oils are different from each other and you need a variety of fatty acids found in a variety of fats and oils.

❦   *Don't save oils that have become rancid* even if they were expensive. Rancid fats and oils are dangerous to consume: throw them away.

❦   *Don't consume any products containing partially hydrogenated vegetable fats and oils*: they contain the *trans* fatty acids, which have been identified as the major nutritional cause of coronary heart disease.

❦   *Don't believe the story that there are plenty of people around the world who eat and thrive even though they consume no animal products.* All healthy groups of people seek to provide growing infants and children with milk first from humans and then from animals, and eggs from birds or reptiles or fish.

Note: Individuals with food allergies may need to make exceptions to some of the recommendations above.

Chapter 4

The Many Sources of
Fats and Oils

Commonly Used Fruit/Seed Oils

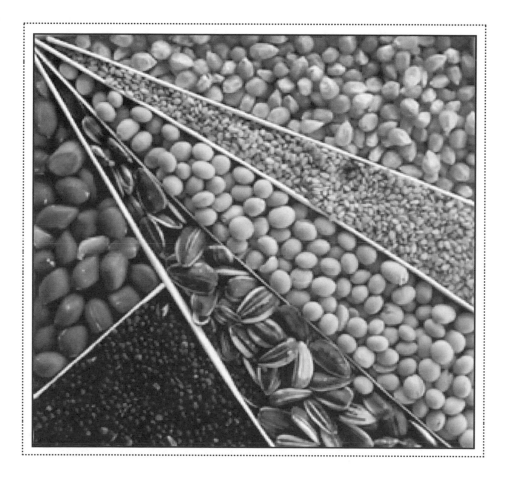

Canola oil (see **Rapeseed Oil**; also see **General Glossary**)

Cocoa Butter

Cocoa butter is the fat that is pressed out of the cocoa bean (*Theobromo cacao*). It is very pale yellow in color, very firm at room temperature, has the odor of chocolate, and melts at body temperature. The official melting point is 34.1°C (93.4°F). The triglycerides of cocoa butter have a unique blend of fatty acids. These fatty acids are the 16 carbon saturate palmitic acid (24 percent), the 18 carbon saturate stearic acid (35 percent), and the 18 carbon monounsaturate oleic acid (38 percent). The remaining 2 percent of the fatty acids are primarily the 18 carbon polyunsaturated fatty acid linoleic acid. Cocoa butter is a very stable fat that does not become rancid under normal conditions of use.

Typical tocopherol and tocotrienol (vitamin E) values are 11 mg/kg α-tocopherol, 170 mg/kg γ-tocopherol, 17 mg/kg δ-tocopherol, and 2 mg/kg α-tocotrienol for a total of 200 mg/kg.

Cocoa butter is a rather unique fat that cannot be totally replaced by other fats and oils for chocolate candy manufacture without changing the physical properties of the candy. Cocoa butter equivalents or replacers that are used for candies and confections include illipe butter, shea butter, fractionated and/or hydrogenated coconut, palm and palm kernel oils, and partially hydrogenated soybean and/or cottonseed oils.

Coconut oil

Coconut oil comes from the fruit/seed of the coconut palm tree (*Cocus nucifera*), which is grown in all parts of the tropics and subtropics. The tree appears to have originated in the islands of Southeast Asia and spread to other parts of the world floating on water or carried by man. Coconuts, in the form of extracted coconut oil or as the whole coconut, fresh or desiccated, have provided an important source of nutrients for people where this fruit tree is grown.

Coconut oil is pressed out of the fruit of the coconut (called the copra). Approximately two-thirds of the dry matter of the fruit is oil. There are currently several methods for extracting the oil. Small-scale extraction from the wet copra is used for specialty and organically produced oil. Larger-scale extraction from the dried copra is the major form of commercial extraction, and the resulting oil is usually refined by deodorization and removal of free fatty acids. The resulting oil has a pale yellow to white coloration, has the odor of coconut, is very stable, and does not become rancid even on long storage. Its melting point is 24-25°C (75-76°F).

The stability of coconut oil has made it very popular with the baking industry as well as with the candy and confection industry where it competes to an extent with palm kernel oil and cocoa butter (see **Cocoa butter, Palm kernel oil**). A large portion of coconut oil is used for nonfood products such as soaps and cosmetics. For example, in addition to soaps and shampoos, such products as toothpastes have as their major ingredient a detergent made from the lauric acid portion of coconut oil.

Other major uses of coconut oil in some parts of the world are for making oleomargarine and for deep fat frying. Coconut oil is also used today as the source of lauric acid, which is important for infant formulas; this fatty acid is found in human milk where it plays a very critical role in infant nutrition. Lauric acid has antimicrobial properties and is the precursor to monolaurin, the antimicrobial active lipid. Coconut oil is also the major source of the fatty acids found in the medium-chain triglycerides oil called MCT oil. MCT oil is approximately 75 percent caprylic acid (C8:0) and 25 percent capric acid (C:10). It has been used for special medical formulas during the past several decades (see also Chapter 1).

Coconut oil is sometimes called a "lauric fat" because approximately 49 percent of its fatty acids is the 12 carbon saturated fatty acid, lauric acid. (Other lauric fats include palm kernel oil and some lesser known fats, such as babassu oil and cohune oil.) The remaining fatty acids in coconut oil include 8 percent caprylic acid, 7 percent capric acid, 18 percent myristic acid, 8 percent palmitic acid, 2 percent stearic acid, 6 percent oleic acid, and 2 percent linoleic acid. The typical tocopherol and tocotrienol content is 5 mg/kg α-tocopherol, 6 mg/kg δ-tocopherol, 5 mg/kg α-tocotrienol, 1 mg/kg β-tocotrienol, and 19 mg/kg γ-tocotrienol for a total of 36 mg/kg.

Corn Oil

Corn oil comes from the whole corn (*Zea mays L.*), an annual herbaceous plant native to Central America. The oil makes up approximately 5 percent of the whole corn. Corn can be either wet milled to produce corn starch, corn sweeteners, and corn oil, or it can be dry milled to produce grits, flakes, meal, and oil. The crude corn oil that is obtained from the corn germ is further refined by deodorization and removal of free fatty acids. It is yellow in color with a mild but usually identifiable odor.

Refined corn oil is used as a salad and cooking oil or in making margarine. The refined oil has good flavor stability, and it resists rancidity quite well even though it is highly unsaturated. Almost half of the world's corn oil is produced in the U.S., corn oil ranks above all domestically produced oils except soybean oil (1990-91 data). Corn oil has been promoted as a food oil for at least 75 years in the U.S.

A typical fatty acid composition for corn oil is 12 percent palmitic acid, 2 percent stearic acid, 28 percent oleic acid, 57 percent linoleic acid, and 1 percent α-linolenic acid. Typical tocopherol levels in unrefined corn oil average 112 mg/kg α-tocopherol, 50 mg/kg β-tocopherol, 602 mg/kg γ-tocopherol, and 18 mg/kg δ-tocopherol for a total of 782 mg/kg. There is no reported tocotrienol content.

Cottonseed Oil

Cottonseed oil is a by-product of the cotton industry. The oil is extracted from the meat of the cottonseed (*Gossypium hirsutum*). Approximately 40 percent of the oil is recovered by screw pressing; the remainder is recovered by various types of solvent extraction. Originally, cottonseed oil was all extracted by the hydraulic press method. About 17 percent of the seed is crude oil. This crude oil is subjected to various forms of refining, including bleaching, deodorizing, and/or winterizing. These refining steps are necessary to remove antinutritional components present in the crude oil. Whether or not insecticide residues remain in significant amounts is not clear.

Cottonseed oil is used unhydrogenated as a salad and cooking oil; for use in margarine and shortening production it is usually partially hydrogenated.   Cottonseed oil was the first vegetable oil used commercially in the U.S.; its production started in the mid-nineteenth century. Currently, cottonseed oil ranks third after soybean oil and corn oil in the U.S.

Cottonseed oil is considered an important, high-quality, relatively stable cooking oil that is used as such for frying (especially potato chips) or as a component of shortening. The stability and mild flavor of cottonseed oil is due to its lack of the omega-3 alpha-linolenic acid. The crystalline qualities that make it popular for use in shortenings, especially in combination with soybean oil, are because of its high content of palmitic acid (~26 percent). The other fatty acids include 1 percent myristic acid, 1 percent palmitoleic acid, 2 percent stearic acid,

18 percent oleic acid, and 53 percent linoleic acid. Typical tocopherol levels are 389 mg/kg α-tocopherol and 387 mg/kg γ-tocopherol for a total of 776 mg/kg.

Olive Oil

Olive oil comes from the fruit of the evergreen olive tree (*Olea europaea*) and is one of the oldest known oils used by man. It is the major edible vegetable oil today in Greece, Italy, Portugal, and Spain. Many of the fruit-bearing trees are hundreds (100-500) of years old.

Olives are crushed between stone or steel rollers, and the oil is pressed from the crushed pulp. The oil content of olives ranges from 30 to 70 percent of the fruit on a dry weight basis. The first pressing yields an oil referred to as virgin oil that is considered as the top grade. Several repeated pressings yield additional grades of oil. Virgin oil is usually darker in color and contains more flavor components than the other grades. Preference for the "stronger" oil is more frequent in countries other than the U.S. Most oil is pressed from green olives and is of a greenish yellow color. Olive oil pressed from ripe olives is yellow in color.

Olive oil is commonly used as a salad oil or for cooking Mediterranean foods. Except for several specialty breads, it is not generally used in baking because of its strong flavor. Due to its content of natural antioxidants that are retained because it is extracted without solvents, olive oil has good keeping qualities and does not readily become rancid. Oil from the olive pit does not have the same composition as oil from the olive fruit.

The fatty acid composition of the average olive oil is 14 percent palmitic acid, 1 percent palmitoleic acid, 2 percent stearic acid, 71 percent oleic acid, 10 percent linoleic acid, and less than 1 percent α-linolenic acid. Typical tocopherol values are 119 mg/kg α-tocopherol and 7 mg/kg γ-tocopherol for a total of 126 mg/kg. Other antioxidants present in the virgin oil, including carotenoids and various phenolic compounds, promote long-term keeping properties.

Palm Oil

Palm oil is extracted from the fruit flesh of the oil palm (*Elaeis guineensis*) and is one of the most important edible oils in the world as well as an important oil source for products such as soap. The yield of oil palm per acre is greater than any other vegetable oil source. Palm oil has been used for more than five thousand (5000) years in parts of the world such as west Africa where it originated. Today the major countries producing palm oil are Malaysia, Nigeria, Indonesia, China, and Zaire. The oil palm grows wild in Africa, but it has been developed into a commercial plantation crop. Modern extraction is accomplished with steam. Because 30 to 70 percent of the fruit is oil, solvent extraction is not needed nor is it generally used.

The palm fruit, which grows in bunches, is usually hand harvested. Hand processing involves fermenting of the fruit, boiling and crushing with collection of the oil that floats on the surface of the pot. The oil content of the fruit ranges from 74 to 81 percent on a dry weight basis. The crude fat that is extracted from the fruit is very colorful, either red or orange, and is highly flavored. Palm oil is known to have high levels of β-carotene (the precursor to vitamin A), other carotenes, the antioxidant tocopherols (vitamin E), and the antioxidant tocotrienols. Some of the palm oil of commerce remains yellow due to high carotene content. As a source of oil, the palm fruit is similar to the olive fruit in that the oil is contained in the flesh of the fruit. The fatty acid composition, however, is different.

Fractionated and refined palm oil has superior functional properties as a bakery shortening and is used extensively in the manufacture of baked goods in Europe. It is also used in the manufacture of margarine (in Europe and Japan), in manufacture of vanispati (in India), and as a frying oil throughout eastern Asia.

Typical fatty acid composition of palm oil is 1 percent myristic acid, 45 percent palmitic acid, 5 percent stearic acid, 39 percent oleic acid, and 9 percent linoleic acid. Fractionation can increase levels of palmitic acid to approximately 54 percent. Typical tocopherol and tocotrienol (vitamin E) values are 256 mg/kg α-tocopherol, 316 mg/kg γ-tocopherol, 70 mg/kg δ-tocopherol, 146 mg/kg α-tocotrienol, 32 mg/kg β-tocotrienol, 286 mg/kg γ-tocotrienol, and 69 mg/kg δ-tocotrienol for a total of 1,172 mg/kg.

Palm Kernel Oil

Palm kernel oil is obtained from the nuts of the palm fruit (*Elaeis guineensis*). As such, palm kernel oil is a by-product of palm oil production. It is usually recovered by expeller and solvent extractions. In physical appearance, the kernel is approximately the size of a hazelnut with a white interior that resembles a miniature coconut. Like coconut oil, palm kernel oil is a lauric oil and has physical and chemical properties that superficially resemble coconut oil. In the U.S. and Europe, palm kernel oil is used extensively as a confectionery fat, either as a cocoa butter extender or a cocoa butter substitute.

The usual fatty acid composition of palm kernel oil is 4 percent caprylic acid, 4 percent capric acid, 50 percent lauric acid, 16 percent myristic acid, 8 percent palmitic acid, 2 percent stearic acid, 14 percent oleic acid, and 2 percent linoleic acid. Typical tocopherol and tocotrienol values are 13 mg/kg α-tocopherol and 21 mg/kg α-tocotrienol for a total of 34 mg/kg.

Peanut Oil

Also called groundnut or monkey nut oil, **peanut oil** comes from an annual legume (*Arachis hypogaea*). The plant is believed to have originated in South America. The peanut plant was first carried to Africa and then to parts of Asia. Today it is a major crop in Africa, India, China, and the U.S. The peanut kernel contains approximately 45 to 55 percent oil. Peanut oil is extracted from peanuts that are not of good enough quality for use as nuts or in peanut butter. Extraction is typically done by expeller press followed by solvent extraction.

The typical fatty acid composition of unrefined peanut oil is 12 percent palmitic acid, 5 percent stearic acid, 46 percent oleic acid, 31 percent linoleic acid, 1 percent arachidic acid, 1 percent gadoleic acid, 3 percent behenic acid, and 1 percent lignoceric acid. Typical tocopherol values are 130 mg/kg α-tocopherol, 216 mg/kg γ-tocopherol, and 21 mg/kg δ-tocopherol for a total of 367 mg/kg.

As a cooking and frying oil, peanut oil is often considered superior because of the quality of flavor imparted to foods. It is one of the more expensive cooking oils in the U.S. and is quite resistant to rancidity when handled properly. The typical composition of peanut oil is somewhat different from other oils because of its 4 to 5 percent content of very long-chain saturated fatty acids that are from 20 to 24 carbons long.

Rapeseed Oils (Regular High-Erucic Acid, Low-Erucic Acid, Canola; Laurate Canola)

Rapeseed oil comes from various plants of the *Brassica napus, B. rapa,* *and B. campestris* genus, which are members of the mustard (*Cruciferae*) family. The seeds contain 40 to 45 percent oil and are grown successfully worldwide. The primary types come from Asia and Europe. Rapeseed oil has been very popular in India and China for centuries. The characteristic rapeseed oil contains high levels (40 to 50 percent) of the very long-chain monounsaturated fatty acid, erucic acid, which is currently considered nutritionally undesirable for the average human. Nevertheless, it had been used as a primary food oil for many centuries prior to the research in Canada that resulted in its removal from Western markets. (Erucic acid has been used as a speciality fatty acid for treatment of leukodystrophies.)

Typical fatty acid composition of standard rapeseed oil is 3 percent palmitic acid, 1 percent stearic acid, 16 percent oleic acid, 14 percent linoleic acid, 10 percent α-linolenic acid, 6 percent gadoleic acid, and 50 percent erucic acid.

Because rapeseed is very adaptable to genetic manipulation, plant breeders have been able to develop varieties of rapeseed that have, for example, high levels of oleic acid instead of erucic acid. This variety of rapeseed oil is now known as **canola oil** (*B. campestris or B. napus*) but it originally was called LEAR oil, which stands for low erucic acid rapeseed oil. It was developed in Canada and has become popular in the U.S. since the mid-1980s, where it is advertised for its high level of monounsaturated fatty acids. These early varieties were genetically modified from the parent rapeseed by selection mutation breeding; later efforts utilized genetic engineering using recombinant DNA technology with various microorganisms as vectors. (see below)

The oil is obtained from the rapeseed by mechanical pressing, solvent extraction, or most frequently by the technique of prepress solvent extraction. The crude oil requires further refining. In part, because of its high levels of the omega-3 fatty acid α-linolenic acid, it is partially hydrogenated for many applications. Margarines made with canola oil and hydrogenated canola tend to have a grainy texture because of the slow crystallization rate exhibited by these oils.

Unhydrogenated canola oil that has been refined by steam distillation loses a substantial portion of its omega-3 α-linolenic acid and some of its omega-6 linoleic acid due to isomerization. Typical fatty acid composition of the totally unrefined canola oil is 4 percent palmitic acid, 2 percent stearic acid, 56 to 64 percent oleic acid, 19 to 26 percent linoleic acid, 10 percent α-linolenic acid, and 2 percent gadoleic acid. Typical tocopherol values are 210 mg/kg α-tocopherol, 1 mg/kg β-tocopherol, and 42 mg/kg γ-tocopherol for a total of 253 mg/kg.

When the high erucic acid rapeseed oil has been totally hydrogenated, a 22 carbon saturated fatty acid called behenic acid is formed. When this fatty acid is removed from the hydrogenated rapeseed oil and then combined with the medium chain fatty acids caprylic and capric acids (C-8 and C-10), a new fat called **Caprenin** is formed. This new fat was promoted as a lower-calorie confectionary fat. The designation of lower calories was related to the lack of absorption of the behenic acid part of the fat in some, but not all, people. There is very little current usage of this man-made oil.

The newest genetically engineered rapeseed oil is **laurate canola**. This oil has been developed by inserting a gene (from the California Bay Laurel tree) responsible for producing lauric acid into the rapeseed canola. According to the Calgene Company, developers of the proprietary product laurate canola, it "...was developed ...as an alternative to imported lauric oils."

The typical reported fatty acid composition of Laurical™ is 37 percent lauric acid, 4 percent myristic acid, 3 percent palmitic acid, 1 percent stearic acid, 33 percent oleic acid, 12 percent linoleic acid, 7 percent α-linolenic acid, and less than 1 percent gadoleic acid. Typical tocopherol values are 227 mg/kg α-tocopherol, 500 mg/kg γ-tocopherol and 46 mg/kg δ-tocopherol for a total of 773 mg/kg.

Safflower Oil

Safflower oil comes from the seeds of a plant (*Carthamus tinctorius*) also noted for its flowers from which dye is produced. The plant has been grown for thousands of years as both an oilseed crop and for its colorful flowers. It is a relative to the thistle. Safflower originated in Southeastern Asia and was carried to China, India, Egypt, and North Africa where it is extensively cultivated. Spanish explorers carried it to the New World and Mexico is currently a major producer, occupying second place between India, who ranks first, and the United States. Safflower is a plant that is adapted to a dry climate and is tolerant of salty water or soil. The seeds resemble sunflower seeds but are about half the size. The dehulled seeds have between 36 to 43 percent oil. The oil is obtained by expeller or solvent extraction.

There are two varieties of safflower, one a high linoleic variety and the other a high oleic variety. The high linoleic variety was the primary one used commercially in 1978 according to USDA, and the

Institute of Shortening and Edible Oils listed only the high linoleic variety among the principle oils in 1988; the high oleic variety has become popular in the last several years especially among producers for the health food industry. Safflower oil is yellow in color and has practically no odor. The high oleic varieties were developed through selection mutation breeding in the 1970s.

The typical composition of the high linoleic variety is 6 percent palmitic acid, 2 percent stearic acid, 13 percent oleic acid, and 78 percent linoleic acid. The typical composition of the high oleic variety is 5 percent palmitic acid, 2 percent stearic acid, 80 percent oleic acid, and 12 percent linoleic acid. Typical tocopherol values reported are 387 mg/kg α-tocopherol, 174 mg/kg γ-tocopherol, and 240 mg/kg δ-tocopherol for a total of 801 mg/kg.

Sesame Oil

Sesame oil comes from an annual herb (*Sesamum indicum*). The plant is a warm weather plant that grows from the tropics to warm temperate regions. The major producing countries are China, India, Sudan, and Mexico. The seed is 40 to 60 percent oil and is used directly for food purposes when it is cold pressed. The oil is also recovered by combined expeller and solvent extraction. Sesame paste is a popular food in the lands along the eastern Mediterranean.

Sesame oil has very good oxidative stability, which is thought to be related to sesamin or another unknown antioxidant in the native oil. When sesame oil is added to other oils for use in frying, the oxidative properties of the recipient oil are improved. The oil is pale yellow and without odor after refining, but also is sold in a darker version for use in Asian cooking.

The fatty acid composition has some similarities to peanut oil in that the levels of oleic acid and linoleic acid are very similar. Typical composition of sesame oil is 10 percent palmitic acid, 5 percent stearic acid, 41 percent oleic acid, and 43 percent linoleic acid. Typical tocopherol values are 136 mg/kg α-tocopherol and 290 mg/kg γ-tocopherol for a total of 426 mg/kg.

Soybean Oil

Soybean oil comes from an annual legume (*Glycine max.*) This legume has been cultivated by man for thousands of years in China. The plant was originally used as a soil conditioner since the soybean plant is like other legumes and clover and "fixes" nitrogen. The commercial production of soybean oil in the United States dates from the early 1940s. Currently soybeans are the major oilseed crop in the world. In addition to being a source of oil, they are a source of meal for animal feed as well as the major source for hydrolyzed protein isolates. Soybeans contain approximately 17 to 27 percent oil. This oil can be obtained by expeller pressing, but more frequently it is obtained by hexane extraction. Because of its high linolenic acid content, the unhydrogenated oil has a tendency to develop oxidative flavor reversion. Research conducted by companies such as Dupont has recently produced genetically modified soybeans with higher levels of oleic acid and stearic acid and lower levels of linolenic acid in a effort to produce an oil with greater oxidative stability.

Most of the vegetable oil and shortening in the U.S. food supply is soybean. Approximately 70 percent of the oil used for food in the U.S. is estimated to be soybean oil. Until recently even household salad and cooking oils made from soybean oil were partially hydrogenated. New technology has eliminated this need for most of the household oil. Refining such as deodorization isomerizes a portion of the omega-3 linolenic acid. Soybean oil is still extensively partially hydrogenated for most applications such as commercial cooking oils, margarines, and shortenings. (See Chapter 1) The unrefined oil is brownish yellow with a strong odor. Refined soybean oil is pale yellow and has a mild odor. Crude soybean oil is a major source of phospholipd emulsifiers such as food grade lecithin.

Typical fatty acid composition of unrefined, unhydrogenated soybean oil is 11 percent palmitic acid, 4 percent stearic acid, 23 percent oleic acid, 53 percent linoleic acid, and 8 percent linolenic acid. Typical tocopherol values are 101 mg/kg α-tocopherol, 593 mg/kg γ-tocopherol and 264 mg/kg δ-tocopherol for a total of 958 mg/kg.

Sunflower Seed Oil

Sunflower seed oil from the native American sunflower (*Helianthus annus*) is a popular oil in many parts of Europe where the plant has been cultivated since its introduction in the 16th Century. The former Soviet Union has been a major producer for many years. The plant is a fast growing annual (70 days to 4 months), and there are many varieties with different heights as well as varieties with different oil composition. Both high linoleic acid (approximately 65 percent) and high oleic acid (approximately 82 percent) varieties exist, but sunflower oil is not a source of more than trace amounts of linolenic acid. High oleic varieties are the result of mutation breeding, which produced seeds whose fatty acid composition was stable to varying growing temperatures. Original varieties varied in levels of linoleic acid (higher in northern climates such as Canada) and oleic acid (higher in southern climates such as Florida).

Oil content from sunflower seed varies from 20 percent to 40 percent. High quality oil is used as a table oil with the inherent waxes removed by winterization; lower quality oils are used for industrial purposes. Commercial sunflower seed oil with added sesame oil and rice bran oil (the latter two for their antioxidant content) is being promoted in Europe as a stable frying oil. The refined oil is yellow and has a slight nutty odor and flavor.

Typical fatty acid composition of unrefined regular sunflower seed oil is 7 percent palmitic acid, 5 percent stearic acid, 19 percent oleic acid, 68 percent linoleic acid, and less than 1 percent linolenic acid. Typical composition of unrefined high oleic sunflower seed oil is 4 percent palmitic acid, 5 percent stearic acid, 81 percent oleic acid, 8 percent linoleic acid, and trace amounts of linolenic acid. Typical tocopherol values are 487 mg/kg α-tocopherol, 51 mg/kg γ-tocopherol, and 8 mg/kg δ-tocopherol for a total of 546 mg/kg.

Selected Characteristics of Commonly Used Fruit/Seed Oils

Fruit/Seed	Percent crude oil in seed	Major fatty acid
Cocoa	40-50%	Stearic acid (35%)
Coconut	62-69% dry weight basis	Lauric acid (45-50%)
Corn	5%	Linoleic acid (57%)
Cottonseed	17%	Linoleic acid (53%)
Olive	30-70% dry weight basis	Oleic acid (71%)
Palm fruit	74-81% dry weight basis	Palmitic acid (45%)
Palm kernel	46-57% dry weight basis	Lauric acid (45-50%)
Peanut	45-55% dry weight basis	Oleic acid (46%)
Rapeseed		
regular	40-45% dry weight basis	Erucic acid (50%)
canola	40-60% dry weight basis	Oleic acid (56-64%)
Safflower		
regular	36-43% dry weight basis	Linoleic acid (78%)
hybrid	"	Oleic acid (80%)
Sesame	40-60% dry weight basis	Linoleic acid (43%)
Soybean	17-27% dry weight basis	Linoleic acid (53%)
Sunflower		
regular	20-40% dry weight basis	Linoleic acid (68%)
hybrid	"	Oleic acid (81%)

Less Commonly Used Fruit/seed Oils (Known as Gourmet or Specialty Oils)

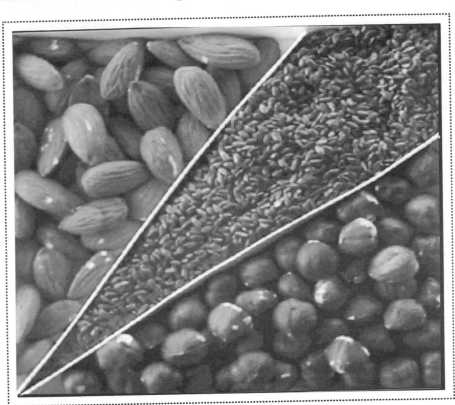

Almond Oil

Almond oil is extracted from the nut of the almond tree (*Amygdalus communis*). This tree originated in central Asia and has been known since biblical times as an important nut bearing tree. Almond is currently the fourth leading nut crop in the world. Major growing areas are the United States, Italy, and Spain. Almond oil is considered a gourmet oil and is found in specialty stores. It is considered a flavorful, stable oleic-rich oil. It has a yellow color and an odor that is readily recognizable.

Typical fatty acid composition of the oil is 7 percent palmitic acid, 2 percent stearic acid, 61 percent oleic acid, 30 percent linoleic acid, and less than 1 percent alpha-linolenic acid. Typical α-tocopherol content is reported as 392 mg/kg.

Avocado Oil

Avocado oil is pressed from the fruit of the avocado tree (*Persea americana*). The fruit from this subtropical evergeen is also called an alligator pear. Avocados are usually used as whole food in sauces, salads, or soup. They have a range of fat between 9 and 25 percent of the whole food (35 to 70 percent on a dry weight basis) and are used as speciality oils in cosmetics as well as for food. The oil is pale yellow and has a mild odor.

Typical fatty acid composition varies depending on the variety. Composition of oil from California avocados is 17 percent palmitic acid, a trace (less than 0.1 percent) of stearic acid, 3 percent palmitoleic acid, 68 percent oleic acid, 12 percent linoleic acid, and less than 1 percent alpha-linolenic acid. Composition of oil from Florida avocados is 21 percent palmitic acid, less than 1 percent stearic acid, 9 percent palmitoleic acid, 51 percent oleic acid, 17 percent linoleic acid, and 1 percent alpha-linolenic acid. Typical α-tocopherol content is reported as 13.4 mg/kg.

Black Currant Oil, Borage Oil, and Evening Primrose Oil

Several oils are currently under cultivation and production as sources of gamma-γ-linolenic acid (GLA). These include **borage oil**, which contains about 20 to 25 percent GLA, **black currant oil**, which contains about 15 to 19 percent GLA, and **evening primrose oil**, which contains about 7 to 10 percent GLA. These oils have become popular for use as medicinal oils because of their content of GLA, a fatty acid considered beneficial in certain disease states (see Chapter 1 and the General Glossary for discussion of the functions of GLA).

Black currant oil comes from the seeds of the black currant berry bush (*Ribes nigrum*). This perennial shrub is thought to have originated across northern Europe and northern Asia where it grows wild, and it has been cultivated beginning in the Baltic area in northern Europe since the 15th century. It is grown commercially in Europe, which supplies more than 80 percent of the world production. It has not been grown commercially in many parts of the United States since the end of the 1800s due to incompatibility of the black currant plant and white pine trees. The berry is used for its juice, jam, and a liqueur (crème de cassis), and the seeds are a by-product of the manufacture of the juice and jam.

The oil is yellow in color and has an odor resembling the fruit.

Typical fatty acid composition of black currant seed oil is 7 percent palmitic acid, 2 percent stearic acid, 11 percent oleic acid, 47 percent linoleic acid, 17 percent gamma-linolenic acid, 13 percent alpha-linolenic acid, and 3 percent stearidonic acid (C18:4 n-3). Typical tocopherol values are not available for this oil.

Borage oil is extracted from the seeds of a flowering plant (*Borago officinalis*). Borage is reported to have originated in the Mediterranean area and spread to Europe where it became a popular herb growing in gardens. The leaves and flowers are used in salads or soups. Borage also grows all over North America. The oil is pale yellow with an odor of the herb.

Typical fatty acid composition of borage oil is 10 percent palmitic acid, 4 percent stearic acid, 16 percent oleic acid, 38 percent linoleic acid, 23 percent gamma-linolenic acid, and 8 percent gadoleic acid, erucic acid, and nervonic acid (C20:1, C22:1, C24:1). Total tocopherol values are reported as 0.02 percent for this oil.

Evening primrose oil is extracted from the seeds of a flowering plant (*Oenothera biennis*). It is a biennial plant that originated in North America and was introduced into Europe in the 17th century, where it grows wild. The oil was first produced in China where it was used for its medicinal properties. Today, the oil is obtained from seeds grown primarily in North America, Europe, Israel, and New Zealand. The seeds contain 22 to 28 percent oil, and the oil is typically marketed in capsule form. The oil is pale yellow in color with a specific odor.

Typical fatty acid composition of the oil is 7 percent palmitic acid, 2 percent stearic acid, 9 percent oleic acid, 72 percent linoleic acid, and 10 percent γ-linolenic acid. Total tocopherol values are reported as 0.05 percent for this oil.

Flaxseed (Linseed) Oil

Flaxseed oil from a herbaceous annual (*Linum usitatissumum*) is also frequently referred to as "food-grade" linseed oil. It is obtained from that strain of the plant known as common flax with high oil content in the seed (35 to 44 percent) as opposed to the strain that produces mainly linen flax fiber. Flax is a warm temperature (subtropical) crop that is grown principally in Argentina, India, the former USSR, the USA, and

Canada at this time. Flaxseed is reported to have originated in Asia or the Mediterranean region and has been used as both food and medicine since antiquity. Ground flaxseed has been used as a food for more than 3000 years in Ethiopia. Several bakeries in the USA use flax seed in their products. Its use as a food oil today is mostly restricted to the health food establishment.

Because of the very high content (greater than 50-60 percent) of alpha-linolenic acid, flaxseed oil requires extra care in handling to prevent oxidation if it has been refined and stripped of its native antioxidants. Although flaxseed oil is not recommended for use in cooking, it is known to be used in China for low-temperature stir frying. Unrefined flaxseed oil has a golden yellow color and a grassy odor. The refined oil is pale yellow.

Typical fatty acid composition of the oil is 6 percent palmitic acid, 3 percent stearic acid, 17 percent oleic acid, 14 percent linoleic acid, and 60 percent alpha-linolenic acid. Typical tocopherol content is not reported.

Grapeseed Oil

Grapeseed oil from the seed of the grape (*Vitis vinifera*), a by-product of the wine industry, is not widely used in the U.S. The oil is pressed and solvent extracted from dried grape seeds. The amount that can be retrieved from the seeds ranges from about 6 to 20 percent depending on the variety of grapes. The oil is a greenish color.

The fatty acid composition of grapeseed oil is not unlike most high linoleic oils, and typically is 7 percent palmitic acid, 4 percent stearic acid, 16 percent oleic acid, 72 percent linoleic acid, and 1 percent alpha-linolenic acid. Typical tocopherol content is reported as 250 mg/kg..

Hazelnut Oil (Filbert)

Hazelnut oil is extracted from the nut of the hazel tree (*Corylus avellana*), which is native to Europe, Asia, and North America. Principal growing areas are Turkey, Italy, and Spain. In the United States, most commercial growing of filberts is along the west coast. Hazelnut oil has a history of being manufactured nearly 2000 years ago in Japan where it was used for lighting purposes. Current usage is as a gourmet oil. It has a yellow color and a nut-like odor.

Typical fatty acid composition values for this oil vary

considerably depending on the source of information. They are 5 to 7 percent palmitic acid, 2 percent stearic acid, 69 to 81 percent oleic acid, 10 to 21 percent linoleic acid, and less than half a percent alpha-linolenic acid. The oil is reported to be rich in α-tocopherol.

Hemp Seed Oil

Hemp seed oil has recently been introduced into the health food market in the United States and Canada. The hemp plant (*Cannabis sativa*) has a long history of use as raw material for rope and as bird seed. It is well-known as a source of the psychoactive substance marijuana. The oil is extracted from seeds, either sterilized or fresh, and has been reported in toxicology journals to contain cannabinoids in sufficient quantity so that they have been identified in drug testing of individuals who consumed the oil. Hemp seed oil is highly unsaturated and requires careful storage. It is not an appropriate oil for cooking use

Typical fatty acid composition of the oil is 6 percent palmitic acid, 2 percent stearic acid, 12 percent oleic acid, 57 percent linoleic acid, 2 percent gamma-linolenic acid, and 19 percent alpha-linolenic acid. Typical tocopherol content as vitamin E (alpha-tocopherol only) is reported as 10 mg/kg, which seems quite low for a highly unsaturated seed oil.

Perilla Seed Oil

Perilla seed oil comes from the beefsteak plant (*Perilla frutescens*). It is common in east Asian countries and was in common use in Japan in the 9th century. It is not found at this time in west except as it is imported for Korean food stores. The composition of perilla seed oil is similar to that of flax seed oil (approximately 60 percent alpha-linolenic acid and 15 percent linoleic acid) and it too would require careful handling to prevent oxidation.

Rice Bran Oil

Rice bran oil comes from the major cereal crop *Oryza sativa* of Asia but has never been a major oil of commerce because of technical and logistic problems with its recovery. When the oil is extracted promptly following the milling of the rice, it has good quality and good oxidative stability in large part due to its native antioxidants. The oil has equal amounts of monounsaturated and polyunsaturated fatty acids and is a source of the antioxidants gamma-oryzanol and cycloartenol as well as tocopherols, which give this oil good oxidative stability.

Typical fatty acid composition of the oil is 16 percent palmitic acid, 2 percent stearic acid, 42 percent oleic acid, 37 percent linoleic acid, and 1 percent alpha-linolenic acid. Typical α-tocopherol content is reported to be 323 mg/kg. The oil is pale yellow and without specific odor.

Walnut Oil

Walnut oil is extracted from the nut of the *Juglans regia* tree. Originally from Persia, it is grown in temperate areas of Europe, Asia, and North America. Walnut oil is very flavorful, and it is used primarily as an oil for salad dressings. It requires careful storage because it has high levels of alpha-linolenic acid. The oil is yellow in color and has a specific odor.

Typical fatty acid composition of the English or Persian variety of this oil is 7 percent palmitic acid, 2 percent stearic acid, 23 percent oleic acid, 54 percent linoleic acid, and 12 percent alpha-linolenic acid. Typical fatty acid composition of the Black variety (*Juglans nigra*) of this oil is 4 percent palmitic acid, 3 percent stearic acid, 22 percent oleic acid, 62 percent linoleic acid, and 6 percent alpha-linolenic acid. Typical α-tocopherol content is reported to be 26.2 mg/kg.

Wheat Germ Oil

Wheat germ oil is extracted from the seed germ of the common grain *Triticum vulgare*. It is used as a salad oil or a nutritional supplement. It is favored by some because of its content of octacosanol, a 28 carbon high molecular weight fatty alcohol thought by some to have healthful properties. Unrefined wheat germ oil has a very high vitamin E content, but because of its high levels of polyunsaturated fatty acids, it is also one of the oils prone to rancidity depending on how carefully it is handled. The oil has a yellow color and a specific odor.

The typical fatty acid composition of wheat germ oil is reported as 13 percent palmitic acid, 2 percent stearic acid, 19 percent oleic acid, 60 percent linoleic acid, and 5 percent alpha-linolenic acid. Typical tocopherol and tocotrienol values are 1330 mg/kg α-tocopherol, 710 mg/kg β-tocopherol, 260 mg/kg γ-tocopherol, 271 mg/kg δ-tocopherol, 26 mg/kg α-tocotrienol, and 18 mg/kg β-tocotrienol for a total of 2615 mg/kg.

Other Nut and Fruit Oils

Oils are also pressed from other nuts such as brazil nuts, cashew nuts, macadamia nuts, pecans, and pistachio nuts. These oils, which are categorized as oleic-rich or having nearly equal amounts of oleic acid and linoleic acid are appearing in specialty catalogues or in specialty food stores. Apricot kernel oil, argan oil, passion flower oil, peach kernel oil, or mango kernel oil are some of the more exotic oils available in some areas. One of the older high linoleic acid oils is poppy seed oil, which is occasionally used as a specialty oil. Sorghum oil is popular in many parts of the world, and although about 25 percent of the world's sorghum is grown in the US, the oil is not currently in use in the US. See Table 4.4 and Appendix 3 for composition data.

There are also several lauric rich oils, in addition to coconut oil and palm kernel oil, such as babassu oil, which is native to Brazil, cohune oil, murumuru butter, ouricuri butter, and tucum oil grown in South America.

Selected Characteristics of Specialty Fruit/Seed Oils

Fruit/Seed	Crude oil in seed	Major fatty acid
Almond	52%	oleic (61%)
Avocado	35-70% dry weight	oleic (51-68%)
Flaxseed	35-44%	alpha-linolenic (~60%)
Grapeseed	6-20%	linoleic (72%)
Hazelnut	63%	oleic (69-81%)
Hemp	36%	linoleic (57%)
Perilla	?	alpha-linolenic (~60%)
Rice bran	20%	oleic (42%)
Walnut	57-62%	linoleic (54-62%)
Wheat germ	10%	linoleic (60%)

(Black currant, borage, and evening primrose oils are known for their content of gamma-linolenic acid, but their major fatty acid is linoleic.)

Commonly Used Fats from Animal and Marine Sources

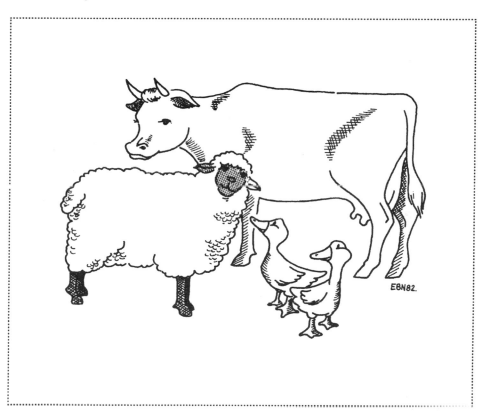

Butter (Milk) Fat

Butter is one of the oldest fats from animal sources used as a food. Typically in the U.S., butter is obtained from cows (***Bos***). Butter from the milk of other animals such as buffalo (***Bubalus bubalis***), goats (***Capra***), sheep (***Ovis***), camels (***Camelus***), and other domesticated ruminant animals has been used all over the world for centuries. Although not common in the United States, butter from goats' milk is sold in Canada along with other butter and cheese. Butter is used as a table spread, for general cooking, and for pastries and other baked goods.

European butter is typically 82 percent fat and is usually unsalted. Butter in the United States is usually 80 percent fat and 20 percent water with milk solids, salted or unsalted. Butter oil, also called ghee in Africa and Asia (especially in India), is 100 percent fat; it is a very stable form of butter.

Butter is known for its content of short-chain and odd-chain fatty acids. Milk fat is considered one of the most complex natural fats in existence. Butter made from cream from animals grazing on grass contains high levels of vitamin A and other factors such as conjugated linoleic acid, which are known to have special health benefits. (See also General Glossary for milk fat.)

Typical fatty acid composition of butter is 4 percent butyric acid, 2 percent caproic acid, 1 percent caprylic acid, 2 percent capric acid, 3 percent lauric acid, 12 percent myristic acid, 26 percent palmitic acid, 12 percent stearic acid, 2 percent palmitoleic acid, 28 percent oleic acid, 3 percent linoleic acid, less than 1 percent alpha-linolenic acid, and 2 to 3 percent odd-chain fatty acids. Typical α-tocopherol content is reported to be 16 mg/kg.

Chicken, Duck, Goose, and Turkey Fat

Rendered fat from poultry such as chicken (*Gallus gallus*), duck (*Anatifdae*), and geese (*Anatidae*) has a long history of use for cooking. Chicken fat is used extensively in some ethnic dishes. It was a popular fat in the U.S. a hundred years ago where it was used as a pastry fat. Goose and duck fat have been more popular in Europe. Turkey (*Meleagris gallopavo*) is a popular bird in the United States, but not generally known for its fat.

Poultry fat is a source of the antimicrobial fatty acid, palmitoleic acid. Chicken fat usually has more of this fatty acid (6-8 percent of the total fat) than duck (4 percent), goose (3 percent), or turkey (6 percent). Poultry fats are relatively unsaturated. The actual fatty acids depends somewhat on the feed given the birds. The level of saturated fatty acids is approximately a third or slightly less of the total fatty acids, and monounsaturates are around half of the total fatty acids, except that turkey fat is lower in monounsaturates and higher in omega-6 polyunsaturates.

Typical fatty acid composition of **chicken fat** in the United States is less than 1 percent lauric acid, 1 percent myristic acid, less than 1 percent myristoleic acid, 23 percent palmitic acid, 6-8 percent palmitoleic acid, 6 percent stearic acid, 42 percent oleic acid, 19 percent linoleic acid, and 1 percent linolenic acid. Total tocopherol is reported as 27-29 mg/kg of fat.

Typical fatty acid composition of **duck fat** in the United States is less than 1 percent myristic acid, 26 percent palmitic acid, 4 percent palmitoleic acid, 8 percent stearic acid, 46 percent oleic acid, 13 percent linoleic acid, and 1 percent linolenic acid. Total tocopherol is reported as 30 mg/kg of fat.

Typical fatty acid composition of **goose fat** in the United States is less than 1 percent myristic acid, 22 percent palmitic acid, 3 percent palmitoleic acid, 6 percent stearic acid, 56 percent oleic acid, 10 percent linoleic acid, and less than 1 percent linolenic acid. Total tocopherol is reported as 30 mg/kg of fat.

Typical fatty acid composition of **turkey fat** in the United States is less than 1 percent myristic acid, 22 percent palmitic acid, 6 percent palmitoleic acid, 6 percent stearic acid, 38 percent oleic acid, 22 percent linoleic acid, and 1 percent linolenic acid. Total tocopherol is reported as 29 mg/kg of fat.

Lard

Lard is the rendered fat from the pig (*Sus scrofa*). There are numerous parts of the world where lard has been a major food fat for centuries. These include China, parts of Europe, and until recent times the United States. Lard has been a popular fat for pastry and for frying potato chips. In the U.S., it can still be found in these foods in spite of the inappropriate consumer activist pressure to replace it with partially hydrogenated vegetable shortenings. Lard can be either a firm fat or a soft fat depending on what the pig is fed.

Lard is more or less the equivalent of tallow in its usage, except that is has more unsaturates and can become rancid if not handled properly. Usually it is about 40 percent saturated, 50 percent monounsaturated, and 10 percent polyunsaturated fatty acids. (This fat should be considered as a monounsaturated fat.) Lard has between 2 and 3 percent palmitoleic acid, which as noted above possesses antimicrobial properties. Most lard is home rendered or sold in certain ethnic stores (e.g., stores catering to Hispanic peoples).

Typical fatty acid composition is 1 percent myristic acid, 25 percent palmitic acid, 3 percent palmitoleic acid, 12 percent stearic acid, 45 percent oleic acid, 10 percent linoleic acid, and less than 1 percent linolenic acid. Typical tocopherol and tocotrienol content is reported to be 12 mg/kg α-tocopherol, 7 mg/kg γ-tocopherol, and 7 mg/kg α-tocotrienol.

Tallow and Suet

Tallow is the rendered fat from ruminant animals including cattle (*Bos*) and sheep or lamb (*Ovis*). **Suet** is the form of beef or lamb fat that is incorporated into foods without prior rendering. Both tallow and suet have been used for centuries. They are stable fats that do not normally become rancid -- no free radicals are formed from normal usage. Tallow had been a popular fat in the U.S. for deep frying potatoes until the mid-1980s. Foods fried in tallow have a lot of taste and usually lower amounts of fat than the same foods fried in liquid plant oils. (See Chapter V for discussion of the anti-saturated fat agenda.)

Tallow is 100 percent fat and suet is 94 percent fat. The composition is about 50-55 percent saturated, 40 percent monounsaturated, and 3-6 percent polyunsaturated fatty acids. Tallows have several percent of an antimicrobial fatty acid palmitoleic acid.

Typical fatty acid composition of beef tallow is 3 percent myristic acid, 25 percent palmitic acid, 3 percent palmitoleic acid, 22 percent stearic acid, 39 percent oleic acid, 2 percent linoleic acid, and less than 1 percent linolenic acid; additional fatty acids include 2 percent margaric acid (17 carbons) and other odd chain fatty acids. Typical tocopherol level is reported as 27 mg/kg α- tocopherol.

Typical fatty acid composition of lamb tallow is 5 percent myristic acid, 24 percent palmitic acid, 2 percent palmitoleic acid, 25 percent stearic acid, 33 percent oleic acid, 4 percent linoleic acid, and 1 percent linolenic acid; additional fatty acids also include 2 percent margaric acid (17 carbons) and other odd chain fatty acids. Typical tocopherol level in lamb tallow is reported as 2.2 mg/kg α- tocopherol.

Cod Liver Oil

Cod liver oil is obtained from soft-finned saltwater fish including cod (*Gradus morrhua*) and other related fish with large livers. Cod liver oil is extracted from the fresh livers of the fish and processed for sale as a liquid oil or in capsules. It is a well-known source of vitamin A and vitamin D as well as some of the elongated omega-3 fatty acids such as EPA and DHA. It is also a fair source of vitamin E. Each 100 grams of cod liver oil provides approximately 85,000 IU of vitamin A, 8,500 IU of vitamin D, and 20 mg of vitamin E. Cod liver oil was part of the ancient diet of the Vikings in Norway for centuries, and was used as "medicine" prior to the discovery of vitamins.

Typical fatty acid composition for cod liver oil is 4 percent myristic acid, 14 percent palmitic acid, 12 percent palmitoleic acid, 3 percent stearic acid, 22 percent oleic acid, 1 percent linoleic acid, 1 percent stearidonic acid, 12 percent gadoleic acid, 7 percent eicosapentaenoic acid, 11 percent cetoleic acid, and 7 percent docosahexaenoic acid. Typical tocopherol content is reported to be 220 mg/kg α-tocopherol.

Herring Oil

Herring oil is obtained from *Clupea harengus*. This fish is found in the north Atlantic along the coasts. On the European coast it ranges from Gibraltar to Ireland and the White Sea. On the American coast it is found from Cape Hatteras north to Greenland. The herring usually has a very high fat content, which makes it a suitable source of oil. It is also used extensively for smoking and pickling for human foods and the oil is used for making margarine and in animal feed.

Gunstone (1996) reports the typical composition for unhydrogenated herring oil from Nova Scotia as 25 percent saturated fatty acids, 62 percent monounsaturated fatty acids, and 7 percent polyunsaturated fatty acids, of which 6 percent are omega-3. Ackman (1982) found somewhat higher levels of omega-3 fatty acids, of 14 percent, in herring oil from the North Sea.

Specific fatty acid composition of unhydrogenated herring oil from Nova Scotia is 9 percent myristic acid, 15 percent palmitic acid, 7 percent palmitoleic acid, 1 percent stearic acid, 16 percent oleic acid, 1 percent linoleic acid, 16 percent gadoleic acid, 3 percent eicosapentaenoic acid, 23 percent cetoleic acid, and 3 percent docosahexaenoic acid. Typical tocopherol level is reported as 92 mg/kg α-tocopherol.

Menhaden Oil

Menhaden oil is obtained from the large herring-like fish of the genus *Brevoortia tyrannus* and *Brevoortia patronus*. The fish is found along the east coast of North America, including in the estuaries. Menhaden are an important forage fish for whales and porpoises, large fish, and seabirds. Because of their high fat and oil content, they are an important commercial fish in the eastern United States. They have used for fish meal, industrial oil and fertilizers, and recently have been promoted for food use.

Typical fat composition of the unhydrogenated menhaden oil

varies somewhat but is reported (RG Ackman 1982) as 35 to 42 percent total saturated fatty acids, 26 to 30 percent total monounsaturated fatty acids, and 28 to 38 percent total polyunsaturated fatty acids. Levels of the omega-3 polyunsaturated fatty acids are reported to be 24 to 29 percent. The composition of partially hydrogenated menhaden oil is quite different: up to approximately 50 percent saturated fatty acids, varying amounts of *trans* fatty acids, and none of the omega-3 fatty acids.

Typical fatty acid composition of unhydrogenated menhaden oil is 8 percent myristic acid, 22 percent palmitic acid, 11 percent palmitoleic acid, 3 percent stearic acid, 21 percent oleic acid, 2 percent linoleic acid, 2 percent gadoleic acid, 14 percent eicosapentaenoic acid (EPA), 2 percent cetoleic acid, and 10 percent docosahexaenoic acid (DHA). Typical tocopherol levels in the unhydrogenated menhaden oil is reported as 75 mg/kg α-tocopherol.

Other Fish Oils

Fish oils such as tuna oil, sardine oil, capelin oil, anchovy oil, and shark oil are sold in capsule form or as oil for adding to animal foods. Capelin is a small fish in the smelt family, which is about 13 percent total omega-3 fatty acids. Anchovy and sardine oil are about 32 percent and 37 percent omega-3 fatty acids, respectively. Tuna oil from the central Pacific is reported to be about 30 percent omega-3 fatty acids; tuna from other areas is reported to have less. Shark oil is usually sold in capsules for its vitamin A content.

Fish as a Source of Elongated Omega-3 Fatty Acids

Many people are of the mistaken idea that all fish are able to supply the same amount of omega-3 fatty acids. This is not correct. There is a great deal of variability both in the amount of fat among individual species of fish and also within a species depending on both the subspecies and the area of the oceans, lakes, or rivers where the fish grow.

Table 4.1 a-c gives some information for most of the commonly seen fish in the United States and Canada. In this table, the amount of energy in kilocalories (kcal), the grams of fat, the milligrams of cholesterol, and the grams of omega-3 fatty acids are given for the categories of low fat fish, medium fat fish, and higher fat fish. The more complete fat composition for these fish can be found in the composition tables in Appendix C.

Table 4.1-a Low Fat Fin Fish

with less than 2 g fat per 100 g serving of fish	kcal	fat, g	chol, mg	omega3 g
Atlantic Cod Fillet-Raw	82	0.67	43	0.185
Pacific Cod Fillet-Fish-Raw	82	0.63	37	0.217
Sole/Flounder Fillet-Fish-Raw	91	1.19	48	0.207
Grouper Fillet-Fish-Raw	92	1.02	37	0.257
Haddock Fillet-Raw	87	0.72	57	0.187
Atlantic Ocean Perch- Fillet-Raw	94	1.63	42	0.348
Perch Fillet-Mixed Species-Raw	91	0.92	90	0.265
Northern Pike Fillet-Raw	88	0.69	39	0.128
Walleye Pike Fillet-raw	93	1.22	86	0.325
Sea Bass Fillet-Mixed Species-Raw	97	2.00	41	0.595
Snapper Fillet-Mixed Species-Raw	100	1.34	37	0.315
Fresh Skipjack Tuna Fillet-Raw	103	1.01	47	0.256
Whiting Fillet-Mixed Species-Raw	90	1.31	67	0.258

ESHA Food Processor®

Table 4.1-b Medium Fat Fin Fish,

between 2 and 10 g fat per 100 g serving of fish	kcal	fat, g	chol, mg	omega3, g
Freshwater Bass Fillet-Raw	114	3.69	68	0.706
Striped Bass Fillet-Fish-Raw	97	2.33	80	0.769
Bluefish Fillet-Raw	124	4.24	59	0.771
Carp Fillet-Fish-Raw	127	5.60	66	0.622
Channel Catfish Fillet-Wild-Raw	95	2.82	58	0.435
Farmed Channel Catfish Fillet-Raw	135	7.59	47	0.370
Atlantic Croaker Fillet-Fish-Raw	104	3.17	61	0.229
Atlantic/Pacific Halibut Fillet-Raw	110	2.29	32	0.428
Atlantic Herring Fillet-Raw	158	9.04	60	1.672
King Mackerel Fillet-Raw	105	2.00	53	0.303
Pacific/Jack Mackerel Fillet-Raw	158	7.89	47	1.491
Spanish Mackerel Fillet-Raw	139	6.30	76	1.373
Striped Mullet Fillet-Raw	117	3.79	49	0.350
Atlantic Salmon Fillet-Wild-Raw	142	6.34	55	1.733
Pink Salmon Fillet-Raw	116	3.45	52	1.037
Sockeye Salmon Fillet-Raw	168	8.56	62	1.264
Seatrout/Steelhead Fillet-Mx Spec-Raw	104	3.61	83	0.376
Rainbow Smelt-Raw	97	2.42	70	0.742
Fresh Bluefin Tuna-Raw	144	4.9	38	1.171

Data from ESHA Food Processor®

Table 4.1-c Higher Fat Fin Fish,

greater than 10 g fat per 100 g serving of fish	kcal	fat, g	chol, mg	omega3, g
Pacific Herring Fillet-Raw	195	13.9	77	1.713
Atlantic Mackerel Fillet-Raw	205	13.9	70	2.457
Chinook Salmon Fillet-Raw	180	10.4	66	1.441
Farmed Atlantic Salmon-Raw	183	10.9	59	1.907*
Sable fish-Raw	195	15.3	49	1.489

*Only with high-omega-3 feed; Data from ESHA Food Processor®

Nuts - Foods High in Fat

Nuts are very high in fats/oils. Not all nuts have the same fatty acid composition in their oils. Some like hazelnuts are very high in monounsaturates (~78 percent), not unlike olive oil. Some like nutmeg -- used for nutmeg butter -- are very high in saturates (~90 percent). On the other hand, nuts like walnuts are very high in polyunsaturates. Oils from the tropics are always more saturated because of the climate: the plants need to keep a certain amount of firmness in the plant membranes. Table 4.2 gives fatty acid composition of tropical nut oils; Figure 4.1 lists categories of nut fats.

The amount of fat and the fatty acid composition for nuts and their oils is found in Table 4.3.

Table 4.2 Tropical Nut Oils

Fatty Acids g/100g food

	Saturates			Unsaturates		
	Short Chain C4-8	Medium Chain C10-12	Long Chain C14-22	*cis* Mono C16-18	*cis* Poly omega6	*cis* Poly omega3
Babassu	6.2	49.0	26.0	11.4	1.6	--
Cocoa butter	--	--	58.7	32.8	3.0	--
Coconut	8.1	50.6	27.8	5.8	1.8	--
Palm kernel	3.5	50.7	27.3	11.4	1.6	--
Cupu Assu	--	--	53.2	38.7	3.8	--
Shea nut	0.2	1.5	43.3	44.0	5.2	--
Nutmeg butter	--	3.1	86.9	4.8	--	--

Sources: USDA Handbook 8-4;

High in Monounsaturates
        Acorn (24)
        Almond (52)
        Cashew (46)
        Hazelnut[1] (63)
        Hickory (64)
        Macadamia (73)
        Peanut[2] (49)
        Pecan (68)
        Pilinuts-Canarytree (80)
        Pistachio (50)

High in Polyunsaturates
        Butternut (57)
        Soybean[2] (24)
        Sunflower (50)
        Walnut (57-62)

Nearly Equal in Monounsaturates/Polyunsaturates
        Beechnut (50)
        Brazilnut (66)
        Chestnut (2)
        Ginkgo (2)
        Pinenut (51-61)
        Pumpkin (19)
        Sesame (50)

---

[1] Same as filbert nut
[2] Legumes used as nuts

USDA Handbook 8-4

Figure 4.1 Categories of Nuts (Percent Fat)

Table 4.3 Fat and Fatty Acid Composition of Commonly Consumed Nuts/Seeds (weight percent)

Fatty acid	Acorn	Almond	Butternut	Brazil	Cashew	Filbert*
C6:0 (caproic)	–	–	–	–	–	–
C8:0 (caprylic)	–	–	–	–	0.3	–
C10:0 (capric)	–	–	–	–	0.3	–
C12:0 (lauric)	–	–	–	–	1.2	–
C14:0 (myristic)	–	0.6	–	1.0	0.8	0.2
C16:0 (palmitic)	1.1	6.9	1.6	15.0	9.8	5.2
C18:0 (stearic)	12.5	2.0	0.8	9.0	6.7	2.1
C18:1 (oleic)	66.2	66.8	19.0	35.4	60.5	81.5
C18:2 (linoleic)	20.2	21.1	61.9	37.6	17.3	9.8
C18:3-γ (linolenic)	–	–	–	–	–	–
C18:3-α (linolenic)	–	0.8	16.0	0.1	0.4	0.4
Others	–	0.7	–	0.6	–	0.5
% Fat	31.40	52.21	56.98	66.22	46.35	62.64

*also Hazelnut

Table 4.3 Fat and Fatty Acid Composition of Commonly Consumed Nuts/Seeds (weight percent)

Fatty acid	Macademia**	Pecan	Pinenut	Pistacio	Pumpkin	Walnut
C6:0 (caproic)	–	–	–	–	–	–
C8:0 (caprylic)	–	–	–	–	–	–
C10:0 (capric)	–	–	–	–	–	–
C12:0 (lauric)	–	–	–	–	0.1	–
C14:0 (myristic)	0.7	–	–	0.1	0.1	0.3
C16:0 (palmitic)	8.9	6.4	7.6	11.6	12.8	7.2
C18:0 (stearic)	3.8	1.6	3.5	1.4	6.4	1.8
C18:1 (oleic)	58.4	64.0	37.1	69.3	32.3	22.6
C18:2 (linoleic)	1.8	24.8	42.9	15.2	47.2	53.9
C18:3-γ (linolenic)	–	–	–	–	–	–
C18:3-α (linolenic)	–	–	–	0.5	0.4	11.6
Others	22.6	1.0	1.4	1.1	0.2	0.9
% Fat	73.7	67.6	50.7	48.4	45.8	61.9

**C16:1 (palmitoleic)

Physical and Chemical Characteristics of Fats and Oils

Fats and oils in the form of triglycerides or other glycerides such as phospholipids, when combined with proteins and carbohydrates, are the principal structural components of all living cells, both in animal cells and plant cells.

Fats and oils form crystal structures that vary in part because of the melting characteristics of the component fatty acids. They also vary in form because the different triglycerides have different shapes depending on which fatty acid is predominant in which position on the triglyceride. The solidifying (solid fat index) and melting properties of fats and oils impart important functionality to their use in food products such as bakery products. See Table 4.4 for melting points of various fats and oils. Also see Table 4.4 for smoke points of various fats and oils. Light duty frying oils are reported to be stable for 10 hours and to have a smoke point of 225°C. Oils that are considered high-stability frying oils are supposed to be stable for 25 hours and have a smoke point of 235°C. None of the cooking oils in Table 4.4 meet the temperature requirements for high-stability frying oils.

Ranges of iodine values (IV) and saponification values for commonly used vegetable fats and oils and commonly used animal fats are given in Table 4.5. These are physical characteristics that are useful in analysis of fats and oils. The iodine value is used to determine the number of double bonds in a fat or oil. The saponification value is used to determine the length of the fatty acids in triglycerides. See also Appendix A: the General Glossary.

Fats and oils are not soluble in water. Because they are lighter weight than water soluble molecules such as carbohydrates and proteins, they float on top of water. As noted in Chapter 2, the lack of water solubility is the reason fats and oils are carried on molecules called lipoproteins in the serum of biological systems.

Fats and oils can undergo changes because of their chemical structures. The lipid oxidation that occurs from autooxidation of unsaturated fats and oils in the presence of oxygen is a typical free radical reaction, which leads to oxidative deterioration of lipids.

Table 4.4 Physical Characteristics of Fats and Oils

Melting points	°C (°F)
Babassu	26 (78.8)
Beef tallow	50 (122)
Borneo tallow	38 (91.4)
Butterfat	37 (98.6)
Cocoa butter	36 (96.8)
Coconut oil	26 (78.8)
Cottonseed oil	11 (51.8)
Lard, prime	45 (113)
Palm oil, refined	40 (104)
Palm kernel oil	29 (84.2)
Peanut oil	13 (55.4)
Castor oil, hydrogenated	60 (140)
Sardine oil, hydrogenated	57.5 (135.5)
Soybean oil, hydrogenated	66.5 (151.7)

(Source: T.H. Applewhite, Kirk-Othmer Encyclopedia of Chemical Technology, 4th Edition)

Smoke Points for Selected Cooking Oils*	°C (°F)
Corn oil	204 (400)
Cottonseed oil	220 (428)
Palm oil	233 (451)
Peanut oil	218 (425)
Olive oil	138 (280)
Rapeseed (Canola) oil	227 (440)
Safflower oil	159 (318)
Soya oil	228 (443)
Sunflower oil	232 (450)

* Refined oils 0.05% FFA content
(Source: ISEO)

Table 4.5 Ranges of Iodine Values and Saponification Values for Commonly Used Vegetable Fats and Oils

Oil/Fat	Iodine Value	Saponification Value
Cocoa butter	32-40	190-200
Coconut oil	7-13	248-264
Corn oil	110-128	186-196
Cottonseed oil	99-121	189-199
Olive oil	76-90	188-196
Palm oil	45-56	195-205
Palm kernel oil	14-24	243-255
Peanut oil	84-102	188-196
Rapeseed oil		
regular	97-110	168-183
Canola	110-115	188-193
Safflower oil		
regular	138-151	186-198
hybrid	85-93	185-195
Sesame oil	104-118	187-196
Soybean oil	125-138	188-195
Sunflower oil		
regular	122-139	186-198
hybrid	81-91	--

Ranges of Iodine Values and Saponification Values for Commonly Used Animal Fats

Oil/Fat	Iodine Value	Saponification Value
Butter fat	25-42	210-240
Chicken fat	76-80	194-204
Lard	53-68	192-203
Tallow (beef)	33-50	190-202
Tallow (lamb)	35-46	192-198

(Source: Durkee Industrial Foods)

The following flow chart lists the typical steps for extracting oil from the numerous seeds, nuts and/or fruits that are currently in common usage today.

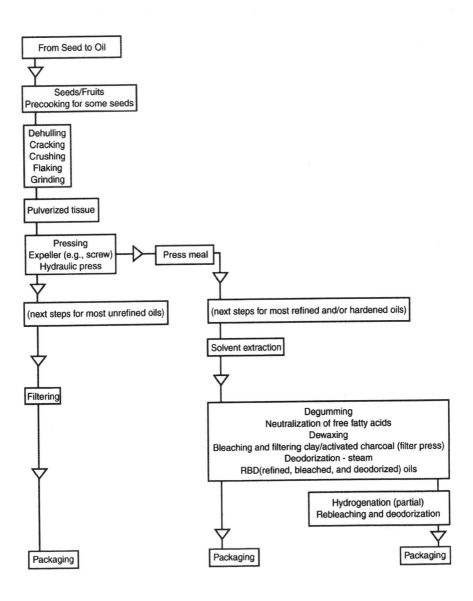

Oil Presses in Antiquity

Oil pressed from fruits, nuts, and seeds has a very long history. In many of the less industrialized countries, some of the ancient methods of pressing oils are still being used. Some of the small oil pressing companies in the United States and Canada have tried to emulate some of the older methods, which do not use solvents.

There are several museum quality books on historic oil mills published in the United States by Carter Litchfield's OLÉARIUS EDITIONS. These include:

Seiyu Roku: Oil Manufacturing in Japan in 1836 by N. Okura and N. Matsukawa, is a charming reproduction and translation of an authentic style Japanese book, which describes the ancient process of producing rapeseed oil with many beautiful old illustrations.

Ghani: The Traditional Oil Mill of India by K. T. Acahya, illustrates and describes the wooden ghanis used for grinding oilseeds of groundnut, mustard, safflower and sesame; these ghanis were based on the mortar and pestle principal and powered by various animals (or occasionally by man).

The Bethlehem Oil Mill 1745-1934: German Technology in Early Pennsylvania by C. Litchfield, H.-J. Finke, S. G. Young, and K. Z. Huetter describes in story and picture the combination oilseed, hemp, and tanbark mill built by the Moravian community artisans. The oil mill was a stamping mortar built of wood and was used both for cold pressed oil and oil pressed from heated cake, usually of flaxseed, but also of hempseed, cottonseed, and sunflower seed.

The History and Technology of Olive Oil in the Holy Land by R. Frankel, S. Avitsur, and E. Ayalon describes the ancient techniques for producing olive oil by both mortar and pestle and screw press methods. The book includes many drawings and photographs of ancient sites and oil presses that date back about nine centuries to the iron age.

Sources of Information on Fats and Oils: Which Ones Are Most Accurate?

If you have gotten this far in this book, and have not been able to find specific information in the glossary or listed in the index, there are a number of professional journals, and a number of textbooks that should be considered as reliable sources of technical information on fats and oils.

Currently, there are not many popular books on fats and oils that are accurate enough to be used as resource material. So if a book is not listed here, assume that it has sufficient inaccuracies so that it should not be used. If you find a statement in this book and it contradicts something you see in another book, check a resource journal or text to sort out any discrepancy. You will likely find *Know Your Fats* to be accurate since the author is scientifically trained in fats and oils.

Some of the unacceptable books are written by well-meaning but clearly ill-informed clinicians (e.g., naturopaths, medical practitioners, veterinarians). Some are written by fats and oils salesmen with an agenda but without any adequate basic scientific training in lipids.

This author has a real problem with individuals who pretend to have credentials, whose influence is widespread, and whose information is often inaccurate. In nutrition, a Ph.D. from an accredited university does not guarantee an adequate education in all of the nutritional sciences, but a purchased "Ph.D." from a non-accredited "college" or "university" is a sure guarantee of inadequate training in the valid sciences. Always ask for the author's credentials -- and check them. Someone with a valid degree is proud of that degree because the work involved to earn the degree was a real apprenticeship. Any book that lists a degree for the author but no credentials is suspect.

Some of the books that are written by reliable individuals on topics such as the prostaglandins may be old enough so that the latest finding is not included. Nonetheless, books or articles of this sort are valid for use as long as you recognize the limitations imposed by age of the writing. Always check the date of publication.

Technical information on fats and oils can be found in scientific libraries connected with universities and colleges, and sometimes in very large municipal libraries. The books that would be available in such places include the famous *Bailey's Industrial Oil and Fat Products, 5th Edition* published by Wiley, Gunstone's *The Lipid Handbook* published by Chapman Hall/CRC Press, and the numerous books listed in the references for this chapter. A classic, *The Lipid Handbook* by Gunstone,

Harwood, and Padley was published in 1986 (first edition) and again in 1994 (second edition). The only problem with this classic book is its price, which most individuals would find they cannot afford, but it is well worth a trip to the library to browse through its many pages if you seek technical information on fats and oils. A greatly shortened version of some of its parts is the 1996 book *Fatty Acid and Lipid Chemistry* by Gunstone, which is published by Blackie Academic & Professional, an imprint of Chapman and Hall, for a smaller price. The *Fats and Oils Handbook* by Bockisch was published by the American Oil Chemists Society in 1998.

There are a number of textbooks that can be used as resources for more extensive technical information than you can find in *Know Your Fats*, which is intended as a primer. The well-known textbook *Lipid Biochemistry: An Introduction*, written by Gurr and James in its earlier editions and by Gurr and Harwood in the most recent editions, is also published by Chapman and Hall.

The many publications of the American Oil Chemists' Society and the International Fats and Oils Society are comprehensive and their journals are filled with ongoing research in fats and oils. Those journals are dedicated to the topics of fats and oils, and they can supply technical resource information. The most readily available lipids journals include: *Lipids, Journal of the American Oil Chemists' Society, Journal of Lipid Research, Inform,* and *Journal of Lipid Technology.* Many of the food and nutrition journals also include research articles on food fats and lipids, and these articles would be identified in library searches. Occasionally there are methodology errors in some of the research papers where the group involved in the research is not sufficiently trained in lipid biochemistry, and as a result, the articles are collectively sometimes contradictory.

Books on lipid topics, in addition to being published by the American Oil Chemists' Society, The Oily Press (in England), and Chapman Hall, are also published by the CRC Press, Academic Press, Plenum Press, Elsevier, and other publishers of scientific material. These books, in addition to being highly technical, are also usually more expensive than the average reader is prepared to pay. Unfortunately, there are also errors in some of these books.

There are numerous companies in the business of selling fats and oils and many maintain information sheets and/or booklets on fats and oils. An outstanding example of this, which is no longer available, was Alban Muller International, a French company, which supplies edible fats and oils products to the health and cosmetic industry. This company did maintain a web site with a rather encyclopedic blend of information on most of the edible fats and oils. It had information on oils ranging from unusual oils such as argan oil and milk thistle oil to the more common oils such as corn oil and soybean oil. The site gave such information as the geography and history of the plant from which the oil is extracted as well as the typical composition values and analytical data sheets.

Unfortunately some of the health food companies who maintain web sites and advertise the oils they sell over the Internet have numerous inaccuracies in their information pages. There are also a number of specialized web sites with information on foods whose pages on fats and oils are rather blatantly inaccurate.

A word of caution about even some of the technical journals, as there are occasionally some errors-of-fact in articles from technical magazines and journals about fats and oils. An example of this is found in a recent technical journal cover story in which the author, an associate editor, writes that "...stearic acid, a combination of medium- to short-chain saturated fatty acids, has been shown..." Now, stearic acid is an 18 carbon saturated fatty acid and is not a combination of anything except carbons, hydrogens and oxygen; and you could combine medium- and short-chain fatty acids until the cows come home, but the only thing you could get from that is a collection of medium- and short-chain free fatty acids or, if they were combined and esterified with glycerol, a combination of triglycerides containing medium- and short-chain fatty acids.

Chapter 5

Labeling Fats and Oils for the Marketplace

An Example of Fats and Oils Labeling in the Days of Mark Twain

Though there has probably been more misinformation given out about dietary fats and oils during the past forty years than at any other time in history, consumers have also been lied to in the past about which fat was in the tub or which oil was in the bottle.

A classic example of this is the story told by the hero Mark Twain in *Life on the Mississippi* (by the late Samuel Clemens). We are told that Mark overhears two men who are called drummers (salesmen) exclaiming about their ability to fool the consumer with cheap replacements for butter and olive oil. The drummer from Cincinnati, Ohio extolls the virtues of his product that is imitation butter, and he proudly claims all "houses" (hotels) to the west are using this oleomargarine. The drummer from New Orleans explains how they are able to bottle cottonseed oil with a phoney label saying it is olive oil. In early times, he notes, they shipped the actual bottles to Italy and France and back again to obtain a customs stamp. When that was stopped by French and Italian customs, they resorted to using imported stamped labels for a bottle of "cottonseed olive" oil that never left the U.S.

Of course, this type of overt fats and oils fraud should no longer be able to exist; presumably the Food and Drug Administration or the Federal Trade Commission are on the lookout for just such fraud. Such mislabeling and/or misbranding, however, has been replaced by a more insidious mislabeling/misbranding. The "cheap replacement for butter" is now selling quite openly, but on a trumped-up health-benefit marketing approach. The current olive oil replacement is being promoted on its own merits because of its own relatively high level of monounsaturates and Greek and Italian cuisines that would normally be cooked with olive oil are made with the cheaper replacement. This is unknown to most consumers who assume their oil and vinegar is olive oil and vinegar. Since most of the canola oil is partially hydrogenated, the replacement oil adds *trans* fatty acids to the diet where the olive oil would not.

Never mind that the supposed benefits of "heart healthy" polyunsaturated spreads and monounsaturated oils will not stand the test of time. The industries benefitting from this modern agenda will continue to propagandize the public and the professionals in order to keep their multibillion dollar markets.

Labeling of Fats and Oils During the Past Three Decades

As noted in Chapter 1, we generally know the composition of *unprocessed* fats and oils since they do not vary significantly most of the time. The fatty acid composition of the *processed* vegetable fats, however, is not always known or reported with any degree of accuracy. For example, the incomplete fatty acid composition declaration (incomplete because there is no declaration of *trans* fatty acids) usually listed on the back or side of certain popular cracker packages bears no relationship to the correct fatty acid composition determined by chemical analysis (see Figure 5.1 for a label declaration along with comparison to the chemical analysis performed by the author at the University of Maryland Lipids Research Laboratory).

Even foods that do not contain partially hydrogenated fats and oils contain incomplete or inaccurate fatty acid profiles on their labels. The incomplete fatty acid composition declarations find their way into many of the data banks used by universities and government agencies and then into the data banks of the popular computer programs for dietary analysis. Unfortunately, these latter data banks are starting to be used by nutritionists and dietitians for counseling the public on what to eat.

In Table 5.1, there is a list of the compositional findings of the USDA, the Durkee fats and oils company, the University of Maryland (UofMD) lipids research laboratory analyses (by the author and colleagues), and the data base for the National Health and Nutrition Examination Survey (NHANES) II of the Public Health Service. You can see that the USDA Handbook 8 composition values, the UofMD analyses, and the Durkee analyses are almost identical or so close that they are basically the same. However, the data used by the NHANES II for their analyses is so totally different that you have to wonder where they obtained such data.

Table 5.1.

Data Source	n	avg Sat(SE) wt %	avg Oleic(SE) wt %	avg Linoleic (SE) wt %
Soybean oil				
USDA 8-4	68-70	14.1 (0.1)	22.8 (0.3)	51.0 (0.3)
Durkee	?	15.0	23.4	53.2
U of MD	10	14.8 (0.2)	23.2 (0.4)	54.8 (0.5)
NHANES II				
01401 (688)*	?	9.96	28.03	53.03
Cottonseed oil				
USDA 8-4	120	27.1 (0.2)	17.8 (0.3)	53.9 (0.4)
Durkee	?	27.9	17.6	53.9
U of MD	4	29.1 (0.7)	18.5 (0.7)	52.0 (1.2)
NHANES II				
05463 (707)	?	17.5	21.0	51.3
Safflower oil				
USDA 8-4	90	8.9 (0.1)	12.1 (0.2)	77.5 (0.3)
Durkee	?	8.9	13.1	77.7
U of MD	1	9.1	10.8	80.0
NHANES II				
91830 (690)*	?	9.0	75.0	14.0
Corn oil				
USDA 8-4	298	13.3(0.0)	25.3(0.0)	60.7(0.1)
Durkee	?	14.4	27.5	57.0
U of MD	3	13.1(0.9)	24.1(1.1)	62.4(1.6)
NHANES II				
91825 (689)	?	12.7	24.2	58.0

n - number of samples
* (Typical of composition of 50% of oils listed by NHANES II)
**(The composition used for 40% of respondents for salad and cooking oils)

For example, soybean oil always had about 15 percent saturated fatty acids, but NHANES II used 10 percent. Soy also always had about 23 percent oleic acid, but NHANES II listed 28 percent. The value for the saturates in cottonseed oil is not accurate for the NHANES II data, and the value for oleic acid is higher than normally seen. The most unusual composition listed by NHANES II, though, is the one for safflower oil. The data are for high oleic safflower oil, which is the 1970s was not the safflower oil that was being used -- the high linoleic oil was the one. Also, the safflower oil value was used by NHANES II for calculating the salad and cooking oils intake for 40 percent of the respondents. When this author wrote about this gross error for several FASEB presentations in 1988, the interesting response came from Dr. Fred Mattson, who was formerly with the fats and oils industry, in the form of a paper published in the Journal of the American Dietetic Association in 1989 in which he "retrofitted" the presence of high oleic safflower oil into an earlier date when it was still being developed.

All the current data bases are inadequate for purposes of constructing recommendations about dietary fats if the data bases are used without recognizing that the typical fatty acid composition readily available to the professional nutritionist or dietitian frequently uses the prototype of the original oil (before it is hydrogenated) or the prototype of the wrong oil. The possibility of another kind of confusion exists because USDA Handbook 8 collapses the fatty acid data (for any foods that contain processed fat) in a way that makes application of the data impossible for conscientious clinicians.

The consumer, and, to a large extent, the food and dietetics professional, assumes that the information on the food label is accurate. If we examine the information about fat that has been included on the labels of typical snack foods, we see many examples of misinformation about the amounts and types of fat/oil and fatty acids. Most people do not have the expertise needed to discern when the amounts listed are not correct.

Several examples of this type of misinformation is given in the next set of figures. The example given in Figure 5.1A is typical of many of the labeled snack crackers from a nationally distributed brand. The label indicated that the product serving had a total of 9 grams, of which 2 grams were polyunsaturated (Poly), 5 grams were mono-unsaturated (Mono), and 2 grams were saturated (Sat). A chemical analysis of the crackers determined that the composition was quite different than what was represented. The actual levels of Poly and Mono were far from what was declared. The Poly was 0.5 grams instead of 2 grams and the Mono was 2.7 grams instead of 5 grams. Only the Sat was accurate. The balance of the 9 grams of fat was 3.7 grams of *trans*. At the time of this analysis, the company would not have labeled the *trans* fatty acids, but the regulations said that if the Mono and Poly were labeled (they were voluntary) they must be accurate, and since the *trans* could not be included in those categories, the amount of fatty acids would not add up to the total.

The examples given in Figures 5.1B and 5.1C represent either carelessness in labeling or actual lack of understanding of what is supposed to be labeled.

In Figure 5.1B, we see that the potato chips were labeled as having been cooked in either or both cottonseed and safflower oil. These two oils have very different fatty acid compositions. Based on the grams of fat per serving (9g) which translates to 31.75 grams per 100 grams of product, of which the fatty acids are determined as being 96.5 percent (30.353 grams per 100 grams), we can do the arithmetic and realize that the numbers only allow for 4.6 percent of the total fatty acids to be monounsaturated. Since there is no fat or oil in existence with that composition, it becomes apparent that there is something very wrong with the composition that is listed. Actual analysis of the potato chips gave the correct composition and the correct label was calculated.

In Figure 5.1C, we view another package of potato chips made with either cottonseed oil, peanut oil, or corn oil - or some of two of them or all of them. When we look carefully, paying attention to the amounts of polyunsaturated fatty acids (PUFA) and saturated fatty acids that were listed on the label, and then calculate the monounsaturated fatty acids by difference, we see that there is no combination of the oils that could provide the labeled composition.

In the following tables, the information that was included on the labels is in *italics*. The balance is a discussion by the author based on chemical analysis and compositional evaluation.

Sandwich crackers w/Cream Cheese & Chives

Fat ingredients according to package label:

Grams:	*Total fat*	9
	Poly	2
	Mono	5
	Sat	2

Actual fat ingredients based on analysis by capillary gas chromatography (U of MD)

Grams:	Poly	0.5
	Mono	2.7
	Sat	2.0
	(*Trans*	3.7)

Analysis of several additional products manufactured by this company gave the following information on *trans* levels in addition to the other major fatty acid classes:

Saturated fatty acids:	17.3 - 20.2%
Trans-monounsaturated fatty acids:	33.7 - 38.0%
Cis-monounsaturated fatty acids:	32.6 - 34.3%
Polyunsaturated fatty acids:	9.8 - 10.0%

These products typically have approximately one-third of the fat as *trans* fatty acids.

Figure 5.1A   Example of Typical Mislabeling of Fat Components

Supermarket Brand "Natural Potato Chips"

Label ingredients:　　　*Potatoes, cottonseed and/or safflower oil, salt.*

Fat g/serving	*9g/1 oz.(28.35 g)*	= 31.750g/100g	
PUFA	*6300mg/1 oz.*	= 22.222g/100g	= 73.3%
Saturated	*1900mg/1 oz.*	=　6.702g/100g	= 22.1%

Total fatty acids　　　　　　　　= 30.353g/100g
Monounsaturated (by difference)　= 1.429g/100g　= 4.6%

Question:　　　What oil or combination of oils could be labeled as

22.1% saturated fatty acids,
 4.6% monounsaturated fatty acids, and
73.3% polyunsaturated fatty acids?

Answer:　　　There is none, based on the following standard compositions (from the Durkee Table) for the labeled oils

How do we know?

Fatty acid classes		Cottonseed*	Safflower*
Saturated	(wt%)	27.9	9.0
Monounsaturated	"	17.6	13.1
Polyunsaturated	"	53.9	77.7

*Durkee Table

Fatty acid classes		(Avg/2 oils) (50:50)	(Avg/2 oils) (90:10)	Proper Label
Saturated	(wt%)	(18.5)	(26.0)	22.1
Monounsaturated	"	(15.4)	(17.2)	4.6
Polyunsaturated	"	(65.8)	(56.3)	73.3

Figure 5.1B　Mislabeling of Fat Contents

Supermarket Potato Chips (continued)

Actual chemical analysis* showed the fat in the potato chips to be a 90:10 blend of cottonseed oil and safflower oil

		Total fat g/100g = 24.6
		Fatty acids g/100g = 23.5
Saturated	(wt%) 26.0	Saturated g/100 g = 22.36
Monounsaturated "	16.7	Monounsaturated g/100g = 14.36
Polyunsaturated "	56.8	Polyunsaturated g/100g = 48.85

*Analysis by glass capillary GLC SP-2340 at University of Maryland, December 1989

Therefore the correct label would be:

Fat g/serving	7.0g/1 oz.	(24.6g/100g)
PUFA	3.8g/1 oz. (or 3787mg)	(13.3g/100g)
Saturated	1.7g/1 oz. (or 1733mg)	(6.1g/100g)

Thus the chips have 9% less saturated fatty acids, 40% less polyunsaturates, and 22.5% less total fat than the label indicates

The person responsible for the label numbers should have been able to figure out the correct amounts if that person understood fats and oils composition

Figure 5.1B (continued)

Supermarket Brand Peaks'n dips Potato chips [C-P9120]

Label ingredients: *Potatoes, vegetable oil (contains one or more of the following: cottonseed oil, peanut oil, corn oil), salt.*

Fat g/serving	*6g/1 oz. = 6g/28.35g*	*= 21.2g/100g*
PUFA	*4g/1 oz. =*	*13.5g/100g = 66.5%*
Saturated	*1g/1 oz. =*	*3.4g/100g = 16.7%*

Therefore: total fatty acids   =   20.3g/100g
Monounsaturated (by difference) =   3.4g/100g = 16.7%

Question: What oil or combination of oils could be

16.7% saturated fatty acids,
16.7% monounsaturated fatty acids, and
66.5% polyunsaturated fatty acids?

Answer: There is none, based on the following standard compositions (from the Durkee Table) for the labeled oils

Fatty acid classes		Cottonseed*	Peanut*	Corn*
Saturated	(wt%)	27.9	20.3	14.4
Monounsaturated	"	17.6	46.5	27.5
Polyunsaturated	"	53.9	31.4	57.0

*Durkee Table

(Average/3 oils)	Label
(20.9)	16.7
(30.5)	16.7
(47.4)	66.5

Figure 5.1C Mislabeling of Fat Contents

Peaks'n dips (continued)

Actual chemical analysis* showed the fat in the potato chips to be cottonseed oil:

			Total fat g/100g	= 26.5
			Fatty acids g/100g	= 25.3
Saturated	(wt%)	28.1	Saturated g/100 g	= 7.1
Monounsaturated "		17.6	Monounsaturated g/100g	= 4.4
Polyunsaturated "		54.3	Polyunsaturated g/100g	= 13.7

*Analysis by glass capillary GLC SP-2340 at University of Maryland, December 1989

Therefore the correct label would be:

Fat g/serving	7.5g/1 oz.	(26.5g/100g)
PUFA	3.9g/1 oz.	(13.7g/100g)
Saturated	2.0g/1 oz.	(7.1g/100g)

Thus the chips have 100% more saturated fatty acids and 21% more total fat than the label indicated!

Figure 5.1C (continued)

Since there is variation of the types of fat and the amounts of fat used within brands and between brands, the consumer (or the clinician) doesn't get any real information from the currently used listing of the different types of fats and oils that may be in the product. More realistic for the consumer (or the clinician) would be the accurate listing of the amounts of the major fatty acids present in the fats or oils in the product. This is not a difficult number for the food industry to acquire because the different blends of fats and oils, which are used in various food products, can be easily analyzed. For example, typical corn snack chips made in unhydrogenated corn oil would have the same basic fatty acid composition as corn oil, and the hypothetical nutrition label could reflect that information as seen in Figure 5.2.

For serving size		100 g
Fat		33.0g
Saturates		
Short/medium chain		0
Long chain		4.6g
Trans		0
Monounsaturates		8.4g
Polyunsaturates		19.8g
Omega-6	19.8g	
Omega-3	0	
Cholesterol		0 mg

Figure 5.2   **Example of Hypothetical Fat Labeling for Corn Chips Made with Unhydrogenated Corn Oil**

Another type of snack corn chip is frequently made with partially hydrogenated soybean oil so it would have the basic composition that reflected the partially hydrogenated oil as the major source of the fat. The nutrition label could reflect that information as seen in Figure 5.3.

For serving size		100 g
Fat		25.2g
Saturates		
Short/medium chain		0
Long chain		4.0g
Trans		7.7g
Monounsaturates		7.2g
Polyunsaturates		5.4g
Omega-6	5.4g	
Omega-3	0	
Cholesterol		0 mg

Figure 5.3   Example of Hypothetical Fat Labeling of Typical Tortilla Chips Made with Partially Hydrogenated Soybean Oil

Still another type of snack chip made with peanut oil would have the basic composition that reflected the unhydrogenated peanut oil and the extremely small amount of corn oil inherent in the ground corn used to make the chips as seen in Figure 5.4.

For serving size		100 g
Fat		25.0g
Saturates		
Short/medium chain		0
Long chain		5.5g
Trans		0
Monounsaturates		11.5g
Polyunsaturates		7.8g
Omega-6	7.8g	
Omega-3	0	
Cholesterol		0 mg

Figure 5.4   Example of How Tortilla Chips Made with Unhydrogenated Peanut Oil Could be Labeled

The composition of the chips made with the unhydrogenated oils would not vary enough to warrant different labels from batch to batch. There is always the possibility of producing very small amounts of *trans* fatty acids in extrusion processes. The levels are so low, however, that they would usually not have to be included on the label, and they are more an analytical curiosity than they are a biological problem unless they are consumed in extremely large amounts.

Substitution for Tropical Oils?

An example of what happens when misinformation is given to both the public and the professional can be seen in the attacks a decade ago against the tropical oil markets in the U.S. Started in 1986, apparently as the brainchild of consumer activists groups, including the Center for Science in the Public Interest (CSPI), this campaign of misinformation was expanded upon by the domestic soybean oil industry, the economic beneficiary of the campaign, and was intensified during 1988-1989.

The anti-tropical oils campaign originated with a petition from CSPI to the FDA in 1986 to add singularly pejorative anti-tropical oils labeling, and when the FDA did not approve the petition, CSPI and the soybean oil industry then asked the Congress to introduce legislation requiring singularly pejorative anti-tropical oils labeling. (Instead of requiring a full fat labeling declaration for **all fats and oils**, which are needed, the petition and proposed legislation would have singled out tropical oils.) Fortunately, this latter effort also failed.

The amount of misinformation written about food fats in this campaign was dangerously misleading to the public. The old adage "a little knowledge is a dangerous thing" applies here. For example, CSPI, an organization that had no fat analysis capability at the time (it currently hires laboratories to do analysis for certain projects), had been selling a booklet "The Saturated Fat Attack" that told the public what kinds of fats were in the different foods. Chemical analysis at the University of Maryland of a random sampling of some of the foods listed by CSPI indicated that these foods **did not contain the fats that CSPI said they did** (see Figure 5.5).

Charles Mitchell, a CSPI staff attorney is quoted on page 160 of the June 1989 issue of *Vogue* magazine as saying: "If the ingredients say 'contains partially hydrogenated cottonseed, palm, and/or soybean oil', your guess is as good as mine about what's in the product." Well, the labels at that time did say "and/or" but that apparently didn't stop CSPI from guessing what fats were in the food in "The Saturated Fat Attack," and it didn't stop CSPI from finding palm oil in all of them.

The tropical oils such as palm oil, palm kernel oil, and coconut oil have made up a minuscule part of the U.S. food fats in the recent past, and have gotten even smaller as a result of that anti-tropical oils campaign. Generally the tropical oils had been used to blend with other oils to lend good baking or frying properties. These natural oils have been used for thousands of years in many parts of the world.

Under a heading *Saturated Fats in Processed Foods* in the booklet "Saturated Fat Attack," a 1988 report sold by the Center for Science in the Public Interest (CSPI), the following foods from Nabisco have been listed as containing a "Type of Saturated Fat"; University of Maryland (U of MD) chemical analyses were done 1987-1988

Product	Type of Ingredient Fat	
	According to CSPI	**By Analysis U of MD**
Wheatsworth crackers	Palm	Partially hydrogenated soybean oil
Premium saltine cracker	Lard	Partially hydrogenated canola oil
Almost Home cookies	Palm	Partially hydrogenated soybean oil
Cheese Tidbit crackers	Palm	Partially hydrogenated soybean oil
Chips Ahoy cookies	Palm	Partially hydrogenated soybean & cottonseed oils
Brown Edge wafers	Lard, palm, butter	>95% partially hydrogenated soybean oil

Figure 5.5 Example of Ingredient Misbranding by CSPI

The palm kernel oils were used in candies, and if they were replaced *for misguided health reasons* with partially hydrogenated soybean oil, then the overall product contained **more** fat and what were termed the saturate-equivalents (saturated fatty acids plus *trans* fatty acids) were about equal (because of the *trans* fatty acids contained in the replacement shortenings), so the consumers at that time were not getting what they were led to believe they were getting, i.e., less "so-called saturated fat."

In addition, coconut oil and palm kernel oil provided more than half of their fat as lauric and capric acids, two medium-chain fatty acids, which have significant and desirable functional properties because they are used by the human body to make antimicrobial (antiviral, antibacterial, and antiprotozoal) derivatives. (See discussion on lauric acid and capric acid in Chapter 1, Chapter 2, Chapter 4, and the General Glossary.)

Palm oil is used alone as a frying oil or as a baking shortening, and also for blending with soybean oil into shortenings. When palm oil is added to soybean oil for making shortenings, *less* hydrogenation is needed and the levels of *trans* fatty acids are lower. A 50/50 blend by weight of palm and soybean oils has approximately 30 percent saturates. If you consider that an unhydrogenated cottonseed oil also has approximately 30 percent saturates, then from the standpoint of levels of saturates, it hardly makes any difference which oil is used for snack chips, etc. In actual practice, blends using palm oil have only about 25 percent palm oil, so the contribution of saturates is even less. The overall level of saturates with a 25/75 (palm oil/soybean oil) blend would be about 21 percent -- which has less saturates than the cottonseed oil, and apparently about the same amount as typical soybean oils has recently been shown by analysis (Lichtenstein et al 1999).

Replacement of Coconut Oil and Palm Kernel Oil By Other Oils Means More Calories for Consumers

In an October 1987 letter to the Food and Drug Administration, (Food Chemical News 12 October 1987), the National Confectioners Association (NCA) noted that a switch from tropical [coconut and palm kernel] oils to domestic [U.S.] oils [e.g., soybean, cottonseed] for confectionery coatings and coatings for baked goods would of necessity result "in higher fat levels and increased caloric density." NCA noted that since "confectionery manufacturers are bound by technological constraints" this would result in an increase in fat content of the product because the manufacturers would have to use a higher weight of domestic oils to achieve the high viscosity levels required. (This author's calculations show that this increased caloric density will be between 4.6 and 5.6 percent.)

Actually there are two reasons for the increase in caloric density in a food item when coconut and palm kernel oils are abandoned in favor of replacement types of oils such as soybean and/or cottonseed and/or safflower. One, as noted above, is because the manufacturers need to use 2-3 percent more of the replacement fat to get the same textural properties normally provided by the tropical oils; the second is that the tropical oils such as coconut and palm kernel oils actually have at least 2.56 percent fewer calories per gram of fat. This latter fact is apparently not well-known. The reason for the fewer calories is related to the short- and medium-chain fatty acid content of these two oils, and to their lower heats of combustion.

Coconut oil has 63.4 percent short- and medium-chain fatty acids and only 36.6 percent long-chain fatty acids; 28.5 percent are saturated. The corresponding percentages for palm kernel oil are 57.8 percent, 42.2 percent, and 26.4 percent. The replacement oils on the other hand have 100 percent long-chain fatty acids (which are mixtures of saturated and unsaturated fatty acids). The caloric value of the short- and medium-chain fatty acids is considerably less than the caloric value of the longer chain fatty acids.

Coconut oil and palm kernel oil have only 3910 kilocalories per pound compared to soybean, cottonseed, or corn oil, for example, which have 4010 kilocalories per pound. This means there are 100 fewer kilocalories per pound for these tropical oils, and since the confectionery manufacturers must use more of the replacement fats to get the same product, the end result is more calories per item for the consumer. Since the consumer today is being told to cut down on calories and to cut down on fat, the switch away from coconut oil and palm kernel oil does a major disservice to the consumer.

The domestic oils must be partially hydrogenated to perform satisfactorily as replacements for coconut and palm kernel oils. As a result of that process, the levels of long-chain saturated fatty acids are higher in the replacement fats than in coconut and palm kernel oils. Coconut and palm kernel oils have at most 28.5 and 26.4 percent long-chain saturated fatty acids. Chemical analyses of partially hydrogenated soybean and/or cottonseed oils used as confectionery fats show anywhere from 30.9 to 46.9 percent long-chain saturates or from 57.9 to 66.5 percent long-chain saturate-equivalents (long-chain saturate-equivalents include the *trans* fatty acids formed in the partial hydrogenation process since the *trans* fatty acids are recognized as physically equivalent to long-chain saturated fatty acids).

A History of the Current Label: 1990 to 1999

Unfortunately for consumers and professionals who do not know better, the current labels provide misinformation rather than good useful information.

Up until the signing of the food labeling law passed by Congress in 1990, the type of labeling of fats and oils listed only polyunsaturated fatty acids and saturated fatty acids if a breakdown of the fat was included; these were labeled as "polyunsaturated" (or "PUFA") and "saturated," respectively. The labels were supposed to give equal prominence to the amounts in grams per serving, and the order was "polyunsaturated" first, followed by "saturated." The labeling was permitted as long as the food contained more than 10 percent of the dry weight as fat and a serving contained more than 2 grams of fat.

For purposes of labeling, the polyunsaturated fatty acids were defined as *cis-methylene interrupted* and they then could include linoleic acid (18:2) and α-linolenic acid (18:3), as well as the longer chain polyunsaturates such as arachidonic acid (20:4), eicosapentaenoic acid (20:5), and docosahexaenoic acid (22:6).

The saturated fatty acids were defined to include lauric acid (12 carbons (12:0)), myristic acid (14:0), palmitic acid (16:0), and stearic acid (18:0); not included were saturated fatty acids shorter than lauric acid (i.e., 10:0, 8:0, 6:0, 4:0), or longer than stearic acid (i.e., 20:0, 22:0, 24:0). Also not included were the odd-chain saturates of microbial origin (i.e., 15:0, 17:0, 19:0).

The original purpose of labeling polyunsaturated and saturated fatty acids was to enable the consumer to find foods that had twice as much polyunsaturates as saturates, since at that point in food labeling history certain organizations (e.g., National Heart, Lung, and Blood Institute (NHLBI), American Heart Association (AHA)) had decided that eating twice as much polyunsaturates(P) as saturates(S) was desirable for cholesterol lowering. This was the era of the P/S ratio, and the marketing of oils and margarines, etc., as having high P/S ratios was continued until it was realized that high levels of polyunsaturates were linked with cancer, gallstones, and other undesirable health effects. As a result, the desire to identify the PUFA on the label became less important, and the emphasis was shifted to the saturates. (The quiet back-pedaling of the agencies such as NHLBI and AHA eventually brought the P/S ratio down to a one-to-one and eventually even to a 0.8:1.0 -- the latter being the effort of the National Academy of Sciences.)

Subsequently, the 1990 labeling law shifted the emphasis entirely to saturated fatty acids because of the mistaken belief that these fatty acids are the main ones to be decreased in order to lower serum cholesterol as part of a policy of changing risk factors for heart disease. Research published in 1990, however, showed that fatty acids called *trans* fatty acids had an even more undesirable effect on the serum cholesterol values (Mensink and Katan, 1990). Further research reported in 1991 by the same group confirmed the 1990 report. These research findings had been predicted by relevant animal studies a decade or more earlier, but were mainly ignored. These *trans* fatty acids are found in large amounts in many foods that are, as a result of the current labeling law, considered low in saturates. **This certainly presents a dilemma for those individuals who recognize the undesirable effect of the *trans* fatty acids but have been unable to determine their levels in the foods because they are not listed.**

As a Faculty Research Associate involved in the ongoing analyses of the fatty acid composition of many foods conducted at the University of Maryland by the Lipids Research Group of the Department of Chemistry and Biochemistry, this author determined the fatty acid composition of more than 500 foods. These compositions have been published in part, and/or have been reported at various scientific meetings and, on two occasions, to the FDA at the invitation of the Bureau of Foods in 1979 and 1988. These compositions became part of the USDA food composition data base and have been included in the provisional *trans* fatty acid table (Dickey and Caughman 1995).

On those occasions when we compared the fatty acid composition of the food that was chemically analyzed with the label declaration, we almost always found the label declaration in substantial error. The errors related in part to the label's failure to acknowledge the existence of *trans* fatty acids, which at times made up as much as 50 percent of the fat, but it also related to faulty listing of the saturated and other components. Frequently, for foods containing partially hydrogenated vegetable oils, the faulty labeling of fatty acids included hiding the *trans* fatty acids under the "monounsaturates," which was a violation of the labeling law. To the informed, it was obvious that the only reason for not including the *trans* fatty acids in the label was because the edible oil industry was afraid to let the consumer know these fatty acids even existed, let alone the actual amounts of them in the foods!

The Canadian government and the British government both have recognized the *trans* fatty acids as separate components and *by definition* do not allow these fatty acids to be hidden in the categories called monounsaturates or polyunsaturates (which are both defined as *cis* only). Further, the Canadian government has specifically stated that *trans* fatty acids should not be increased in the Canadian diets. Labeling as originally proposed in Canada and the United Kingdom would have allowed the consumer to judge the amounts of *trans* fatty acids in diets. (The British labeling initiative died and the Canadian labeling became voluntary for a time and currently (as of August 1999) is being revisited.)

In the U.S., by labeling only the saturates, the implication was that the remainder of the fat was composed of monounsaturates and polyunsaturates; this type of labeling is deceptive and non-informative to the consumer and the professional.

Methodology for analysis of fats was originally defined and developed by the FDA as it was related to the P/S ratio agenda, and compliance was according to the methods published by the FDA. Appropriate methodology for the analysis of all fatty acids including *trans* fatty acids is available, and these methodologies have been published in peer-reviewed journals. The University of Maryland's lipid research group has utilized published methodologies for all of its analyses.

A public health agenda that equates dietary intake of foods and their individual components with prevention and/or treatment of diseases and that uses database information to generate relationships between food components and disease (and/or health) must have accurate, quantitative information about those components. To use anything less is truly scandalous. The evaluations of dietary fat (fatty acid) intake and health outcomes (e.g., NHANES) have been very inaccurate with respect to fatty acid components.

At about the time this book was going in for printing, the Food and Drug Administration made an announcement (12 November 1999) that the recommended regulations for labeling the *trans* fatty acids were being released for 90 days of public comments before making its final rules. The announcement is presented in the following boxes. What final recommendation will be made is hard to predict. The FDA proposes to include the *trans* fatty acids under the saturate category, but with an asterisk specifying the actual amount of *trans*. A regulation that would include the *trans* fatty acids in the category of saturated fatty acids is not appropriate inasmuch as such inclusion implies that they are similar. The biological effects of the saturates and the *trans* are entirely different, and in most instances they are the opposite of each other. (See Chapters 2 and 3)

FDA Proposes New Rules for *Trans* Fatty Acids in Nutrition Labeling, Nutrient Content Claims, and Health Claims

"The Food and Drug Administration (FDA) proposed today to amend its regulations on nutrition labeling to require that the amount of *trans* fatty acids in a food be included in the Nutrition Facts panel. Included in this proposal is a new nutrient content claim defining "*trans* fat free" and a limit on *trans* fatty acids wherever there are limits on saturated fat in nutrient content claims or health claims.

"*Trans* fatty acids, also known as trans fat, are made through the process of hydrogenation that solidifies liquid oils. Hydrogenation increases the shelf life and flavor stability of these oils and foods that contain them. *Trans* fat is found in vegetable shortenings, and in some margarines, crackers, cookies, snack foods and other foods.

"FDA based its proposal on recent studies that indicate that consumption of trans fatty acids contributes to increased blood LDL-cholesterol ("bad" cholesterol) levels, which increase the risk of coronary heart disease (CHD). Recent information from the American Heart Association indicates that CHD causes about 500,000 deaths annually, making it the number one cause of death in the United States. FDA is proposing to provide for information on trans fatty acids in nutrition labeling and for limits on *trans* fatty acids for content claims and for health claims in response to this important public health matter. This proposal also responds to a petition submitted by the Center for Science in the Public Interest.

"The Nation's experience with the new food label has shown that it can be a powerful tool for consumers. By requiring information about *trans* fatty acids, this proposal should assist individuals in their efforts to reduce their risk of coronary heart disease," said Jane E. Henney, M.D., FDA Commissioner.

"FDA is soliciting comments from the public on this proposed rule. "

FDA Announcement 12 November 1999

FDA FACT SHEET 12 November 1999

TRANS FATTY ACIDS IN NUTRITION LABELING, NUTRIENT CONTENT CLAIMS, AND HEALTH CLAIMS

The FDA's proposed rule on *trans* fatty acids (also called "*trans* fat") would require that the amount of *trans* fat per serving be added to the amount of saturated fat per serving so that the amount and percent Daily Value (%DV) per serving on the Nutrition Facts panel will be based on the sum of the two. When *trans* fatty acids are present, an asterisk (or other symbol) would be required after the heading "Saturated fat" to refer to a footnote stating that the product "*Includes __ g trans fat." This footnote would be optional on foods that contain no *trans* fat (i.e. less than 0.5 gram per serving, as analytical methods cannot reliably measure lower levels), except when a fatty acid or cholesterol claim is made.

The FDA has proposed limits on *trans* fat on several nutrient content claims found on food labels. Restrictions on *trans* fat will change the nutrient content claims as follows:

- "Low saturated fat" claims would be permitted to be made only when there is less than 0.5 grams of *trans* fat per serving in addition to the current requirement of 1 gram or less of saturated fat.

- "Reduced saturated fat" claims would be permitted to be made only when there is at least 25 percent less saturated fat and *trans* fat combined in addition to the current requirement of at least 25 percent less saturated fat.

- Cholesterol claims would be permitted only on food containing 2 grams or less of saturated fat and *trans* fat combined, instead of the current requirement of 2 grams or less of saturated fat.

FDA FACT SHEET (continued)

- "Lean" claims would be permitted when, in addition to meeting limits on total fat and cholesterol, the food contains 4.5 grams or less of saturated fat and *trans* fat combined, instead of 4.5 grams or less of saturated fat.

- "Extra lean" claims would be permitted when, in addition to meeting limits on total fat and cholesterol, the food contains less than 2 grams of saturated fat and *trans* fat combined, instead of less than 2 grams of saturated fat.

- The proposed new "*Trans* fat free" claim would be permitted in the labeling of foods that contain less than 0.5 grams of *trans* fat and less than 0.5 grams saturated fat per serving.

In addition, the labeling of foods containing more than 4 grams of saturated fat and *trans* fat combined per serving would not be able to carry health claims (e.g. sodium and hypertension, calcium and osteoporosis). However, the labeling of such foods would be permitted to bear nutrient content claims (e.g. "low sodium") if they have the following statement by the claim: "See nutrition information for saturated fat content." This statement would not have to accompany nutrient content claims when the food contains 4 grams or less of saturated and trans fat combined.

The FDA notes that it is not proposing a *trans* fat limit for the claim "Saturated fat free" because the agency has already defined that claim as less than 0.5 grams of saturated fat and less than 0.5 grams of *trans* fat.

Labeling Regulations Regarding Foods For Children

The following information has been excerpted from the Food and Drug Administration 1999 document for labeling regulations as they apply to fats and cholesterol.

With respect to modifications of the labeling format, in some circumstances, variations in the format of the nutrition panel are allowed, and sometimes there are mandatory modifications. For example, compared to the label information meant for adults, the labels of foods for children under the age of 2 (except infant formulas, which have their own special labeling rules under the Infant Formula Act of 1980) may not carry information about saturated fat, polyunsaturated fat, monounsaturated fat, cholesterol, calories from fat, or calories from saturated fat.

The reason for this regulation is to prevent parents from wrongly assuming that infants and toddlers should restrict their fat intake, when, in fact, they should not. Fat is very important during these years to ensure adequate growth and proper development. See Chapter 3, Figure 3.6.

The labels of foods for children under the age of 4 may not include the percent Daily Values for total fat, saturated fat, or cholesterol. They may carry percent Daily Values for protein, vitamins and minerals, however, because these nutrients are the only ones for which FDA has set Daily Values for this age group.

Chapter 6

An Overview of Dietary Fat Intake Recommendations

How Sound Is the Advice on Fats Currently Being Given to the Public?

All the advice being given to people about making changes in the amounts of saturated, monounsaturated, or polyunsaturated fatty acids they should consume in their diets is supposed to be based on the need to improve the kinds of fat we are eating in order to improve our health. This kind of thinking supposes that we really know what kinds of fatty acids people have been eating in the past and that there also was a proven connection between what they were eating and some level of good health or ill health that was resulting. There is also a presumption that those people giving the advice and those following the advice really know what the present fatty acid composition of the foods is.

Hopefully the information in this book will be of help to the reader in making his or her decision to accept or reject advice from the vocal media or the various consumer groups and government agencies.

What Have "Experts" Been Recommending?

The intense rush in the United States to promulgate dietary recommendations for food fats and oils has resulted in a lot of shifting by the various government agencies over the years.

For example, in 1977 the recommendation from the National Heart, Lung and Blood Institute of the National Institutes of Health was that people should consume two times (twice) as much polyunsaturates as saturates. Monounsaturates were treated as if they didn't exist. Then a few years later there was a shift to a recommendation that everyone should consume equal amounts of saturates, monounsaturates, and polyunsaturates, i.e., to consume 10 percent of the kilocalories for each class, with a total of 30 percent of the kilocalories in the diet as fats. (This of course assumed that there were only three classes of fatty acids existing in foods.) The most recent recommendations coming from the National Academy of Sciences (1989) are to consume up to 10 percent of the kilocalories as saturates, 12-13 percent as monounsaturates, and no more than 7-8 percent as polyunsaturates (the total fat kilocalories again being no more than 30 percent of the total energy intake, and again assuming the existence of only the 3 classes of fatty acids).

As you can see, that is quite a change in a decade with respect to the recommendations for polyunsaturates. The reason for abandoning the earlier recommendation for higher intakes of polyunsaturates was that the high levels of omega-6 polyunsaturates had been implicated in promotion of cancer, they were known to cause gallstones, and they have recently been shown to alter unfavorably the body's immune response. Additionally, the high omega-6 polyunsaturated fatty acid intake has been shown to increase whole body cholesterol, and especially liver cholesterol, and although it lowers the so-called "bad" LDL serum cholesterol, it also lowers the "good" HDL serum cholesterol levels. Also, new evidence shows that it is the altered forms of the excess polyunsaturates in the serum lipoproteins (e.g. oxidized LDL) that actually are one of the causes of heart disease.

Food Industry Influence

A former FDA official has documented the extent of the influence the food industry has had on the nutrition policy in the United States (Forbes 1994). The same food industry influence is seen in other parts of the world, although not to the extent that we experience it in this country. In the United States, many billions of dollars go to support extensive public relations efforts. This is sometimes combined with, and sometimes in addition to, the typical advertising of foods, such as the advertisements found in newspapers and magazines for individual brands of food. The food industry has developed many councils and associations to support its agenda, which of course is to sell its various products at any cost.

An example of the food industry influence in the fats and oils area can be seen by examining the information put out on fats by the International Food Information Council (IFIC), an organization supported financially by the large food industries. The information papers, booklets, and newsletters from this group are aimed at the media and the consumer as well as the dietetic profession. The trickle-down effect of the misinformation emanating from this group is substantial.

The misinformation is at times so subtle that it takes years to realize the extent of this influence. Specific examples of the bias can be appreciated when we compare the IFIC writings on fat in general, which defends the partially hydrogenated fats, and criticizes the so-called saturated fats such as dairy fat, meat fats, and tropical fats (oils) in particular. According to IFIC, natural fats are no good, but manmade fats are just fine.

The American Dietetic Association (ADA) has been a major supporter of the processed food industry propaganda regarding food fats. This support has been needed by the industry in order to push the fabricated fats. The ADA is the largest dietetics and nutrition organization in the United States. The current ADA recommendations regarding dietary fat intake is to select "...lower-fat versions of ...dairy products, such as skim milk and skim milk-based cheeses....to [skim fat off the surface of soups and stews]...to choose low-fat or non-fat versions of...sour cream...to use polyunsaturated or monounsaturated oil [instead of] melted shortening or butter...[and]...to use vegetable oil margarine in place of butter or lard." In the December 1998 fact sheets published on the official ADA internet website, where fats and the hydrogenation of oils is discussed, there is no mention of the *trans* fatty acids formed by this process. Advertisements in this organization's journal are predominantly for processed foods.

Dietary Fat Intake Recommendations in the 1930s

The essential fatty acids were recognized in the 1930s. Nutrition and dietetics texts wrote that among the eight listed functions of fat "..aside from their energy-producing function...[and]...padding around the vital organs, holding them in place and absorbing the shocks to which they might otherwise be subjected..." were those that are important for use to "...conserve body heat...[as]...sparers of body protein...[as] ...carriers of vitamins A, D, and E...[and as well that]...certain fats, act as body-regulators and protective agents..." (Note the similarity to a modern listing given in **Chapter 2**.)

The fat requirements during this period were based on the knowledge that "since every cell in the body must contain some fat, the daily intake of fat must be adjusted to the individual. The amount of fat needed by the average adult is from 1 to 2 grams per kilogram of body weight per day (depending upon the amount of exercise taken), or the amount of fat to furnish approximately from 30 to 40 percent of the total calories required per day" (Proudfit 1942).

The Current U.S. Government-Sponsored Dietary Fat Intake Recommendations

The latest (1989) recommendations (from the National Academy of Science-National Research Council), when applied to the current 30 percent of calories as fat recommendation, translate to an average (of the total) fat intake that is 33 percent saturated fatty acids, 40-43 percent monounsaturated fatty acids, and 23-27 percent polyunsaturated fatty acids. This goal can be readily accomplished with a typical mixture of animal, dairy and all types of vegetable oils **as long as the vegetable oils are either unhydrogenated or minimally hydrogenated. There would be absolutely no reason to exclude any of the natural fats or oils.**

However, if the typically hydrogenated commercial fats and oils, such as are used in restaurants, (and which have 42 percent *trans* fatty acids and 20 percent saturated fatty acids) are used for a **major** portion of an individuals' fat intake, the amount in the saturated fatty acid categories as defined by the FDA in the proposed (November 1999) *trans* labeling regulation, would be well above the latest recommendation. See comments in Chapter 5.

USDA Pyramid

The Food Guide Pyramid is a tool used to teach people to eat a balanced diet from a variety of food portions without counting calories or any other nutrient. The USDA expanded the four food groups used earlier used as a guide to six groups and then expanded the number of servings in each group to meet the calorie and protein needs of most persons. These recommendations have their origins in the dietary guidelines that came out of the McGovern Committee hearings in the 1970s.

The pyramid's daily recommendations, starting at the bottom of the pyramid, are to consume 6 to 11 servings of bread, cereal, rice, and pasta, 3 to 5 servings of vegetables, 2 to 4 servings of fruits, 2 to 3 servings of milk, yogurt and cheese, 2 to 3 servings of meat, poultry, fish, dry beans, eggs and nuts, and to use fats, oils and sweets sparingly.

Know Your Fats suggests that individuals who are carbohydrate sensitive need to exert caution regarding the use of the pyramid as a guide for selecting from mostly refined food products. This is especially true if they are consuming their bread and cereal servings as refined products. The entire set of recommendations is best used with food products *only* in their original, natural state with all the original fats intact. This means that cereals should come with their normal fats. Meat should come from animals fed foods historically appropriate for them, which results in normal levels and types of saturated and monounsaturated fats. Fish should come from a native habitat and thus have its normal fat composition, which would include omega-3 fats if the fish comes from the ocean. Milk should be whole and should come from grass-fed cows or other appropriately fed milk-producing animals. Eggs should come from free-range fowl for the most natural fat composition. Any oils added to the human diet should be unrefined, protectively stored, and selected for flavor or function.

Current Canadian Dietary Fat Recommendations

Canadian dietary fat recommendations are similar to the recommendations in the United States and are found in the document "Canada's Food Guide to Healthy Eating," which is based on "the 4 food groups and other foods" as outlined in the guidelines from the Canadian federal agency Health Canada.

These guidelines are listed as: 1. Enjoy a VARIETY of foods. 2. Emphasize cereals, breads, other grain products, vegetables and fruit. 3. Choose lower-fat dairy products, leaner meats and food prepared with little or no fat. 4. Achieve and maintain a healthy body weight by enjoying regular physical activity and healthy eating. 5. Limit salt, alcohol and caffeine.

There is similar emphasis on lower fat versions of foods, as there is in the United States. Nonetheless, restaurant foods have similar high fat cooking methods, and many of the foods are made with the same partially hydrogenated vegetable fats and oils that are used in the United States. As noted above, labeling issues have included *trans* fatty acids as part of the core components for several years.

Future Dietary Fat Recommendations

It would be nice to have a crystal ball to look into the future as this book goes to press at the end of 1999. There is a public meeting scheduled for May 30-31, 2000 for the "National Nutrition Summit." This is the successor to the 1969 "White House Conference on Foods and

Nutrition,"which had continued to meet in the early 1970s, and which produced the *imitation foods*-promoting "New Foods Document." This conference also brought about the Senate Hearings and the "Dietary Goals" that emanated from the McGovern Committee.

A preliminary conference held by the organizers of the National Nutrition Summit meeting was held on 9 December 1999 at the USDA

Prepared Statement of oral input for the Summit at the public meeting on December 9, 1999 by Mary G. Enig, Ph.D., F.A.C.N, L.N., C.N.S., Consulting Nutritionist, Enig Associates, Inc.; President of the Maryland Nutritionists Association, Silver Spring, MD 20904

I want to address the topic of food fats and oils and their impact on health, because fat represents an important nutrient that was negatively impacted by the forerunner to the planned National Nutrition Summit, namely, the 1969 White House Conference on Foods and Nutrition and the resulting McGovern Committee hearings in the 1970s, which produced the Dietary Goals. These Dietary Goals and later Guidelines have been largely responsible for promoting an unbalanced intake of the fat components of our diets.

Natural fats such as butter, tallow, lard, and palm and coconut oils have been relegated to the garbage heap, and the manmade fats such as the widely-used partially hydrogenated shortenings and margarines, and excessive polyunsaturated oils have been promoted as if they were magic medicine. That is just the opposite of what we should be doing because those natural fats and oils have components found only in them, which are health-promoting, and their replacements are now known to be disease-causing.

The 1969 White House Conference produced the New Foods Document, which promoted the acceptance of imitation foods as if they were real foods. This has led to a major decline in the quality of our foods, and especially in the quality of food fats. It has led to the open promotion of genetically-modified foods that suits the production of processed fats, and has also led to a decline in quality and uses of our farm produced fats.

Now, 30 years later, there may be an opportunity to correct some of the mistakes. It is necessary, however, for those who will be in charge of the forthcoming Summit to make an effort to become properly educated as to the changes in the diet that occurred during the intervening 30 years, which have resulted in the situation we have today. We are confronted with the problems of widespread obesity, runaway diabetes in adults, ever increasing cancer incidence rates, immune dysfunction, a continuing increase in heart disease rates, and growth and development problems in our young.

(Continuation)

In 1970, the FDA prepared an internal memo that said the *trans* fatty acids in the food supply should be identified. Thirty years later the FDA has proposed the cloudy labeling of the *trans* fats under an unsuitable saturated fats umbrella. In the intervening 30 years, in my former position as a fats, oils, and lipids researcher in a university lipids laboratory, I have frequently pointed out to various agencies, through reports to the appropriate dockets, that ignoring the levels of *trans* fatty acids in foods has prevented us from having accurate data on fat composition of our diets. As a result of being misled, we have a consuming public terrified of natural fats and oils -- a public, which, by its avoidance of these natural fats and oils, and consumption of fabricated, man-manipulated fats and oils replacements such as the *trans* fats and the unstable polyunsaturates, is becoming increasingly obese and ill.

This attempt by the FDA to tar the wholesome saturated fats with the sins of the *trans* fats so as to promote in the minds of consumers the idea that they are both the same, is not supported by real science. Biologically, the saturates and the *trans* have totally opposite effects; the effects of the saturates are good and those of the *trans* are undesirable. Actually, the FDA is just responding favorably to a petition by the Center for Science in the Public Interest (CSPI), which is a transparent and ingenious effort by CSPI and its mostly vegetarian nutritionist staff to beat on the dairy and meat industries by having consumers incorrectly connect animal products with *trans* fat.

Many of you at this meeting may not have been born by 1969. Those of us who were adults at that time know the extent to which the "new foods" really are imitation foods even though they are not labeled as such.

headquarters in Washington DC. Interested individuals were given an opportunity to present a three-minute comment to this group. The statement made by this author, which gave a brief overview of the effects during the intervening 30 years is included in this chapter.

What will be the outcome for dietary fat recommendations? Will they be as wrong as those recommended in the past 30 years? Who knows. It will likely depend on how much those in charge understand about food fats and oils and the correct biological effects of natural fats and oils versus the commercial creations that have been guiding the bureaucrats. Maybe some of them will have read this book by that time. In which case, there may be some hope for promotion of better fats in our future and our children's and grandchildren's future.

Different people harbor different beliefs, and as long as there is no scientific proof for or against their beliefs, there is not much one can do to challenge these beliefs. When there is absolute scientific proof against a belief, however, it seems foolish to maintain the belief. This is somewhat of the situation with regard to beliefs about the fats and oils.

In the meantime, those individuals who have the ability to make those changes to their diets that favor the inclusion of adequate amounts of the natural fats could have some influence with their pocketbooks. If you do not purchase the kinds of imitation foods that are made with the less appropriate fats and oils, the industries will eventually get the message.

Chapter 7

Small Summaries of Dietary Fat Facts

Summarizing Some Important Facts About Fat

What is fat really? Fat is a collection of high-energy molecules (each molecule formed from three fatty acids and glycerol). Fat is found in food and in our bodies. In food, fat can be solid fat or liquid fat (oil); but solid or liquid it is still fat. In our bodies, fat is also in a solid or liquid form but which one is not so apparent because the fat is mostly locked into our cells and other structures. Whether any fat is solid or liquid depends on the proportion of the individual kinds of fatty acids and their melting points.

The most common fatty acids come in varying lengths (3 to 24 carbons long) and range from saturated (no double bonds through monounsaturated (one double bond) to polyunsaturated (two or more double bonds). Plants make fatty acids and our bodies make fatty acids. The plants make the whole range of fatty acids, e.g., saturated, monounsaturated, and polyunsaturated; the latter are called omega-6 or omega-3.

While our bodies can only make saturated or monounsaturated fatty acids from scratch, our cells can alter the plant polyunsaturates (and monounsaturates) that we eat (making them longer and/or giving them more double bonds). Basically, our bodies make plenty of stable saturates and then make the "good" monounsaturates out of these saturates; but we can also make not-so-good polyunsaturates or monounsaturates out of the *trans* fatty acids that we consume.

Properly formed, properly nourished bodies are quite adept at dealing with small insults from our environments. Larger insults require some extra work on the part of our mechanisms that maintain homeostasis. This is where active lipids such as eicosanoids (prostaglandins, thromboxanes, leukotrienes) or monoglycerides play a role.

Microorganisms make fatty acids with odd-number carbon lengths, and some put *trans* double bonds into existing fatty acids with a process called biohydrogenation. The edible fats and oils industry also puts *trans* double bonds into fatty acids with a process called partial hydrogenation.

The partial hydrogenation process is used to turn liquid vegetable fats (oils) into solid (unsaturated) fats to compete with the natural solid fats, since solid fats have better functional characteristics for cooking and baking and also are more stable for long-term storage. These oils made solid by man, however, have up to 60 percent *trans* fatty acids. These *trans* fatty acids are mostly the unnatural kind that accumulate in our bodies and cause disease.

Some representatives of the food industry would have us believe that there really are not very many *trans* fatty acids in most of the foods. This is not true, and if we look at some of the research, we can see how untrue it is.

Some of the writers who are not trained in the science of fats and oils have tried to turn the essential fatty acid connection to sulfur-containing proteins into something magical to support the sale of highly unsaturated fatty acid oils. The enzymes involved in elongation and desaturation of the essential fatty acids have coenzymes that are sulfur-containing, so there is nothing unusual about such a connection.

Some Important Cholesterol Facts

Cholesterol is sometimes called a fat, but in reality it is a special kind of alcohol. Cholesterol is perhaps the most misunderstood and wrongly maligned biological molecule in existence.

Our brains (when they are well-formed) are largely cholesterol (and saturated fat). Infants who don't get enough cholesterol in their diets during the first years when their brains are developing risk a loss of cognitive function. As noted in Chapter 2, cholesterol has been reported to be necessary for the part of the brain in the fetus that allows the eyes to develop. Research has recently identified the cyclopian eye as the result of inadequate cholesterol in certain tissues. (Strauss 1998)

Our hormones are made of cholesterol, our cell membranes are protected from free-radical attack by cholesterol, and our body heals itself using cholesterol. If we don't make quite enough, and we don't eat very much, we risk running short. Fear of cholesterol is truly unwise.

What about dietary cholesterol? Feeding dietary cholesterol raises serum cholesterol in healthy normal people whose cholesterol levels are low, and lowers serum cholesterol in hypercholesterolemics whose cholesterol levels are high. In the former group, where not enough cholesterol is being manufactured by the body, adding dietary cholesterol raises the amounts to more adequate (normal) levels. In some individuals whose serum cholesterol levels are high, there is some overproduction that is turned off when the dietary cholesterol is consumed; this results in the same levels of serum cholesterol or sometimes a reduction of serum cholesterol.

If we put serum cholesterol and dietary cholesterol into the same equation (and consequently into perspective), we find that since the blood volume is 5 to 7 liters, or 50 to 70 dL (remember a dL is 100 milliliters), we can calculate that 200 mg per dL of circulating cholesterol is the equivalent of 10,000 to 14,000 mg of circulating cholesterol in the blood. If we eat 400 mg of cholesterol per day, and we absorb 50 percent of that cholesterol, we are tossing 200 mg into a pool of 10,000 to 14,000 mg and we can calculate that the serum cholesterol could increase from 200 mg per dL to 203-204 mg per dL. That is an amount so small it probably can't be measured accurately.

Since the total body cholesterol pool for a 70 kg man is equal to 145,000 mg, and the metabolically active pool is equal to 100,000 mg, the concerns and worries about a few milligrams here and there seem overblown.

There are many reasons why serum cholesterol levels are higher in some people than in others. Some reasons are related to genetics, and some are related to things like increased cholesterol production in response to increased stress. (See Chapters 1 and 2 for more details)

What About Fat and Heart Disease?

The claim that saturated fat leads to heart disease is simply false. This claim was initiated as a marketing tool to sell oils and margarine (in competition to butter, lard and tallow). Eventually the idea became dogma as it was repeated year after year. The major fatty acids in the cholesterol esters in the atheroma blockages are **unsaturated** (74 percent of total fatty acids). Proportionally, there are, by far, many more polyunsaturates (41 percent) than saturates (26 percent) in these lesions. (Felton et al 1994)

What About Fat and Weight Gain and/or Loss?

Obesity is a major problem in the United States. The gain of excess adipose is being studied all the time without any success in understanding why it is becoming so prevalent. Foreign populations that do not have an obesity problem are usually found to consume only natural fats.

Switching from a diet of imitation foods, such as those found in the typical low fat and high carbohydrate diets or those imitation foods high in partially hydrogenated vegetable fats, to a diet of real foods with normal levels of natural fats in the foods will result in a gradual and sustained weight loss in most overweight people. Sometimes it is as simple as using home processed foods instead of factory processed foods. (See also Chapter 2)

What Constitutes a Low Fat, Medium Fat, or High Fat Diet?

Stubbs et al (1995a) from the well-known Rowett Research Institute in Aberdeen, Scotland studied food intake regulation using diets reported as "low fat" (20 percent of calories as fat), "medium fat" (40 percent of calories as fat), and "high fat" (60 percent of calories as fat). The fat in the food was hidden by the use of casserole-type dishes.

There was no difference in the amount of the total food taken in by the different groups over the study period, but the higher fat dishes provided higher energy intake. This is not surprising since the purpose of higher fat diets has always been to increase the caloric intake. What is interesting is that these researchers recognized 40 percent of energy as medium [moderate] fat and 60 percent of the energy as high fat.

In a second study covering 14 days (Stubbs et all 1995b), there was a small weight loss on the low fat diet (1.6 pounds over 2 weeks), a slight weight loss on the medium fat diet (1.1 pounds over 2 weeks), and a 3 ounce gain over the same time period on the high fat diet. If this type of effect could be extrapolated to long term, the low fat diet of the sort utilized might result in about a 41 pound weight loss in a year's time; the high fat diet would produce a 5 pound weight gain, while the medium fat diet would produce a 29 pound weight loss.

What Happens When You Include Coconut Oil in a Phase I National Cholesterol Education Program Diet?

Adding coconut oil to this kind of dietary regimen **improved** the measures of those serum lipids considered important for risk of coronary artery disease.(Howard et al 1995) This is not surprising, since research several decades ago (Hashim et al 1959, Hegsted et al 1965) showed exactly the same thing, and research from Ginsberg et al in 1990 showed that the average American diet with added coconut oil gave better measures of serum lipids than did the AHA diet. What is interesting is that the authors of both of the recent studies made no comment on this part of the results.

What About Dietary Fat and Children?

What about the diets of children? What would you think of a total diet that supplied 53.5 percent of the calories as fat, of which 25.8 percent of the calories are saturated fatty acids, 21.3 percent of calories are monounsaturated fatty acids, and 6.4 percent of calories are polyunsaturated fatty acids? Well, this is the typical diet of the infant fed human milk from a well-fed mother. If you think about it, it makes sense to expect that a two-year old or a three-year old should be consuming a diet that is not much different. And when children between the ages of 7 months and 22 months were put on fat-restricted diets, they suffered severe growth failure, which included linear, weight, and weight-for-height failure. When they are put on fat and cholesterol-restricted diets, even older children with genetic hypercholesterolemia (very high serum cholesterol) develop growth failure with nutritional dwarfing, including failure during adolescence to develop appropriate sexual maturity.

As a result of recognizing the uniqueness of the nutritional needs of children of all ages (up to the cessation of growth), the Canadian government and the Canadian pediatric society established guidelines, which, among other things, recommended that fat should not be restricted until full growth has been achieved.

(See example of proper fat levels for growing children in Figure 3.6 in Chapter 3.)

Why Is There So Much Lactation Failure Today?

Could it be that the fabricated foods have something to do with the problem? We know that the partially hydrogenated vegetable fats with their *trans* fatty acids can decrease the level of fat in milk. This has the effect of lowering the quality of human milk since 53 percent of the calories in milk should be from fat. And, if infants do not receive enough fat during a feeding and are not satisfied they will cry for more food. A typical parental response is to then feed formula, which in turn decreases milk production by the mother.

Are We Eating Too Much Fat?

No one needs or wants to consume *excess* fat, but everyone needs some fat, and many humans, especially growing children, need *substantial* amounts of natural fats in their diets. There is also some evidence that older adults need to have additional fat and cholesterol in their diets. Without the additional cholesterol, the brain doesn't function as well.

Most experts agree that the amount of omega-6 EFAs required is about 2-3 percent of the daily calories, and the amount of the omega-3 EFAs required is about 0.5 to 1.5 percent of the daily calories. It also means, that since the amount of total fat generally accepted for humans to eat is 30 percent of the kilocalories, the amount that should then come from non-EFAs is about 25.5 percent of daily energy., i.e., the saturated fatty acids and the monounsaturated fatty acids.

Miscellaneous Fat Facts

Sometimes when writers don't know the answer to a question about fat they just simply make up an answer. Within the framework of their knowledge about other things, they can be very close in their answers or very far from being correct.

As noted in Chapter 4, there are also too many errors-of-fact in articles from technical magazines and journals about fats and oils. The example that was given above from the November 1995 *Food Product Design* cover story "Translating the Mixed Signals on Trans Fat," concerned what the author of the article, an associate editor, wrote (inaccurately) about the supposed composition of stearic acid.

This same editor also wrote about the classic Dutch clinical study (Mensink and Katan 1990) that "[a] problem with the Dutch study was that subjects were given 33 grams of *trans* fats daily, which is three to six times more than most Americans consume." Single diets that contain up to 57 grams of *trans* fatty acids daily have been documented (Enig 1996), however, and a typical range in the U.S. up to 38.7 grams of *trans* fatty acids per day was reported (Enig et al 1990). As noted in Chapter 3, one teenager consumed more than 30 grams of *trans* fat a day, and an American consuming a McDonalds meal of chicken nuggets, french fried potatoes and a pastry consumed 19 grams of *trans* in just one meal. A nursing mother, whose diet was analyzed by a researcher at the University of Maryland (Dr. B. Teter), consumed 22 grams of *trans* just in snacks. So you can readily see how easy it really is for some people to consume 33 grams of *trans* fats daily when you eat the typical American diet of processed foods.

What Are You to Believe?

Discarding deeply ingrained *mis*information and replacing it with factual information is difficult for anyone. For the consumer who today has been the recipient of nearly 3 decades of fats and oils propaganda that is both false and misleading, the task is doubly difficult since the typical consumer lacks enough basic science training with which to judge the truth. Perhaps this book will help to correct some of the fats and oils misinformation. Read the sections that pertain to some of your questions, look up some of the references. Think about the reasons for some of the misinformation. How much is driven by food industry.

Unfortunately, a current driving philosophy among the food and nutrition scientists is that the food industry can improve on the natural foods. These industry types actually believe that nature did not make adequately healthy foods but that man can improve them. This philosophy has provided the commercial world with multibillion dollar markets. In the current commercial fats and oils area, fats that are artificial or tinkered with by man have been found wanting. The refining causes losses of important components or distortions of the functioning parts of the fats and oils.

The common scenario is that of a highly intelligent person, with one or more advanced degrees, who finds a research task that will lead to funding either from the food and/or pharmaceutical industry or from the industry-controlled government agencies. If that research shows an adverse effect of any of the new foods being studied, this is frequently ignored. Also, if someone else's research shows a problem with a particular food component, the typical response is not to read the information, not to know about it. That apparently helps to prevent one's conscience from interfering with the status quo. Of course, the research that is done by many of the industry-supported scientists is good basic research, and it usually is of great interest so as long as it supports the food industry or avoids a clash with the industry it is promoting.

What seems so ironic, is that the very foods (saturated fats and cholesterol) that people are avoiding are the very foods that are helpful and health-giving. When it comes to fat, this really has become the age of the flat earth.

The healthy and smart bottom line -- use a mixture of natural fats in moderation.

A Mini-Glossary of Food Fats and Oils

Typical Natural "Saturated" Animal Fats

Butter. Used for centuries. Butter is a stable fat made from cream with a wide range of short-, medium-, and odd-chain fatty acids as well as typical saturated, monounsaturated and some polyunsaturated fatty acids. About 15 percent short/medium saturated, 50 percent other saturated, and 30 percent monounsaturated fatty acids. Butter is also recognized as a source of several different kinds of antimicrobial fats. Butter has short chain fatty acids that inhibit growth of pathogenic fungi, medium chain fatty acids such as lauric acid that disable many pathogenic viruses and other organisms, glycolipids that have anti-infective properties, and conjugated linoleic acid (CLA) that has anticarcinogenic properties. All of these are only in the fat part of the milk. Butter is definitely a fat with health-potentiating properties.

Tallow. Used for centuries. Tallow is a stable fat that does not normally become rancid -- no free radicals are formed from normal usage. It is usually rendered from beef or mutton (lamb) fat and is about 50-55 percent saturated, 40 percent monounsaturated, and 3 6 percent polyunsaturated fatty acids. Foods fried in tallow have a lot of taste but usually smaller amounts of fat than foods fried in liquid plant oils. Tallows have several percent of an antimicrobial fatty acid palmitoleic acid.

Typical Natural "Saturated" Vegetable Fats

Coconut oil. Used for centuries. Coconut oil is a stable fat with good baking and cooking properties. It contains mostly medium chain (65 percent) saturated fatty acids, with 28 percent other saturated and about 8 percent mono- and polyunsaturated fatty acids. Coconut oil is a major source of the antimicrobial fatty acids lauric acid and capric acid. Nearly half of its fatty acids are lauric acid, which is why it is considered a lauric fat. Antimicrobial fatty acids are those that the body uses to kill or disable pathogenic viruses, bacteria and protozoa. Lauric acid gives human milk its major antimicrobial properties, and it may be a conditionally essential fatty acid since it cannot be made by mammals other than the lactating female and must be obtained from the diet.

Coconut oil has been prescribed for centuries as a medicinal food by Ayurvedic physicians in India. Both coconut and palm oil are sold in African, Caribbean or Asian food stores. Unfortunately, these oils have been chased out of the U.S. food supply. It would be beneficial to consumers if more crackers and cookies were made with coconut oil so that people would have these foods available as sources of lauric acid. As it is now, only macaroons made with desiccated coconut provide reliable sources of the coconut oil fatty acids.

Palm oil. Used for centuries in Africa and Asia. Palm oil is a source of beta-carotene and antioxidants in its unprocessed state; how much of these antioxidants are still retained depends on the degree of processing. It is a stable fat that has 50 percent saturated, 40 percent monounsaturated, and 10 percent polyunsaturated fatty acids. Palm oil has functional properties for baking and frying similar to the animal tallows and lard.

Palm kernel oil. The inner seed of the palm fruit is the source of palm kernel oil, which is a lauric fat like coconut oil with a nearly identical fatty acid composition. Most of the palm kernel oil in the U.S. is utilized by the confectionary industry in candies or as a coating fat.

Mostly Omega-9 "Monounsaturated" Animal Fats

Chicken, duck, goose, and turkey fat. Poultry fats have been used commercially in the U.S. up until the early part of this century. They are still used in parts of Europe and Asia. Polyunsaturates are higher in turkey fat (23 percent) and chicken fat (21 percent) than either duck fat (13 percent), or goose fat (11 percent). Monounsaturated fatty acids range from about 42 percent (chicken fat) to 57 percent (goose fat). A substantial portion of the monounsaturates in some poultry fat is palmitoleic acid (e.g. 6-8 percent in chicken fat).

Lard. Widely used in the home for centuries. Rendered from pig fat, lard is more or less the equivalent of tallow, except that is has more unsaturates and can become rancid if not handled properly. This fat should be considered as a monounsaturated fat, although it is commonly misidentified as a saturated fat. It usually has about 40 percent saturated, 50 percent monounsaturated, and 10 percent polyunsaturated fatty acids. Lard has between 2 and 3 percent palmitoleic acid, which as noted above possesses antimicrobial properties. Most lard is home rendered or sold in certain ethnic stores (e.g., stores catering to people with Hispanic ancestry).

Mostly Omega-9 "Monounsaturated" Vegetable Fats

Olive oil. One of the oldest, if not the oldest food oil. Olive oil is used selectively because of the flavor it imparts to the foods containing it. It is a very stable liquid oil that contains antioxidants that prevent it from becoming rancid under long-term storage. Over 70 percent of the fatty acids are monounsaturated, 16 percent are saturated.

Hybrid safflower and sunflower oils These oils are high-oleic forms of the original oil developed by selective mutation breeding practices, and are mostly used commercially by the baking, snack chip, and food service industry. They are stable but usually have been solvent extracted unless they are from a natural food oil producer where natural expeller pressed versions are available.

Mostly Omega-9 "Monounsaturated" With Some Omega-6 and Omega-3 Vegetable Fats

Canola oil. The newest major fat in the food supply. This oil was produced by genetically modifying the parent rapeseed so that the monounsaturated fatty acid would be oleic acid instead of another monounsaturated fatty acid called erucic acid. Erucic acid-containing rapeseed oil is considered undesirable as a food by the U.S. and Canadian governments. Nonsolvent extracted (frequently called expeller pressed) canola oil is available, but like any highly unsaturated fat it needs to be carefully handled as it becomes rancid very readily. Native canola oil is about 6 percent saturated, 65 percent monounsaturated, and 30 percent polyunsaturated; 10-15 percent of the polyunsaturates are omega-3 fatty acids. When canola oil is partially hydrogenated, the very high levels (50-60 percent) of *trans* fatty acids make it an undesirable food fat. When canola oil is refined (e.g., deodorized) it loses most of its omega-3 fatty acids.

Mostly Omega-3 "Polyunsaturated" Vegetable Fats

Flaxseed oil. A highly polyunsaturated oil that has seen recent popularity. It has been used for centuries in many parts of the world and recently in Canada and the U.S. As much as 60 percent of its fatty acids are the omega-3 polyunsaturates. Best obtained as cold-pressed and used for salad and non-cooking applications. It requires careful handling and storage.

Mostly Omega-6 With Some Omega-3 Vegetable Fats

Soybean oil. The most commercially abundant food fat in the U.S. (nearly 80 percent of all the seed oils). More than three-fourths of this oil is partially hydrogenated (up to 50 percent *trans*), and only a small amount is nonsolvent extracted. Soybean oil that is refined, even though not hydrogenated, may have some *trans* fatty acids due to the deodorizing process. The cold-pressed soybean oil provides a mixture of both omega-6 and omega-3 fatty acids, but does not make a good cooking oil for most applications; it requires appropriately careful storage and handling. Cold-pressed soybean oil usually has its inherent antioxidants (several forms of vitamin E) intact. Soybean oil is a common ingredient in mayonnaise in the U.S.

Regular Omega-6 Vegetable Fats

Corn oil, cottonseed oil, regular safflower oil, regular sunflower oil. These oils are all sold in supermarkets and used commercially in food manufacturing, food service and restaurants. They are usually solvent-extracted, although cold-pressed varieties can be purchased in natural foods stores. The refined corn, cottonseed, and sunflower oils are used for frying purposes without being partially hydrogenated; they do not have omega-3 fatty acids and consequently do not present the same stability problems that are seen with unhydrogenated canola and soybean oils.

Nearly Equal Omega-9 and Omega-6 Vegetable Fats

Peanut oil, rice bran oil, and sesame oil. These oils are sold in some supermarkets as well as in most health food and specialty shops. Peanut oil and sesame oil have been used for centuries in various parts of the world. They are usually more expensive than most oils. Sesame oil has special stability to heat, as does the newer rice bran oil.

How Should Fats and Oils Be Used?

❧   Natural fats and oils that should not be used for frying or be heated include flaxseed oil, unprocessed, cold-pressed canola oil, and unprocessed, cold-pressed soybean oil.

❧   Natural fats and oils that should only be used for cold preparation are flaxseed oil and any other highly polyunsaturated oil that comes to the market.

❧   Natural fats and oils that are quite appropriate both for cooking and for salad dressing include corn oil, peanut oil, and olive oil.

❧   Natural fats and oils that are safe for most deep fat frying applications include coconut oil, palm oil, lard, tallow, high oleic safflower oil, high oleic sunflower seed oil, and regular sunflower seed oil with added sesame oil and rice bran oil.

❧   Natural fats and oils that are safe for one-time frying include corn oil, olive oil, and peanut oil.

Some Personal Preferences

An all purpose frying oil. A unique blend of oils that can be used for sauteing and light frying is one that is a blend of coconut oil (one-third), sesame oil (one-third), and olive oil (one-third). It is easy to make up in small portions ranging from a single tablespoon measure (one teaspoon of each oil) to a pint and a half size (one cup of each oil).

    This mixture of oils will remain liquid at normal room

temperatures in the U. S. after proper mixing. The coconut oil needs to be warmed to about 80 to 90 degrees F to melt before mixing.

Other oils such as high-oleic safflower or sunflower oils could be substituted for the olive oil. Both the coconut oil and the sesame oil, however, have particular properties that make them non-replaceable in this blend. The coconut oil gives us lauric acid and capric acid and heat stability; the sesame oil provides heat stability from the sesamin.

Oil for snack foods. The best oil to use for making popcorn is straight 100 percent coconut oil. The best kinds of coconut oil to use are the natural cold-pressed coconut oils and the hand extracted virgin coconut oils. Some of these coconut oils are currently sold in the United States and Canada by natural products companies including Omega Nutrition and Carotec.

Fats and oils for baked goods. Since most baked goods require a solid fat for the best product, the most appropriate fats to use are butter, coconut oil, lard, palm oil, and tallow. For those individuals who wish to use only vegetable fats and dairy fats, the lard and tallow would not be appropriate although they are perfectly healthy fats. Freshly extracted and unprocessed poultry fats can be used for some savory pastries as long as a softer fat is acceptable for the product and as long as you know that such a fat requires careful handling to prevent the development of rancidity.

Chapter 8

Frequently Asked Questions and Their Answers

Over the period of many years, this author has received many requests for information on fats and oils from all over the world. In recent years the requests have come mostly by email. Many of these email requests were answered, if there was time and if they seemed important, and gradually they accumulated as many hundreds of "sent" email files.

During the period from mid 1996 through the end of 1999, these requests seemed to come in ever-increasing numbers, especially as the topic of fat became more widely covered by the media, as there was more access to the internet, and as people became aware of my web page on the *trans* fatty acids. Most of the requests fell into several general categories and the most representative of these queries have been collected for this chapter: they are arranged by topic.

The subject line, where there was one, and the correspondents' initials are included; the only editing was to correct some obvious misspellings and to delete full names of individuals, and in the case of students, the names of their schools, etc. Otherwise, the material is just as it came and just as it was answered. When editorial or other comments have been added during the writing of this chapter, because it was felt they were needed, they are enclosed in brackets [ ].

Questions from Consumers Regarding Foods and *Trans* Fatty Acids

Question: Subject: Trans fats in soy oil. Hi. I'm interested in the trans fats in Soy oil. Especially [national brand] Mayonnaise..... Thanks, L.E.
Answer: Not surprised the 800 number was no help. The refined soy oil in mayonnaise has between 0 and 5 % trans depending on the particular batch of oil; and on average about 1.6 % according to 1997 report using USDA data.

Question: (email) Are there any butter substitutes in the US that do not have trans fatty acids?
Answer: There are none [in 1999] on the US market that I am aware of

that I would consider purchasing. A spread that is truly free of partially hydrogenated oils and does not have a myriad of additives could be made, but I do not know of any yet.

Question: ..... Perhaps you can clear up some confusion on my part. Is there any data or research suggesting that the consumption of margarine is any safer than butter?
Answer: There is nothing unsafe about butter; quite the opposite, butter contains healthful components that are not found in anything else (other than real cream). Any reported pro-margarine data or research was done by the very industry that benefits from its sale. Not all margarine is partially hydrogenated in many countries, so that kind of margarine would not present the problem that the fats and oils with trans fatty acids do. The major problem is that butter is a competition to the soybean, canola, or corn oil margarines.

There are numerous studies published within the last ten years that spell out the problems caused by margarine made with partially hydrogenated oil. Names to look for in recent years who are not flacking for the edible oil industry include E. Siguel (USA), B. Koletzko (Germany), W. Willett (USA) and his group at Harvard, Geo. Mann (USA), F. Kummerow (USA), Mensink and Zock, and Katan (Holland), K.Wahle (UK), B. Teter (USA).

Question: In one gram of partially hydrogenated oil...how many mg of transfat? Thanks. Mike
Answer: It depends on what kind of partially hydrogenated oil you are asking about. The levels of trans range from approximately 10% to over 50% of the fatty acids. If the latter, there would be half a gram of trans. However, many popular brands of bakery goods have about 35% trans in their shortenings; in this case there would be about 0.35 grams in a gram.

Question: Thanks for your response. The oil I am interested in is partially hydrogenated soy bean and cottonseed oil. Looking forward to your response. Mike
Answer: Of those products I have personally analyzed, which were labeled as containing only partially hydrogenated soybean and cottonseed oil, the range of trans was from 10.8 to 38.6% for 10 samples. Half were above 20% trans and half were below; three were above 33% trans and four were clustered around 15% trans. Each oil has to be

analyzed as there is no blanket amount for such a combination.

Question: Subject: Nitrite treatment. What effect does treatment of fat meats with nitrite have on trans fatty acid production?
Answer: In a word, none.

Question: Subject: danger of trans fatty acids in a low fat diet. I eat a low fat diet and lately I have noticed that the majority of the foods I consume contain partially hydrogenated oils (breakfast cereal, snack cakes, tortillas etc.). Even though trans fatty acids are not the primary ingredient in these foods should I be concerned with eliminating such foods from my diet? I was also wondering if the percentage of trans fatty acids will be included on food labels in the near future. Thank you, B.S.
Answer: If the fats in low fat foods are partially hydrogenated, they are a source of trans fatty acids. If the portion of trans fatty acids in the individual fat is substantial, as it probably is, then there is a likelihood of accumulating them in the tissues. How soon the FDA will be labeling depends on how much industry control is exerted. Since the Center for Science in the Public Interest (CSPI) wants to cloud the issue by including trans fatty acids with the safe saturated fatty acids on the label, and since some of the people in control at the FDA are either friendly with or related to the people at CSPI, it is unlikely that you will get correct useful information on FDA-controlled labels. This means that it is necessary to avoid such processed foods that contain partially hydrogenated oils if one wants to avoid trans fatty acids. [answer written September 1998]

Question: Subject: Partially Hydrogenated Canola oil. I found your information about trans fats from the internet. I was wondering if you could tell me the Advantages/Disadvantages of ingesting partially hydrogenated canola oil in a protein drink. Yours truly S.S.
Answer: There are, in my opinion, no advantages to consuming partially hydrogenated canola oil and the disadvantages stem from the trans fatty acid content.

Question: Subject: Trans fat. Does I Can't Believe It's Not Butter! contain trans fat? I thought I was ok using this product because I have high cholesterol but a friend told me when her brother had heart by-pass surgery the doctor told him it was the worst product he could use. K.B.
Answer: If the package lists partially hydrogenated oil, it contains trans fatty acids.

Questions Regarding Partial Hydrogenation

Question: Subject: hydrogenated fats. Given a choice between an item with hydrogenated fat and one with partially hydrogenated fat in equal amounts which, if either, would be a less unhealthy choice? Or are they both equally bad? P.S.
Answer: The terms mean the same for all practical purposes on food labels. [Except on labels on peanut butter where the word hydrogenated alone does not mean partially hydrogenated.]

Question: Subject: trans fatty acids/hydrogenation. Thank you for making information on trans fatty acids available on the web. I'm a little confused by the fact that so much of the discussion of this topic seems to consider hydrogenation and trans fatty acid formation as the same when in fact they are not the same at all. Does the formation of trans double bonds from cis double bonds only occur during hydrogenation? My understanding of the edible oil process is that high temperatures and pressures and other rigorous conditions are used in many of the refinement steps, even in processing the so called "natural" oils. Isn't this what converts cis bonds to trans? Can we assume that the refined polyunsaturated vegetable oils have no trans double bonds? I have not been able to find the answer to these questions. If you could give me a brief answer to these questions I would appreciate it. Sincerely, M.D.
Answer: I hope by the end of the year to have a small book - a primer - on fats and oils; I will notify when it is available on my web site in the beginning. In that book, I will list a number of references about the various hydrogenation processes. Meanwhile let me quickly run through what is going on and why it is confusing; the food oil industry has tried to cloud the issue over the years in the popular literature, and even in some of the scientific literature.

Domestic oils (soy, canola, etc.) are highly unsaturated, liquid, and unstable for many of the commercial uses. Thus they are treated in several ways that produce trans fatty acids - from small amounts such as 2 to 4 % to more than half of the fatty acids. Refining, which uses steam, pressure, and certain filters (but no hydrogen) will produce a cis/trans isomerization of one or more of the double bonds in cis,cis- or the cis,cis,cis-polyunsaturates without bond migration. Chemically there are usually still the same number of double bonds in the entire batch of oil and the same iodine value. However, the true omega-3 fatty acids are some times more than half gone, and a small dent is made in the omega-6; this leaves the oil with a lowered essential fatty acid (EFA) value. I have analyzed many refined vegetable oils in the past when I was at the university. If they were not partially hydrogenated, oils such as cottonseed oil, palm oil, coconut oil, peanut oil, and sunflower oil didn't have any trans fatty acids even though they were refined and some most likely were solvent extracted; they did not have any linolenic acid (omega-3) in the original oil. I have analyzed some refined corn oil that had trans and some that did not. The partial hydrogenation process, which is the "ultimate" refining process, uses a catalyst, heat, pressure and the presence of hydrogen. The several types of partial hydrogenation range from brush hydrogenation, which produces smaller amounts of trans fatty acids all the way to major partial hydrogenation for hardstock, which produces up to 60 to 70% trans fatty acids depending on the originating oil and various conditions (most common for uses as liquid and solid shortenings are those that produce fats with 25% trans, 36% trans, 42% trans, or 48% trans). In partial hydrogenation, the individual double bonds that were in the original oil are either totally saturated (but in very small amounts) or geometrically altered (most of the change) to the trans form with massive bond migration and a much lower iodine value; there is also some bond migration of some of the remaining cis double bonds. What was an omega- 3 fatty acid with 3 cis double bonds in the 9,12,15 positions usually becomes a fatty acid with one trans double bond in anywhere from the 4 position to the 16 position. What was an omega-6 fatty acid with 2 cis double bonds in the 9,12 positions becomes a trans containing fatty acid also with the double bond having migrated between the 4 and 13 position. There is another kind of trans fatty acid, which is the result of biohydrogenation in the rumen of all ruminant animals; typically, the trans double bond is mostly in the 11 position and it is a precursor to conjugated linoleic acid. There are also some very odd fatty acids in some plant leaves, etc., that are not much of a diet source but they do have some trans. They come with the plant.

Question: Subject: Hydrogenation Inf. I am looking for vivid descriptions of the process of hydrogenation for the purpose of educating others. Are there any videos, films or photo illustrations of this process? I think that if more people could actually see what happens to these food products they may get the idea. Any other sources would be greatly appreciated. (I have been avoiding trans fats since 1972). I was referred to you by the Solgar Nutritional Research Center. Thank You. R.H.
Answer: In 1995 (22 Feb) the well-known British television weekly

program DISPATCHES on Channel 4 aired a documentary entitled A Matter of Fat. This documentary was developed and produced by Lauderdale Productions (Andrew Forrester, Head of Programmes) and some of the Channel 4 personnel (the one name that I have is Maureen Plantagenet).

The resulting 41 minute film is excellent and three years later it is right on target and still very current; the industry powers-that-be have kept it from being aired in the US. Channel 4 (UK) may have copies of the program available for sale. The British company Whole Earth Foods produces of a non-hydrogenated spread (Craig Sams, Chairman) and they may have copies to distribute or know how you can get one; I believe they were instrumental in initiating the program.

Questions Regarding Partial Hydrogenation and Health Issues

Question: Subject: trans fats. What I do not understand from the Harvard report and the info I've gleaned from the internet is exactly how trans fats affects the heart and diseases of the heart? Does it raise the cholesterol level and lower HDL level? Or does it create a different set of problems altogether? A.H. (university)

Answer: The answer is yes to both of your queries. The research that has been done shows that the trans fatty acids: (1) lower HDL cholesterol, (2) raise LDL cholesterol, (3) raise the atherogenic lipoprotein, Lp [a], especially in individuals who already have Lp[a] levels that are too high, (4) interfere with insulin binding and increase insulin levels, (4) alter cholesterol ester transferase activities, (5) alters the mixed function oxidase enzymes that potentiate undesirable chemicals, and (6) displace the type of protective antimicrobial fatty acids in the food supply that would reduce the viruses and bacteria now known to cause lesions in the arteries.

How many of these different effects are responsible, either singly or in combination, in any one individual case is not known because none of that research has been done, or if someone has done it they have not published it.

There are some researchers who would consider the effect on Lp[a] critical. It is interesting that the trans fatty acids raise Lp[a] and the saturated fatty acids lower Lp[a]!

Question: Subject: partially hydrogenated oils. Does partially hydrogenated oils contribute or cause cancer. Any information. It appears in almost everything we eat. Any way to counteract it if it is bad for us? Is it bad for us? M.R., a cancer survivor trying to stay that way

Answer: In my opinion, and in the opinion of numerous other researchers, the partially hydrogenated vegetable fats and oils have nothing beneficial to offer. Research indicates they are involved in cancer potentiation and heart disease potentiation. This is related to the way these man-altered fats interfere with some of our protective enzymes. Human beings should not be eating fabricated foods or environmentally contaminated foods; an almost impossible feat but worth an attempt. Suggest you might want to get the cookbook Nourishing Traditions by Sally Fallon.... This is more than an ordinary cookbook; it explains proper ways of preparing foods and also has suggestions for avoiding the less desirable fats, etc. [As *Know Your Fats* went to press, the second edition of this cookbook was available at NewTrends Publishing, 1-877-707-1776 and should be in most books stores shortly.]

Question: Subject: tfa. Do cells take up TFA's if you have an adequate supply of EFA's in the diet? C.F.

Answer: In humans, pigs, and mice, TFAs are taken up into cells even with adequate EFAs in the foods; and in fact, only high saturates (SFAs) prevent some of the uptake. In rats, the higher level of EFAs may inhibit some of the uptake of TFAs into cells, although this has been reported primarily by one of the large food company laboratories. TFAs replace SFAs in cell membranes.

Question: Dear Dr. Enig, I have been looking at various HIV resource on the Internet recently. Can you explain to me why HIV+ individuals ought stay away from trans fatty acids in their diet? What is a better source of fat?

Answer: Research has shown that the trans fatty acids interfere with some of the enzyme systems that are important for a well-functioning immune system. In individuals with compromised immune systems, this is not good. One of the fatty acids known to promote a healthy function of the immune system is lauric acid and that fatty acid is no longer found in our foods as it was in past years because its major source is coconut oil, which has been replaced in our diets by the kinds of fats and oils that are partially hydrogenated and thus a major source of the trans fatty acids. In addition to coconut oil being a good fat, the natural fats and oils that were in our foods a hundred years ago are good fats.

Questions Regarding Fatty Acid Composition of Foods

Question: Subject: Tree nuts   Dear Dr. Enig, Can you advise, do tree nuts contain naturally occurring trans fatty acids, particularly walnuts? If so, which fatty acids are impacted and what portion of the fatty acid is converted to trans fatty acids? Thanks for your consideration....R.S.L.
Answer: No, the nuts as they come off the tree do not have trans fatty acids.

Question: Subject: HELP! I have been trying to find a chart that lists the fat content of various foods (vegetables, meats, fruits) with no luck! Could you please lead me to a site that contains this information or tell me where I can write to get such a list? Thank you very much, R.L.D.
Answer: U. S. Department of Agriculture publishes its Agricultural Handbook 8, Composition of Foods in various long and short versions; these handbooks all contain fat content information. There is a version on the net, or at least there was one in the past. Also, various nutrition text books have reproduced a substantial portion of Handbook 8. There is also Handbook 456. These are all available through the various government printing office facilities. Track down USDA on the net.

Questions Regarding Omega-3 and Omega-6 Fatty Acids

Question: Subject: Omega-3 and Lox. I had a question from a friend concerning omega-3s and I haven't been able to come up with a "reliable" or consistent answer. The question involves salmon. I know that regular salmon is a great source of the omega-3s, but is lox (nova) a good source as well. I would think it would be, but the thin slicing and smoking, I thought, might have an influence. Whadda you think? E.B.
Answer: I would expect the omega-3s that were in the tissue to still be there, and I have never noticed a rancid smell on lox - but I have also never noticed a paper on the subject. I will look and let you know if I come up with something. Meanwhile a quick look at Handbook 8 values for smoked salmon appear similar to raw values for the same salmon (chinook) (raw 5.4% 22:6 of total lipid; smoked 6.2% 22:6 of total lipid - that should really have been calculated from total fatty acids but I don't have time to do it now). Never can tell how much of Handbook 8 is imputed data though, and the only people who would know are dead or working someplace else.

Question: Subject: Regarding Essential Fatty Acids. Hi, I was curious if you have done any studies on Omega 3 Fatty Acid? I'm under the impression that it has been virtually depleted from our diet. From my understanding it is essential! Any thoughts? K.S.

Answer: The omega-3 fatty acid alpha-linolenic acid (LNA) is an essential fatty acid. It is found in green leaves in small amounts, in some nuts and grains, and in totally unrefined oils such as flax oil, canola oil, soybean oil, and a few other oils that are not common in the US. It is effectively destroyed by the regular refining and hydrogenation types of processing, and so is missing from most commercial oils. Whether it is depleted from a diet depends on whether or not there are enough unrefined sources remaining in the diet, and whether or not the LNA in the diet is effectively utilized depends on whether or not there is an adequate background of saturated fatty acids in the diet. Some people do not process the LNA very well since they have too much omega-6 oils in their diets.

Question: Subject: ALA and DHA. A simple question hopefully. If someone were taking in their Omega 3's primarily from Alpha-Linoleic Acid aka Flax Seed Oil, and if under the correct conditions can the body convert ALA to both EPA and DHA or just EPA, and if so should the person supplement with a concentrated DHA supplement along with the Flax. I've heard this discussion before on various radio programs and both equations have been made. Thanks for your help- as usual. A.C., CN.

Answer: Both are made.

Question: Subject: omega 3 fatty acids. I recently heard that omega 3 fatty acids can be of value in controlling osteoarthritis. What foods contain omega 3 fatty acids? Can I buy supplements in health food stores? Thank you, L.R.

Answer: Omega-3 fatty acids are reported to have anti-inflammatory properties; this is related to their ability to displace the inflammatory fatty acids. These effects are related to prostaglandins and the response to injury/infection signals. Omega-3 fatty acids are found in the fat part of many whole foods, but usually only in small absolute amounts unless the food is relatively high in total fat and the fat is high in omega-3.

Those foods having the highest amounts of omega-3 in each of their respective food groups, include: for nuts and seeds (e.g., butternuts, walnuts, chia seeds, flax seeds), for fish and seafood (e.g., roe, salmon, mackerel, oysters, anchovies, herring, shrimp, eel), and for meats (e.g., lamb and beef organ parts).

Only those oils that are totally unrefined retain the omega-3 if they had any to begin with; any bleaching or refining causes loss of omega-3 fatty acids. The oils with the highest amount of omega-3 in their natural state are: e.g., flax oil, walnut oil, canola oil, wheat germ oil, and soybean oil. Partial hydrogenation eliminates the omega-3 fatty acids so the typical processed foods made with such oils have essentially none. Flax seed oil and fish oil are commonly sold in capsules in health food stores. Flax seed oil is sold in bottles; fish oil is not except for cod liver oil. Soybean oil and canola oil are reliable sources only if they are totally unrefined.

Question: Subject: Omega-3. I am a commercial salmon fisherman, commercial real estate lawyer and a citizen concerned about the marine environment. I am particularly concerned with the health and environmental effects of the net cage salmon farming business. I believe that wild pink salmon are a very good source of Omega-3 and farmed salmon are a poor source and high in other fat. I would like to have an authoritative source for this belief but have not been able to find one. Do you have any internet address for a scientific paper on this subject and a comparison with other fish species? -- C. McK.

Answer: I suspect you are right, and that the farmed salmon do not have the same fatty acid composition as the wild, but the only paper I could find on the Medline talks about feeding high omega-3 oils to get omega-3. This is somewhat circular, but you may want to get the paper because it seems to have some references to your concerns. Am including the abstract in this email. I remember seeing some papers in one of the various food chemistry journals in recent years but did not pull it out. I avoid buying farmed salmon because I don't care for the way it looks with the wide stripes of white fat or whatever it is, and had planned to find out what was going on but have been too busy. The fat composition would reflect the oil meal (soybean, or other) that is fed. I understand from colleagues that a major problem is that the color of the farmed salmon does not live up to the wild salmon, and the fish are fed some color compounds to make the flesh turn orange. The amount of farmed salmon is so high, that you probably get that type in canned products and restaurants these days.

Follow up email: Thanks for the reply. You are wise to avoid the farm salmon. It has the highest antibiotic residue or any commercially available protein. However, it is not canned. The cost of the product is too high, (US$3.00lb) compared to wild pink salmon (US$.15), for canned farmed to compete.

Almost all restaurant salmon is farmed. Their marketing gimmick is the use of the word "Fresh". In fact the best salmon available is Frozen at Sea (FAS) which is flash frozen on the boat and then glazed with at least 3 separate dips in sea water. Wild salmon fishers can not overcome the prejudice against frozen. Freezing techniques are so much better today but that concept has not been marketed. The salmon farmers will supply color from a chart. The natural color of farm salmon is a dull gray. A buyer can actually order the color he wants and the farmer will adjust the amount of chemical pigmentation to suit. C.McK.

Questions Regarding Saturated Fat

Question: Subject: Animal fat. I have been reading a lot about the various fatty acid-to-eicosanoid metabolic pathways, in particular the LA--GLA-- DGLA--PGE1 chain. There is substantial evidence that autistic people have high AA levels and low PGE1 levels, so naturally we are interested in restoring balance. Obviously, a big part of this is a low insulin load diet. But I have read that saturated fats inhibit the D6D enzyme, thus blocking the LA--GLA step, which sounds like a bad idea. In addition, the saturated fats in beef are high in AA, which also sounds like a bad idea.

Can you comment on this or simply point me to some sources that would help me to understand why saturated fats are not as bad as everyone says they are? T M, PhD

Answer: Saturated fats do not inhibit the D6D enzyme. Trans fatty acids and high linoleic acid in the diet inhibit the D6D enzyme. Feeding fats with AA does not increase AA. There is some interest in the effect of omega-3 fatty acids on autism. You need to find a practitioner who understands what to try.

Question: Subject: trans fatty vs. saturated. Can you explain to me why the saturated fats do not harm humans as much as the trans fatty acids? I'm still a little confused because it sort of sounds like both butter (high in saturated fat) and margarine (high in trans fatty acids) are coming out even in this argument--both equally good & bad. Is there actually a plus to one over the other? If so, what is it? A.S.

Answer: Saturated fatty acids are normal to the human body and are found in, e.g., certain membrane phospholipids at levels of about 50%; when there are not enough saturates in the food supply, the body can usually make all of them except for fatty acids like lauric acid and capric acid. Trans fatty acids are not normally found in the body unless they are consumed in the diet. Trans fatty acids replace the normal saturated fatty acids in the cell membrane structures and sometimes they replace the essential fatty acids in the part of the membrane responsible for the production of prostaglandins; when this happens, the functions of the cells are altered in an undesirable manner. In brief, in the heart disease risk factor arena, saturates lower Lp(a) raise HDL cholesterol, and improve the TC/HDL or LDL/HDL ratio - all good effects. Trans, on the other hand, raise Lp(a) (not good), lower HDL (not good), and change the ratios to less desirable ones.

Question: Subject: Saturated Fats and Bad Eicosanoids. I've got a very important question for you regarding saturated fats. I truly believe that saturated fats are not the culprit that they are alleged to be by the main stream, I'm aware that the "real" villain is Trans Fats and the associated Hydrogenated Oils. But my question about them concerns whether or not the preformed arachidonic acid that occurs in milk fat and red meat is going to be a problem in the long run. It's my understanding that pre formed arachidonic acid will be a direct building block for the "Bad Eicosanoids" such as PGE2 series.

[A popular writer] has a real concern about egg yolks, red meat and full fat dairy for this purpose, I would really love to get your perspective on this as I seem to do very well on red meat and eggs. Thank You. Respectfully, A.C.

Answer: So-called "bad eicosanoids" in the PGE2 series, e.g., thrombox anes, are only bad if the body doesn't have the "good eicosanoids" in the PGE2 series, e.g., prostacyclins, to oppose their action. Since both of these come from arachidonic acid, it should be apparent that the arachidonic acid in and of itself could hardly be a problem. The prostaglandin story is more complex than that though; PGE3 series and PGE1 play a role too.

Question: I thought at one of your web sites you explain how saturated fat was blamed for heart disease? If so, could you send me a reference? Thank you. S.R.

Answer: You are probably talking about the Oiling of America paper that I wrote with Sally Fallon. It was published in an Australian magazine called Nexus in Dec98/Jan99 and Feb99/Mar99 in two parts. Nexus has put it on its website at www.peg.apc.org/ [in the archives].

The references are at the end of the second part. I believe that there is also another website that has the article on its site. A search engine of my name or Sally Fallon's name will give you these sites.

Question: Subject: Unnatural Saturated FAs ? I am curious if there is information on the function of unnatural SFA's as produced during hydrogenation of fats and oils. R.H.

Answer: Basically, any real saturated fatty acid of the normal lengths found in foods whether unhydrogenated or hydrogenated would never be unnatural; but it might be in company with things that are not considered natural. Total hydrogenation of any 18 carbon unsaturated fatty acid forms stearic acid, and stearic acid is stearic acid is stearic acid.

Questions Regarding Coconut Oil

Question: (email) I was interested to know your opinion regarding the deodorizing step used by both Omega Nutrition and Spectrum Oils during the preparation of their coconut oils. The oil is raised to a temperature of at least 200 degrees during this process and I wondered how this affects the properties of the oil and its subsequent nutrition.... Thank you, M.V.

Answer: Commercial deodorization is accomplished at 200 degrees C or greater, and the resultant fat/oil, which is usually called RBD, is, refined, bleached and deodorized. Spectrum Oils are referred to as semi-refined in their literature today. In the past many of their oils were referred to as "refined" and the flow chart (from Spectrum) indicated that they were in fact RBD. Spectrum coconut oil and Omega coconut oil (butter) have very different appearances, smells, and tastes. My understanding is that Omega coconut oil is filtered, but not steam deodorized; it does not look, smell or taste as if it has been steam deodorized, but it is rather like several other brands of high quality and relatively unrefined organic coconut oils I now have, or have had, in my possession, which were "cold pressed" from copra or wet processed from fresh coconut. None of the common processes used to produce an edible coconut oil should alter the fatty acid composition or alter the amount of medium chain saturates such as lauric acid to any extent. Fractionation of the lauric oils can sometimes change the melting points and also alter the composition somewhat.

Question: (email) ..... I need to find out if coconut oil in its crude form at room temp (solid) is naturally white or brown? I[f] brown, why would there be one that's white? Respectfully, TB

Answer: Regular coconut oil that is white in its solid form is extracted from the white meat (copra) of the coconut. Coconut oil that has a brownish coloration has been extracted from the coconut copra but by a technique that includes some of the brown rind, either by accident or on purpose, or it could also have some smoke contamination from the drying process. A high quality coconut oil would be extracted from the white part of the copra, and the best quality could be from either the fresh copra or the dried copra; the former being a more expensive process and the latter being the more common practice.

Question: .....Are pesticides and other harmful contaminants (ex. salmonella) a concern in crude coconut oil? I understand FDA discourages the crude/unrefined/unpasteurized/etc. oil for human consumption. Do these processes not negate any of the desirable healthful properties (ex. lauric acid)? Again thanks! TB

Answer: Any pesticides or other contaminants are not desirable, and I worry less about them being in coconut oil and palm oil than I do in other oils. Most of the typical vegetable and seed oils have pesticide residues according to research published on the topic even when the oils are refined. My experience with coconut oil is that it is usually closer to "organic" than many oils if it comes from small producers. There is no rule that I know of from the FDA regarding the need to "pasteurize" oils that have been extracted for food use. Commercial oils are usually processed by temperatures higher than those used for pasteurization. However, there are plenty of "cold-pressed" oils on the market, which have been extracted at temperatures lower than those used for pasteurization. They are not in need of further heat treatment. I would not expect salmonella in any oil - it could not survive. Salmonella is a problem in dirty moist foods. When salmonella has been a concern in the past regarding coconut it is the raw copra that was contaminated. Raw coconut products come with a spec sheet of the analysis that indicates they are free of salmonella.

Question: Subject: Tropical Oils. Where can you order beef tallow, or non-hydrogenated tropical oils? I live in Japan at Yokota AB, and would like to see some healthy products find their way into the DOD commissary system. Also, there is a world of health professionals who refuse to look into the dangers of the trans fatty acids. I just had a cholesterol check done. Total cholesterol was 215, HDL 160 and LDL 133. I was advised to lower the LDL by restricting meat, and dairy to 1 serving a day, and to substitute stick margarine for butter, and fry only in canola oil. I mentioned your work to several doctors here who refused to even look at it. Before coming to Japan, I read most of your papers that were on file at UC Davis medical library. I found them very convincing. How do we go about educating the medical community? A.B.S.

Answer: I do not currently know of any sources of beef tallow, but companies that process beef products such as Hormel may know; I believe Hormel has a website. The best source at present for coconut oil is Omega Nutrition in the state of Washington and Canada; they have a website on the internet. Hain Foods may have started to carry coconut oil again; they at one time were major providers to the health food stores. General Mills still makes its original Bugles snack chip with coconut oil; they evidently have no plans to drop it, but have done a lowfat baked version made with partially hydrogenated oil.

Question: Hi, My name is S and I have been out of work with Chronic Fatigue for 4 years. Some think that CFS is viral. Obviously no one knows for sure.

Anyway, recently my chiropractor suggested that I try mono-laurine [sp]. I just started taking it and am now looking for information on it. I have found only a few articles and would like more information about monolaurin and the specific different types of viruses that it is suppose to fight. So if you have anymore articles or could point me to some other web sights, that would be very helpful to me.

I have a network of other sick friends and all of us would like to get well. So if you help me, you may be helping many people. Also, most of the hits (for monolaurine) I got on the internet from searches lead me to many web pages having to do with monolaurin and AIDS treatment. Has it really been beneficial for AIDS? And, if it has, why don't more people know about it?

If you have time to write me back, I would really appreciate it. Sincerely yours, S.

Answer: Monolaurin is an antiviral, antibacterial, and antiprotozoal monoglyceride that your body makes from the lauric acid in the fat in mother's milk, cow's milk, and lauric fats such as coconut oil and palm kernel oil. The largest and easiest source of lauric acid is coconut oil (and of course whole coconut products). There is an extensive scientific literature on its efficacy. Lauric acid is turned into monolaurin in the gut and this is what keeps infants fed human milk from getting sick even when they are exposed to lipid coated viruses and various pathogenic organisms. Because researchers have known of the effects of monolaurin, they have manufactured it and put it into capsules. It is useful to many people, but you can get even more benefit from a couple of tablespoons of coconut oil a day than you can from half a dozen capsules. Many people do not consume coconut oil because of the misinformation about it.

The AIDS virus is killed by monolaurin. Why it is not more extensively used is probably related to the fact that most people don't understand what it does and why it does it even when you explain the effects. There have been some reported benefits for several years from both monolaurin capsules and coconut; however, this has all been anecdotal reporting and there have not been any properly conducted clinical trials, although I have been trying to get one started for several years.

If I had CFS I would certainly try regular consumption of coconut such as macaroons made with desiccated coconut or coconut oil for cooking for 3-6 months to see what happened. I also happen to know that there has been some decent research showing that Coenzyme Q is helpful with CFS.

Question: Dear Dr. Enig, I have been diagnosed as suffering from Celiac disease. In other words, I can't consume any foods made with gluten. That pretty much rules out much of the processed foods available at my local grocery store. Can you recommend any good foods that do not contain gluten, and may help in reducing the effects of CD? Additionally, I have read that coconut macaroons are popular among CD suffers, but I'm not sure why? Can you shed any light on that subject?
Answer: It is my understanding that Celiac disease (CD) is a chronic digestive disorder showing up in individuals that are genetically susceptible. In these individuals, eating food containing gluten affects absorption of nutrients by damaging the mucosal surface of the small intestine. Gluten is found in all forms of barley, oats, rye, and wheat, as well as related hybrids such as triticale and kamut. Additionally, other names for wheat include durum, semolina and spelt. Corn, rice, and other grains like amaranth, sorghum, etc. also contain a type of gluten. However, these glutens are not known to cause a Celiac reaction. You can obtain more information about CD from sites like www.ce.iac.org. As for coconut macaroons, they are an clearly a good source of a variety

of fatty acids, including two key antimicrobial components, lauric and capric acid. There is some feeling that antiviral, antimicrobial components may inhibit CD. In the U.S. and Canada, there is only one gluten-free, preservative-free coconut macaroon available that contains sufficient lauric and capric acid. It is produced by Red Mill Farms, Inc. of New York (www.redmillfarms.com).

Question: Subject: Request for info on coconut oil. Noticed your treatise on lauric acid and coconut oil. Unfortunately, from a health standpoint, coconut oil has one of the highest levels of SATURATED FATS among all vegetable oils which would increase the risks of developing heart and vessel diseases/circulatory disorders. Why did you choose to withhold this fact from your essay ?

Answer: You, and the most of the people in the U.S. have been given some unfortunate propaganda regarding the properties of coconut oil and its health effects. Coconut oil contains 27.5% long chain saturated fatty acids, 65% medium chain saturated fatty acids, and the balance unsaturated fatty acids. Of the medium chain saturated fatty acids, approximately 55% are lauric acid and capric acid, which are antimicrobial fatty acids; especially the 48-50% which is lauric acid. Lauric acid is the saturated fatty acid that is in mother's milk and it protects babies from viral and bacterial infections. (Cottonseed oil contains approximately 28.5% long chain saturated fatty acids, but no lauric acid.)

Heart disease is currently recognized to be multifactorial and to be caused by among other things such substances as oxidized fats, cytomegalovirus, helicobacterpylori, homocysteine, and various toxic chemicals, as well as other inflammatory components. The increased cholesterol levels are related to the body's attempt to heal the lesions. As one of the pathologists who is an expert on atherosclerosis pointed out, the cholesterol does not cause an atheroma any more than the white blood cells cause an abscess; they are both trying to heal. Cholesterol is one of the body's major repair substances. Lauric oils (of which coconut is the most widely grown) do not become oxidized (only polyunsaturated fatty acids can become oxidized). The monoglyceride of lauric acid (which the body makes when lauric oils are eaten) kills cytomegalovirus and helicobacter pylori and thus would be an appropriate treatment and/or preventative substance in heart disease. Also, a number of studies showed that heart disease patients who were fed coconut oil got better, so it is clear to me that there was no reason to repeat misinformation. Even Harvard medical school researchers have taken out a patent to use lauric oils to treat disease.

Question: Subject: Question - coconut oil??? Just read your comments on unhydrogenated coconut oil and their apparent beneficial effects on the human body.

For years, I have been led to believe that this was the best way to clog the arteries. Have you made any other discoveries about coconut oil that are consistent with your initial observations?

Answer: What you have been hearing for years is absolutely incorrect. The atheromas that "clog" the arteries have three times more unsaturated fatty acids than saturated fatty acids, and cholesterol synthesis is increased by polyunsaturates. There is no downside to consuming natural coconut oil, and there are many benefits.

Questions from High School and College Students Who Had Projects or Talks to Give and Who Asked for Help

Question: Subject: could you help me. Dear Dr. Enig, ... I am taking a college human biology course and doing my paper on hydrogenated oils. I cannot find the chemical makeup of what various EFA's and trans fatty acids are. I am hoping to find not only the equation, but the long hand version of what it looks like. I found your web site very informative. It is amazing how hard it is to figure out all of the trans, sans, hidden, etc. meanings. Any assistance would be very appreciated. Thank you, J.H.

Answer: Chapter 5 (on Lipids...) in the 1993 textbook Understanding Nutrition, 6th Edition, by Whitney and Rolfes, published by West Publishing Co. has pictures of structures, explanations, etc. This should help you. Also, there is a 1996 Eagan Press Handbook called Fats & Oils written by Clyde E. Stauffer; it should be in most college libraries and it also has structural information, etc.

Question: Subject: Trans Fats. My name is A. E. I am a student at [a] university - I would like to know why Trans Fats are considered worst for people than any other fats- I am doing a presentation in Nutritional Biochem on Trans fats and its link to heart disease. Thanks.

Answer: Trans fatty acids, when eaten in the amounts typical in many diets in the U.S., replace the normal fatty acids in the phospholipid membranes and thus alter the way various enzymes function. If you look up the research reported by SQ Alam et al a number of years ago in

Lipids, you will see some descriptions of altered functions dealing with, eg, digitalis receptors, cyclic AMP, etc. One paper in particular that should be of interest is: Effect of dietary trans fatty acids on some membrane associated enzymes and receptors in rat heart. Lipids. 1989 Jan;24(1):39-44.

Question: Subject: acid value of fats. I am a second year Biochemistry student and need more information on Acid value of lipids. Could you please recommend web sites in relation to this topic or reply the question. Thanking you. S.McC.

Answer: Lipids such as triglycerides would not have an acid value. Fatty acids would be measured only if they are free fatty acids and that would be done to a phenolphthalein end point using standard alcoholic sodium hydroxide solution. See page 22 in the Eagan Press Handbook Series "Fats & Oils" by Clyde E Stauffer for a description. The Bailey's book on Fats and Oils or Gunstone's books would probably also have something. I would expect any university library to have these.

Question: Lately there has been much controversy between the health effects of butter and margarine leaving consumers like myself to wonder which to choose. Because of this, I chose to divert my efforts to find out which spread is better for one's health. Two articles that I have read by you (July 1996 Consumers' Report, "Diet and Heart Disease: Not What You Think." and March 1996 Consumers' Report, "Why Butter Is Good For You?") have indicated that butter should be chosen over margarine. However, I do not seem to recall any mention of non-trans-fat margarine. Do you feel that butter is better than non-trans-fat margarine? In addition, the American Heart Association currently advises that margarine be used as a substitute for butter. They claim that a consumer should opt for soft margarine rather than harder, stick forms. As well, they recommend margarine with no more than 2 grams of fat per tablespoon and liquid vegetable oil as the first ingredient. Do you agree with what the American Heart Association advises? Your expertise on this issue is greatly needed. I feel that a response from you will give my paper the cutting edge. Your time spent reading this letter is much appreciated. I hope to receive a reply from you soon. Thank You! Sincerely, K.T.

Answer: K., I have written an article called "The Oiling of America" with Sally Fallon; it is appearing in two parts in an Australian magazine called Nexus Magazine. The first part appeared in the Dec98/Jan99 issue, which is available in the larger bookstores and should be in libraries; the website address that lists the contents of Nexus is http://www.peg.apc.org/~nexus/601.conts.html ; they are supposed to put the entire article on their website after the second part comes out in the Feb99/Mar99 issue. The first part of the article gives the history of the butter/margarine business, which started in the 1950s and is basically misinformation that has become dogma. If you cannot find the magazine, I could fax the first part to you, but I do not have a copy yet of the second part.

Butter has many components that are not found in other fats; these components are health-giving and those people who have stopped using butter have lost a source of them. There is nothing wrong with a non- hydrogenated margarine if it does not have a lot of additives, but I know of very few that fit this bill. The aspect of any margarine preventing heart disease is nonsense, though, if it is made with coconut oil it might be useful because such a product would provide enough lauric acid to give the body the raw material to make monolaurin; and monolaurin is known to kill the various viruses (eg, herpes, cytomegalovirus) and bacteria (eg, helicobacter pylori) that cause lesions in the arteries, which in turn lead to some of the atheroma. The heart disease business (and it has become a big business) can be understood perhaps by reading a most comprehensive website written by Uffe Ravnskov, MD, PhD (Sweden). Go onto the internet and pull it up; read all 25 or so pages, not just the first page. Dr. Ravnskov has his bio and all the references in addition to the 8 essays. The web site is titled The Cholesterol Myths and the address is http://home2.swipnet.se/~w-25775/. Have you seen my website about the trans fatty acids? If not, the address is http://www.enig.com/trans.html . If you have done a medline search of my name, you will come up with about 8 citations. The paper that I did for the cereal chemists journal called Cereal Foods World in the February, 1996 issue is not listed, but that may be of interest for you to find in the library. The title of the paper is Trans Fatty Acids in Diets and Data Bases; it was the outgrowth of an invited talk and is based on some research done by me and my colleagues when I was still at the University of Maryland and reported in 1988 and 1989 to the various government agencies. Good luck with your paper.

Question: Subject: begging for help! Hello! I am currently a M.S. student working on my thesis on dietary trans f.a. and the effects on cholesterol levels in post-menopausal women. I am located in Champaign, Il., and am wondering how I might obtain a copy of your 1995 book (on loan). Is there a library in the area that might have it that you are aware of? Or a library that would have it available on intralibrary loan? Or even a professor or colleague at U of I who may be willing to let me have a look at it? I have also reached a point in my research where I am trying to analyze my subjects' diets for the amount of trans fats that they are consuming. I have not found this easy to do! I wondered if you might have some feedback for me on this. I have not been able to find a computerized program that can analyze this. The closest thing perhaps that I have encountered in my review of literature is a blurb in Environmental Nutrition (May 1995) that tells us that if we add up all the fats on the labels, that [(total fat)] - [(monos + polys + saturated)] =transfat. Have you heard anything about this? And would this be a legitimate way of analyzing individual diets for the trans fat content? Any feedback, information, or resources that you might have would be greatly appreciated! Thank you sincerely for your time. B.C.R. **Answer:** The person in this office who has the information on people who have purchased the 1995 TFA book is out of town for two days, but I do not recall any mention of someone in the Champaign area. Most of the orders for the 2nd edition have come from overseas; there are probably some 1993 1st editions in the Illinois area and I will ask. Meanwhile if you will send me a fax number I can fax to you the provisional table on trans that the USDA (Lynn Dickey) put together. This data is supposedly on the internet but not in very usable form I am told, but you might want to look. Am not sure if it is ARS Handbook 8 group that is maintaining it, but someone at the USDA/HNIS office should know. Subtracting the sats, monos and polys from total fat will give you a ballpark number, if the printed numbers on the labels are correct. For example, with some of the Nabisco products that list the lipid classes you will conclude that half of the fat is trans; and in fact, Nabisco uses a shortening that is 48-53% trans.   However, for thesis work you want more accurate numbers such as a good data base could generate. You may want to look at my paper on trans and data bases, etc. in the February 1996 Cereal Foods World. I have ESHA and while their trans data is not complete or always correct, you can put your own number in and make it more accurate; am not sure who else has set aside a category for trans; maybe Nutritionist IV has it now. Good luck,

Question: Subject: TFAs Hi, this is R.H. I'm studying Nutrition and

Dietetics, and I have this huge project to make on trans fatty acids and their health hazards, I'm so confused on how to go about doing it. There is just so much info that I don't know how to organize the whole thing. No one knows about these TFAs in my country, and I thought it would be a great topic to discuss to so many people. It's going to take place in my university and so many professors and doctors are showing up along with lots of students. Please could you HELP? What exactly should I talk about, how should I present this issue, taking in mind that the people I'm presenting it to don't know anything about it? Even my Nutrition teachers don't know about all the risks of TFAs which got me shocked?!!!Plus how can I attract more and more people to come and listen to the presentation this is very important to me, and I hope u can help, Plllllease! My seminar is on April 30th, I have 15 days to go! Thank you. Please reply!

Answer: [April 27] Have been out of my office so could not reply to your request. Assume you have solved your organization process by now. Cannot tell from your email where you are located. If you can go onto the internet in such a way that you can reach Medline, you can see what the latest published research is. The website for getting to Medline is http://www.nlm.nih.gov/ . Researchers publishing on trans can be found by doing a search on trans fatty acids. Dr. Willett from Harvard is still publishing. Dr. Koletzko in Germany is publishing. Drs. R. Wolff and J. Sebedio in France are publishing. Drs. Mensink, Hornstra and others in Holland. Dr. Ratnayake in Canada has food and human milk composition papers. Drs. Wahle and James at Rowett Institute in the UK.

Question: Subject: please read/reply. My name is L.S. I am a student at a community college... I have read the articles from your website and they were very helpful when I first did a research paper on trans fats. Now I am doing a research paper on the physical results (positive/negative) for someone who has eliminated trans fats from his/her diet. I would really like to have your input for this paper. For instance, after eliminating trans fats did you lose weight for only a short time and then the weight loss stopped? Did you at first still eat a few types of food (eg crackers, sandwiches) that had trans fats and it was okay on your overall wellness? If you will please find a few minutes to give your story and send it to the email address below. I would GrEatlY appreciate it. Thank you. L.S.

Answer: I started my research concerning the trans fatty acids in about 1976. During the intervening 23 or so years, I have avoided purchasing foods made with partially hydrogenated fats and oils, and have avoided those products known to me to be fixed with such fats and oils when I have eaten in restaurants. In an attempt to be polite, I obviously have probably eaten some trans fatty acids in peoples homes when I consumed small amounts of foods offered to me for which I did not know the preparation history. I probably do not consume enough trans to see any kind of change in health parameters, and I probably was not consuming much in 1976 as I have always eaten butter in preference to margarine and did most of my own cooking while my children were still living at home. Most of the trans fatty acids are found in commercial bakery goods such as cookies, crackers, donuts, pastries, etc., in prepared foods such as frozen dinners, and in those foods deep fried in restaurants, all of which I have avoided for many decades because I preferred to make my own. Good luck with your research project.

Question: From: [K.H. agriculture school] Subject: Trans fatty acids and their uses in food processing. Dear Madam, I am currently studying Food science at [a university in] England. My colleagues and I have been given a project about trans fatty acids and their uses in the food processing industry, and ways of reducing them but still maintaining their functional properties. Information on this is scarce and we would be very grateful for any help you may be able to provide us with. Please could you send any relevant information you may have at this E-mail address:.. OR, fax me on this number : ... Yours sincerely, M.A.J.S.

Answer: You may want to look at papers on high-oleic sunflower oil. Frankel and Huang, 1994 J Amer Oil Chem Soc, 71:255-259 as a start. Papers on the subject of your interest are probably in the JAOCS over the past decade, or the journal Lipid Technology printed in the UK, or some of the food chemistry journals.

Depending on what functionality you are looking at, e.g., baking or deep frying, the replacement would be different. Unilever has done some changing, and patents should be searchable. The author of lipid biochemistry texts, Michael Gurr (Maypole Scientific Services, Isles of Scilly), probably knows what is available in the literature in the UK. Kurt Berger in London works as consultant in food fats. Good-Fry International, N.V. in Holland has developed stable frying oil as a replacement for partially hydrogenated oils. Blending with palm oil or coconut oil (and some of the more polyunsaturated oils, e.g., soybean, canola, sunflower, etc.) can result in reduced trans levels in shortenings used in baked goods. Let me know what you come up with.

Question: From: K.L.S. [state university] Subject: Trans Fat Info Web Pg. What are medium chain triglycerides?

Answer: As you know from [my] web page, triglycerides (TGs) are the fat molecules composed of 3 fatty acids and glycerol; TGs are called medium chain when all of the fatty acids are of medium chain length (8-12 carbons long - caprylic, capric, and lauric).

In the real world of natural fats, only the lauric oils such as coconut, palm kernel and babassu oils would have any amount of triglycerides with only medium chain fatty acids (for all three fatty acids).

In the world of fabricated fats and oils (i.e., structured lipids), there is a medium chain triglyceride oil called MCT oil, which is made with the fatty acid fraction containing mostly caprylic and capric acid that is left over after the soaps and cosmetic industry removes lauric acid from coconut or palm kernel oil. MCT oil was developed years ago primarily by a fats and oils researcher, Dr. Vigen Babayan; it was used originally as a specialty oil for shock and burn patients, etc., and for people who could not digest long chain fatty acids. Additionally it is now being used in ketogenic diets (for treating childhood epilepsy), and in sports diets. Plain coconut oil or palm kernel oil is about 65 percent medium chain fatty acids and should be cheaper than MCT oils.

Question: Subject: hydrogenized fats. My name is J.R. and I am a junior at [a] College. I am currently enrolled in an Advanced Foods class and I have a research assignment concerning hydrogenized fats. I was wondering if you could give me any addresses of sites that would be helpful in information about hydrogenized fats and the link to cancer, or any other good resources that you might know about. I appreciate your help, and I hope that you have a wonderful day. Sincerely, J.K.R.

Answer: Medline can be used to get references on trans fatty acids from partially hydrogenated fats and oils and their connection to cancer. Use the key words "trans fatty acids" and you will get a list of all the 1997 papers that will include the Kohlmeier et al paper and the Bakker et al paper. Use the word "hydrogenated" rather than "hydrogenized" - the latter term will not be found in MeSH Terms.

Question: Subject: Science project. What liquid will pass through (or around) butter in a sieve but not margarine? Thank You! T. B. & L. C.

Answer: Typical butter is a solid mixture with 80% fat and 20% water/milk solids. Regular stick margarine is a solid mixture with 80%

fat and 20% water/emulsified solids if it is that type, or it can be a mixture of gums and emulsifiers with much less than 80% fat.

Nothing should pass through except perhaps a solvent; Cold water should pass around if there is space around the fat item.   Hot water poured over both would probably melt the butter faster than the hardest margarine, but there is such variability in melting properties of the butters and margarines that it would be hard to predict beforehand without knowing some of the physical properties such as, e.g., the solids index of either.

Question: I am a college student from Missouri and my major is Biology and dietetics. I ran across your web page on trans fat and found it very helpful due to the fact that I am writing a paper on this topic. I haven't found a lot information that has been backed by research. Do you happen to have any of your work published in journals or know of any good sources to find information, I would greatly appreciate it. Thank you very much, D. M.

Answer: If you go onto the medline (through PubMed) and do a search on trans fatty acids you should come up with a number of research references. I believe they have about 8 of my papers listed. I have done a review for the Cereal Foods World, February 1996, vol 41, p 58 (trans Fatty Acids in Diets and Databases); it has 26 references, 5 of which are to my work. Most of the work these days is coming out of Europe because the edible oil industry in the US does not support research that may not come out favorably. My 1990 paper (Enig et al, in the Journal of the American College of Nutrition 9:471) may be easy for you to find. Look for research by Dr. Fred Kummerow; he was first to raise a question back in the 1950s, and he has just submitted a new paper, which I am hoping will be published. Good luck.

Question: Subject: I need info on OMEGA. My name is H. Y. and I'm doing a Jr. Biology project on fatty acids. The basis of my project is Saturated fats and oils vs. Unsaturated fats and oils. My teacher told me that I should look up some info about OMEGA. I'm supposed to write up a statement of the source and it's importance but the problem is, I have absolutely no idea what it is. (I think it has something to do with unsaturated fats and oils). I was hoping you could send me some information on OMEGA. Thanks, I greatly appreciate your help. *Please send the information as soon as possible* THANK YOU!!

Answer: Fatty acids have two ends. The term omega refers to the methyl end of a fatty acid. Thus omega oxidation refers to the oxidation of a fatty acid that starts at the methyl end of a fatty acid. The other end of the fatty acid is the carboxyl end and oxidation from that end is called beta-oxidation because the oxidation begins with the second (beta) carbon of the fatty acid chain. Omega is also used to designate unsaturated fatty acid families. Saturated fatty acid families do not have an omega designation. Omega-3 refers to the family of fatty acids where the first double bond (unsaturation) closest to the methyl end is in the 3 position. Omega-6 refers to the family of fatty acids where the first double bond closest to the methyl end is in the 6 position. Omega-9 refers to the first double bond appearing in the 9 position.

There are numerous omega-3 fatty acids with varying numbers of double bonds ranging from three to six depending on how long they are; the basic omega-3 fatty acid has 3 double bonds and it is 18 carbons long; it is called alpha-linolenic acid and it is an essential fatty acid. There are numerous omega-6 fatty acids with varying numbers of double bonds ranging from two to six depending on how long they are; the omega-6 with 2 double bonds is 18 carbons long, it is called linoleic acid and it is an essential fatty acid. The omega-9 fatty acid in not essential because the body can make it; oleic acid is an omega-9 fatty acid. Look up essential fatty acids in an encyclopedia; also look up fatty acids in a big nutrition textbook or recent biochemistry textbook.

Question: Subject: Fat. My classmates and I are doing a project on Fat. I was wondering if you can give me some ideas on how to burn fat out of a meat patty and how to measure how many calories are in it. Thanks... Sincerely, A.N.

Answer: If you are in a high school, you need to ask your chemistry teacher for help. Maybe the teacher can locate an instrument called a bomb calorimeter, which is used for measuring calories, and then show you how to prepare the different fractions that need to be weighed. You need to look up some of the research done by the US Department of Agriculture about 10 or so years ago that says how much fat is found in a meat patty.

For a very crude estimate of the calories in the fat that melts, the meat patty can be cooked and the weight of the melted fat determined. The melted fat would have approximately 9 kilocalories per gram. When you cook a meat patty, some of the loss of weight is from evaporation of the water in the original meat, so just weighing the meat before and after cooking is not enough, because you need an accurate weight of the fat that melts off. But even then you will only know how much fat melted; you will not know how much fat is still left in the patty. Completely accurate determination requires analytical techniques that are probably beyond the equipment available to you. Look up books on food chemistry in your library.

Follow up email: Thank you doctor for the e-mail you sent me. I am now really advanced in my project. I do not have a chemistry teacher but my biology teacher was able to help me to get the bomb calorimeter. A.N

Question: Subject: trans 11-fatty acids. I have just 'visited' your web site: trans fat info web page. I was wondering if you have any more information on the trans-11 C18:1 fatty acid produced by the anaerobic rumen bacteria butyrivibrio fibrivsolvens. I am interested in this because it is part of my Ph.D. studies on conjugated linoleic acid content in cow's milk. Any information you have would be greatfully appreciated. Yours sincerely, A. L.

Answer: You should look at the article on cow's milk fat components (CLA is one) by Peter W. Parodi in the June 1997 Journal of Nutrition (127:1055). His 1977 reference from the Journal of Dairy Science was the first to note the CLA and I believe there are a number of references on the trans-11 C18:1 in that paper (I can't find my copy right now). Other names to look for in J Dairy Sci are Katz and Keeney in 1966; they characterized the C18:1s in rumen, etc. Mark Keeney is no longer living, but Bev Teter at the U of Maryland may have some of the later references. However, I expect that Parodi is on top of all of the research done on the topic. I don't have an email for him but I once tracked him down on the Australian internet, where the Dairy Research & Development Corporation has a website. We have moved our office less than two months ago and I am still not settled from the packing/unpacking and can't find my correspondence with Parodi. Good luck in your search.

Questions from University Faculty and Researchers

Question: Dear Dr Enig Are you aware of any literature/studies that show that consuming oxidized food (which may not be obviously detectable by the taste buds - e.g oxidized/rancid linseed oil, oxidized fruit juices, oxidized bread containing linseed) may be harmful to health/carcinogenic? Yours sincerely Dr K-B Lecturer, Faculty of

Medicine, M University

Answer: Dear Dr K-B, If you go onto Medline PubMed and use the key phrase "oxidized foods and humans" you will find papers with this subject. Paul B. Addis from the University of Minnesota has done a lot of research on oxidized sterols, etc. If you put in his name as "Addis PB" you will come up with some good papers. Included in this email is one example of one of the abstracts I found on Medline that deals with the topic you are interested in. *** Diabetes Care 1999 Feb;22(2):300-6 Effect of oxidized lipids in the diet on oxidized lipid levels in postprandial serum chylomicrons of diabetic patients. Staprans I, Hardman DA, Pan XM, Feingold KR Department of Veterans Affairs Medical Center, San Francisco, CA 94121, USA.

Question: Subject: trans fat article on web Hi. I read your research with interest on the web. I saw another article in a woman's health web site that claimed that "hydrogenated oil" is NOT a trans-fat product. It claimed that [brand] Spread (a kind of tub margarine) has hydrogenated oil and is okay because it is trans-fat free. Is that just a lie? Hydrogenated is the same as partially hydrogenated, isn't it? Thanks for your time. M.C. (university)

Answer: I know the web page you are referring to. Hydrogenated as in totally hydrogenated does not have trans fatty acids because it only has saturated fatty acids. These saturated fatty acids are as hard as wax and cannot be used for food as such except when they are interesterified with a liquid oil that is highly unsaturated. I suspect the [brand] Spread is possibly an interesterified fat. This is done by chemically freeing the fatty acids from the two fats and then mixing them together and chemically reattaching the fatty acids to the glycerol so that there is a random distribution of the different fatty acids with different melting points. The web site says [brand] is keeping its manufacturing a secret, but they probably are using an old patent that could be tracked down.

Question: Thanks for your information! But, does that mean [brand] Spread is healthy, or what? M.C.

Answer: I would not eat it, because it is basically a chemically manipulated fat with the likelihood of organic solvent traces such as hexane, etc. The test would be if the wild birds would eat it. They avoid other margarines and I am told by one of the industry people that it is likely that they can detect the catalysts. It may also have some additives that I object to for personal reasons. In a starving situation, or possibly to be gracious, I might eat it where I would not knowingly eat a partially hydrogenated fat/oil. I use butter because I know how many protective factors it contains and because I prefer the taste. I would eat any margarine that I could make in my own home by blending appropriate fats and oil - and this is something that I have made as an experiment - but I usually prefer things that were around in our food supplies a hundred or a thousand years ago and that knocks out margarine.

Question: Subject: Arachadonic[sp] Acid from meats and dairy. I would appreciate it if you could help me with a concern of mine, I understand that the recommendation of lipid researchers like yourself is to consume full fat dairy products rather than lowfat products. I understand some of the reasoning behind this because of better retention of the nutrients found in whole milk, but my concern is taking in pre-formed arachodonic[sp] acid from these products. According to [a popular author] these are the direct building blocks of the "bad eicosanoids" in the body, and can be a direct link to anti-inflammatory prostaglandins.

    I'm not a believer in a low fat diet as I feel this [is] not natural to our heritage but I'm a bit concerned about the quality of the fats consumed today vs 100's of years ago. I would really appreciate your feed back on this matter, I'm studying to be a nutritionist and I'm a stickler for getting the facts straight. Respectfully, A.C.

Answer: [The popular author] has a lot of mistakes in his book, including the arachidonic acid (AA) story; he lists foods to be avoided because of their content of AA, but okays foods that have much more AA! He is also wrong on his idea that all AA goes only to "bad eicosanoids" since AA goes to both thromboxanes and prostacyclins which have opposing actions.

Question: Subject: Heating oils during cooking. Hi: I just looked at your website and I have a question for which I have been looking for an answer. When using liquid vegetable oils for frying/cooking, does the chemical composition change? Are trans-fatty acids created and in what percent ages? I think this may be a topic to add to your site if it relates to it. Thanks and Regards, G. L. (university)

Answer: High temperature frying will change the quality of liquid vegetable oils by the formation of numerous breakdown products, and these can be very toxic. However, trans fatty acids (TFAs) are not what is being formed. Some articles have said that TFAs are formed. This however is a mistaken interpretation of some of the research that has shown an increase of TFAs during deep fat frying. What is happening is that the TFAs that are in the prefried foods (the shortenings that are used for prefrying have 35 to 50 percent TFAs) are being exchanged during the frying, so that an oil that did not start out with any TFAs would pick up enough TFAs, e.g., 3 to 5 percent, so that analysis of the oil would make it appear that the TFAs had been formed.

TFAs can be formed from oils in extrusion cooking of things like corn chips because there is high pressure, high temperature, and the presence of limestone components, which act in the same way that clay filters act during the refining of oil; the extrusion cooking and this latter refining process usually produce TFAs at levels of 2 to 5 percent.

Questions from Health Professionals; Nutritionists, Dietitians, Physicians and Other Clinicians

Question: As a physical therapist I am treating people with various types of lymphedema. There is a small number of patients who develop a reflux of lymph fluid sometimes into pockets in the intestinal area. They have been advised to avoid foods containing medium and long chain fatty acids, but I am unclear what foods this indicates. Can you clarify? Thanks! S B, PT

Answer: I can understand the reason for avoidance of long chain fatty acids (LCFAs) in such circumstance, because the lymphatic system carries dietary fat on chylomicrons from the place of absorption in the intestines to the point (thoracic duct) where the chylomicrons enter the blood system. However, the interdiction with respect to medium chain fatty acids (MCFAs) makes no sense, because the MCFAs are carried in the portal blood directly from the intestine following their "digestion" and release from the triglyceride matrix. Unless there is overloading, these MCFAs are not found on chylomicrons, and unless someone has published something recent that I have not seen, my reading of the research is that MCFAs are recommended for people who have lymphatic abnormalities.

All fats and oils contain nearly 100% LCFAs except coconut and palm kernel oils, which average 63% and 58% MCFAs respectively, and butter (milk fat) which averages 12-15% short and medium chain FAs. There is a fabricated oil called MCT oil that is 100% MCFAs.

Question: Subject: trans fatty acids Dear Dr. Enig, A lot can happen in a year and a half. Would you kindly direct me to more recent research reports regarding trans fatty acids? The report I found on the Internet is dated November 1997. Thank you in advance for your response. S.D.

Answer: We hope to have another update on our web site within the next few months. Most of what has happened in the US regarding research has revolved around how much trans is in the food - the food industry says it is not much, but a reading of the food labels, etc., would say otherwise. Some of the research has dealt with feeding trans and CHD markers; USDA research found that the trans did lower the HDL and raise the Lp(a), although the industry had not wanted it to turn out this way. Some of the research in Canada indicates that too much trans is getting into breast milk and causing visual acuity problems in the infants.

There are a number of web pages on trans. Most have been sponsored by the food industry, which of course has a particular bias and are more incorrect than correct. Some have been put on by well-meaning, but not scientifically trained individuals; these are usually critical of trans and frequently are more correct than incorrect. We will include both the US, Canadian, and European research when we update our page.

Question: Subject: trans fatty acids. I believe that I read a recent (last month or so) that a company had developed a new process for removing trans fatty acid residues from margarine. I am a chemist and am fascinated because I can not myself think of a practical way to do this. Do you have any information on this (I can not find the article again). J.K.W.

Answer: The only method I can think of for removing trans fatty acids once they are in the fat is the thin layer chromatography using silver nitrate. This is the method I used to separate cis and trans for analysis. Can't imagine it being scaled up to a commercial food product! I ran my plates in chloroform, which is not as GRAS as hexane, but the only solvent that worked. I haven't been at the bench for a number of years though so it is possible someone has done something that I have not heard about, but I somehow doubt it. I try to keep up with articles in JAOCS and don't recall seeing any thing.

I wonder if the article was really referring to combining hardstock (totally hydrogenated and therefore all stearate and palmitate) with an unhydrogenated oil using the process of interesterification. That has been done in the past for one of the Canadian margarines, and I am told that this is being done in Europe. Don't know of any margarines in the US that are done that way but some of the new spreads may very well be such products. If you come across the article let me know. I will ask one of my colleagues at Maryland when she returns next week and if she knows anything I will send you another email.

Question: Subject: Trans Fats in PB? ....Could you give me an idea as to the trans- fatty acid situation in commercial peanut butters? Thanks in advance, K. S., M.D., Ph.D.
Answer: If the label on the peanut butter jar says partially hydrogenated vegetable oil, there is trans in it. I just checked with one of the people at the university where they are still analyzing foods. He said that they had found trans in all of the major brands that use the partially hydrogenated vegetable oils to replace the peanut oil that they take out; he did not remember how much, but enough so that his family stopped using the brand they had originally used.

Question: A similar question from a Canadian reporter regarding peanut butter.
Answer: Except for totally hydrogenated vegetable oil which is sometimes used in peanut butter as a replacement for the peanut oil, the words hydrogenated and partially hydrogenated on labels have the same meaning -- trans fatty acids. Most all commercial canola and soybean oil is partially hydrogenated -- sometimes even if it does not say so -- and the trans levels can be quite high (greater than 50%). Canadian labeling may be somewhat more accurate than a lot of US labeling. The only thing you can assume is that processed foods have rather substantial levels of trans.

Question: Subject: TFA's and cancer. Please tell me where I would find the latest (1997) info on trans fatty acids and cancer? also, new info regarding atherosclerosis? Thank you. S.A., MSRD
Answer: If you go onto the internet site for the National Library of Medicine and go to the Medline site (PubMed is easiest), and put in the terms "trans fatty acids and cancer " you should get the latest papers from Kohlmeier et al and others involved with the EURAMIC study and their findings of cancer tied to trans.

Putting in just the words "trans fatty acids" will bring up most of the papers and you can find the ones on atherosclerosis such as Clevidence et al. Willett's group has a new paper coming out shortly (they have presented at the SER annual meeting) on trans tied to myocardial infarct in women. There are also some papers coming out of KC Hayes group at Brandies that review the latest on trans; they should come up on the medline search.

Question: Subject: saturated fat in dairy products. I am researching an article on proposed regulations that will permit vegetable oils to be substituted for animal fats in cheese. The resulting product would be legally considered cheese for labeling. The changes are part of harmonization in Codex Alimentarius. Would you care to comment on the role of saturated fat and the effects of removing it from cheese? Could you comment on the type of fats used to substitute in, what is currently called, imitation cheese? A few words on each topic would be adequate. The article is for a gadfly dairy publication with wide circulation. It goes to dairy farmers and people in the cheese industry. Thank you, R.K., MS RD

Answer: The kind of fat used for making imitation cheeses has always been partially hydrogenated when I have analyzed it, as I did for the GAO a decade ago. My understanding is that it is still partially hydrogenated, and it is the source of substantial levels of trans fatty acids. Dairy fat has numerous beneficial components in it including CLA, sphingolipids, ether lipids, lauric acid, and butyric acid. The idea that saturated fatty acids, which are the kind your body makes out of excess carbohydrate and protein, are a problem is a piece of misinformation that is very unfortunate because it has taken away the healthy fats and given the consumer a large portion of very unhealthy fats.

Question: Subject: TFA Food List   I am a practicing RD/LD in an Oklahoma hospital where I counsel Cardiac Rehab patients. I would like to request a list of foods and their trans fatty acid content, specifically foods that contain naturally-occurring fatty acids. If you have this available, I would greatly appreciate your sharing this information with me. D.P., RD/LD

Answer: USDA was supposed to come out with a table, but it never materialized. The closest you can come to functional data is probably to use the web site from the University of Delaware, i.e., http://napa.ntdt.udel.edu/trans/ . Regarding the naturally-occurring trans fatty acids, these would be found only in ruminant animals and their products and the levels are on average about 1 to 2 percent of the total fat. Additionally, the naturally-occurring TFAs are mainly a different isomer (delta-11) than the TFAs produced by partial hydrogenation of vegetable oils.

Question: Subject: Non-Hydrogenated Spreads. ......I was wondering if you had any information regarding the new spreads on the market from company's such as Spectrum Naturals, they claim to contain no hydrogenated fats but yet have the consistency of a margarine. Is it still best to stick with real butter as I've been doing for the past 10 years? A.C.

Answer: Spectrum Naturals spread is apparently made like mayonnaise; it contains a number of additives. The advantageous components that are found in good quality butter are not found in any margarines or spreads currently available in the U.S. Butter is still the best bet.

Some General Questions

Question: I am confused about what kind of bottle oil like flaxseed oil and olive oil should be in. There are some bottles on the shelves that are black. Some are green. Some are brown. And the rest are clear so that you can see the oil.

Answer: Initially, when one producer of natural food fats and oils looked for appropriate packaging for their products, they took a page out of nature. Seeds and some fruits frequently have dark brown coats or skins, which are 100 percent protective of the fragile oils contained in their tissues. After years of development, this company settled on black opaque bottles that were inert and which prevented any penetration by light; soon afterward other companies started to follow this example, especially for the more light-sensitive oils. This is why you see highly polyunsaturated oils such as flaxseed oil sold in black containers, and even some coconut oil is packaged to protect it as if it was still in its shell although coconut oil is not as light-sensitive as the polyunsaturated oils. Olive oil is still packaged in metal cans by some companies. The protection of the oil in the original fruit or seed is related to being contained within the opaque part of the plant tissues, of course, and many of the seeds and fruit do not have brown covers. But the important thing to remember is that the highly unsaturated plants and oils are sensitive to light. In past times, the various oils were stored in opaque metal containers or earthenware jars.

Question: (email) I would appreciate your comments on Phophatidyl Seline [Sp] and MNT [Sp] oil. should either or both of these substances be avoided? Would you also comment on M2 growth hormone developed by Ann de Wees? Thank you. GL.

Answer: Phosphatidyl serine is one of the phospholipids found in crude lecithin and in all membranes [in all the cells]; so it is a food item and a body component. Did you mean MCT oil? If so, it is a specialty oil used effectively for shock and burn patients in enteral feeding. It is also used for individuals who have problems digesting regular fat. It is a by-product of the fractionation of lauric oils in the soap and cosmetics industries. It is digested and used for energy in a different pathway than other fats and oils; it does not accumulate in tissues. There is a researcher in Belgium named Annemie deVrees who does aging research. Have not seen paper on M2 growth hormone.

Question: Subject: Fat. Hello, I just wanted to ask you about fat. The fat found in soya milk is higher than fat found in skim milk. Is the fat from soya cholesterol producing and cause weight gain? Thanks, P.P. (from a university)
Answer: The fat found in skim milk is not enough to be useful; the fat found in whole milk has antimicrobial and anticancer properties, so those who drink skim milk instead of whole milk are cheating themselves out of a beneficial fat. The fat in soya milk is the same as the fat in soy oil except that it is not very much; the soya milk has antithyroid components in it though so drinking a lot of it could theoretically disrupt thyroid function and a sluggish thyroid could conceivably lead to weight gain.

Question: Subject: animal fat vs plant fat. Is there a difference in fats found in animals compared to fats found in plants (beans, nuts, soya milk etc). Is there a difference in fats found in whole milk compared to fats in soya milk? Thanks for your first reply! P.P
Answer: All fats/oils are different from each other in the sense that they all have different fatty acid compositions. For example, peanut oil is different from soybean oil; chicken fat is different from lamb fat. Ask USDA for information on composition.

Question: Subject: Egg. Hi, I heard you on radio, could you tell me how many eggs one person could eat daily,,,,,,,, Thanks a lot, Ping
Answer: If you are allergic to eggs, you should not eat any. However, if you are not allergic to eggs and if you like eggs, there is really no specific limit. Some people eat a dozen eggs a day all the time. Most people who recognize that eggs are a very important food seem to eat the equivalent of 2 to 3 eggs a day.

The Following Is an Exchange in 1999 with a European-Based Journalist

Question: Specifically, I would like [a] comment on the veracity and accuracy of this report, which I got off the Internet, from India's Health Education Library for People (HELP) organization. In particular, I would be interested in whether [you agree] that the MCFA v. LCFA distinction gives coconut oil the advantages in digestion that this article says it does and, if so, why experiments have shown it to increase deposits of cholesterol. THANKS....

Here is the text: "Coconut oil is rich in saturated fat, which is why it is bracketed with animal fat by many people. It should be noted that coconut oil has no cholesterol, as the latter is a component of animal fat only. However, intake of saturated fat may result in elevation of the blood cholesterol levels. But all oils are not the same. Coconut oil is a good food, as most of its saturated fatty acids are what we call medium-chain fatty acids (MCFAs). They account for nearly 64% of the fatty acids in coconut oil. It is only coconut oil and palm kernel oil, among all the edible oils, that contain these good MCFAs. All other vegetable oils and the animal oils contain long chain fatty acids (more than 12 carbon atoms). Both saturated and unsaturated fatty acids in all these oils contain long chain fatty acids (LCFAs). The only exception is butterfat, with 12% short chain fatty acids. Unfortunately those who equate coconut oil with other saturated fats do not know that there are different varieties of saturated fats. Coconut oil is, therefore, different from all other oils containing saturated fatty acids. Being a MCFA oil, coconut oil has certain definite advantages over other LCFAs. The digestion of coconut oils is faster and starts almost in the mouth itself and undergoes complete digestion in the stomach and upper intestine not requiring the pancreatic juice lipase for its digestion. It also has better solubility in biological fluids, getting absorbed directly into the portal blood and carried to the liver directly to undergo rapid oxidation to release energy. Other oils and animal fats containing LCFAs need pancreatic lipase for their digestion and do not easily mix with biological fluids, and so are absorbed after being re-esterified inside the intestinal cells into triglycerides. They are first incorporated into large insoluble particles called chylomicrons by the intestinal cells. These then go to the liver via the lymphatics and the circulatory system, thereby going round all parts of the body before going to the liver for final oxidation. They are, therefore, more likely to get deposited as fats and also change the blood fat content. Coconut oil, therefore, does not produce any significant change in the circulating VLDL [very low density lipoprotein], which supposed to be bad for vessel thickening. (Dr. Kritchevsky at Wistar told me that their experiments with mice did show coconut oil to increase deposits...) Because of the above advantages, coconut oil is preferred as medicinal oil in cooking for people who have bad digestion and also in infant feeds to supply fat content. **The addition of coconut oil to infant feeds helps absorption of calcium and magnesium and could help treat rickets in poor nations of the world.** TRUE? Another distinct feature of coconut oil is that it has 2.56 % less calories per gramme of fat than all other LCFA oils."

Answer: I have your request for information forwarded to me by.... Eating real coconut oil does not cause cholesterol deposits; it never did and it never will. The mouse work done by Kritchevsky and others was done using EFA [essential fatty acid] deficient hydrogenated coconut oil; this is not the food oil eaten all over the world. Yes, coconut oil does provide fewer calories because of its high content (65%) of medium chain fatty acids, and yes they are more readily digested than the long chain fatty acids. Coconut oil is added to infant formulas to try to duplicate human milk; the lauric acid provides antimicrobial support and the absorption of minerals is enhanced.

Next Questions: Subject: Re: Re question on coconut oil Dear Mary, Here are a few more questions: is its image being rehabilitated, with growing awareness about difference in saturated fats, and their virtues w/ respect to hydrogenated oils? Confirm why oils are hydro-genated..for longer shelf life? Hydrogenation gets rid of double bonds (EFAs) they are unsaturated. Problem now with supply? Of persons with low total cholesterol counts, [you] wrote that "there may be a rising of serum cholesterol, LDL cholesterol and especially HDL cholesterol." mean that people with high cholesterol should avoid even natural coco oil? N.J. [France]

Answer: I hope it is being rehabilitated because there is nothing adverse about saturated fats. Oils such as soybean and canola can not be used for deep fat frying or for baking (except in very small amounts) when they are in their original liquid form; they need to be partially hydrogenated to get rid of the triple unsaturated alpha-linolenic acid, which is unstable to high temperatures, etc. that you have with deep fat frying, etc. The normalization of cholesterol levels does not mean that those with high cholesterol levels have problems; in fact the research that was done showed that those with high cholesterol levels had a drop in overall cholesterol, sometimes with a slight increase in the HDL cholesterol. Some of the studies from past decades showed that heart disease patients did as well on coconut oil or better than those on safflower oil. I have those references in a number of my papers.

APPENDIX A

GENERAL GLOSSARY of terms that have application to understanding the functions of food fats and oils and of biological lipids

Acetic acid (acetate) is the two carbon organic (fatty) acid that is very important as an intermediate in the body's metabolism. Acetate is also the primary precursor for the synthesis of all of the steroids. The molecular weight is 60.05.

Acetyl CoA is the active form of acetate and it is derived mainly from the oxidation of simple carbohydrate units, the oxidation of amino acids from protein, or the oxidation of fatty acids. Units of acetyl CoA are used for *de novo* fatty acid synthesis, to elongate existing fatty acids, and as the building blocks for cholesterol. The actual structure of acetyl CoA contains, in addition to the acetyl group, a sulfur-containing molecule called beta(β)-mercaptoethylamine, the vitamin pantothenic acid, and the adenine nucleotide adenosine 3'-phosphate 5'-diphosphate. The molecular weight is 809.6.

Acrolein is a breakdown product of overheated fats and oils. It is a small molecular weight (MW 56) substance formed from the glycerol backbone of the triglycerides when fat is exposed to excessively high temperatures. The acrid odor in the smoke when fat is burned is acrolein. From Goodman and Gilman's *The Pharmacological Basis of Therapeutics*, we learn that acrolein is much more irritating than formaldehyde. Acrolein is a major contributor to the irritative quality of cigarette smoke and photochemical smog. The occupational threshold limit value (TLV) for acrolein is 0.1 ppm; 1 ppm causes lacrimation in less than 5 minutes (Committee on Aldehydes, 1981). Acrolein increases airway resistance and tidal volume and decreases respiratory frequency. Aldehydes increase resistance to air flow at concentrations below those that decrease respiratory frequency.

Active lipids are lipids that play important roles in metabolic functions as opposed to playing just structural roles. Molecules such as prostaglandins, thromboxanes, leukotrienes, and monoglycerides are typical active lipids.

Adipose is the name of the tissue in which energy is stored in the form of fat (triglycerides). Fat is stored in adipose tissue with the help of insulin and these fat stores represent the extra dietary fat that is ingested, or the fat that is manufactured by the body from the extra carbohydrates and excess protein that is ingested. Some adipose stores help the body maintain it's proper structure by acting as padding between organs and around some bones and muscles. This kind of adipose is very important for good health.

Adrenoleukodystrophy (ALD) is a genetic peroxisomal disease that results in the accumulation of very long-chain fatty acids because the enzymes that normally break down these fatty acids are deficient in the cells. The myelin sheath in the brain deteriorates and the adrenal glands degenerate. A special oil made of erucic acid and oleic acid, which is called Lorenzo's oil, has been given as a supplement to the diet in an effort to treat this disorder.

Alpha(α)-linolenic acid is the omega-3 (n-3) polyunsaturated fatty acid with 18 carbons and three double bonds. This fatty acid is an essential fatty acid, which is sometimes referred to by the abbreviation EFA. There are various abbreviations used for this fatty acid including: C18:3, C18:3n-3, LNA, ALNA. It is the basic precursor to eicosapentaenoic acid (EPA), docosapentaenoic acid (DPA), docosahexaenoic acid (DHA), and all series 3 eicosanoids. Alpha-linolenic acid is found in high amounts in flax seed oil (approximately 60 percent), walnut oil (10 percent), totally unrefined or unhydrogenated canola oil (10 to 15 percent), and unrefined or unhydrogenated soybean oil (about 7 percent). Other oils that have high levels of alpha-linolenic acid are perilla oil and hemp oil, but they are generally not widely used in the U.S. Alpha-linolenic acid has a systematic name of cis-9, cis-12, cis-15-octadecatrienoic acid, a shorthand designation of $C_{18:3}$, a melting point of $-11\,°C$, and a molecular weight of 278.4. (See also Figure 1.10 for pathway and Figure 1.12 for graphic)

Amino acids are the basic building blocks of peptides and proteins. There are essential amino acids that the body cannot make and non-essential amino acids that the body can make. Not all amino acids are found in protein. Some amino acids are individual metabolites with various metabolic functions; some are combined to form peptides with special functions. There are 20 standard amino acids of which 9 are essential. The essential amino acids are histidine, isoleucine, leucine, lysine, methionine, phenylalanine, threonine, tryptophan, and valine. The nonessential amino acids are alanine, arginine, asparagine, aspartic acid, cysteine, glutamic acid, glutamine, glycine, proline, serine, and tyrosine, but even some of these amino acids may be conditionally essential under certain circumstances.

Antioxidants are compounds that prevent or delay undesirable oxidation (e.g., the reaction of fats and oils with oxygen). Some antioxidants are found in our foods and some are manufactured in factories or laboratories, e.g., butylated hydroxyanisol (BHT). There are water soluble antioxidants such as vitamin C and fat soluble antioxidants such as vitamin E and cholesterol. Some fat soluble antioxidants are abundant in natural oils where they play an important role in preventing rancidity. There are numerous plant compounds that play a role as antioxidants in the body when they are in the diet. The most commonly researched antioxidants being reported on are the tocopherols, the tocotrienols, and selenium. Others include lipoic acid, oryzanol, and numerous plant carotenoids.

Arachidic acid is a saturated fatty acid with 20 carbons and no double bonds. The most common food source of this fatty acid is peanut oil (1 to 2 percent) and it is found in very small amounts (less than 1 percent) in most other oils. It has a systematic name of eicosanoic acid, a shorthand designation of $C_{20:0}$, a melting point of 75.4 °C, and a molecular weight of 312.5. (See also Figure 1.11 for graphic)

Arachidonic acid is the omega-6 (n-6) polyunsaturated fatty acid with 20 carbons and four double bonds. Arachidonic acid is the fatty acid precursor to a number of series E2 prostaglandins (thromboxanes and prostacyclins) and leukotrienes. Arachidonic acid is found in small and varying amounts (usually less than ½ percent) in lard and some other animal and fish fats. Some of the older literature refers to arachidonic acid as an essential fatty acid, but it is made in the normal body from linoleic acid and therefore is not really a dietary essential for humans although it is absolutely essential for cats and other carnivores. It has a systematic name of *cis*-5,*cis*-8,*cis*-11,*cis*-14-eicosatetraenoic acid, a shorthand designation of $C_{20:4n-6}$, and a molecular weight of 304.5. (See also Figure 1.9 for pathway and Figure 1.12 for graphic)

ATP (adenosine triphosphate) is a major carrier of chemical energy to the processes in cells that need energy. It is formed during energy-yielding oxidation of fuel molecules such as fat and carbohydrate.

Behenic acid is a saturated fatty acid with 22 carbons and no double bonds. The most common natural food source is peanut oil (4 percent). Very small amounts (less than half a percent) are found in other oils such as rapeseed, rice bran, and soyabean oils. The total hydrogenation of the 22 carbon monounsaturated fatty acid erucic acid produces behenic acid, which is used as an industrial lubricant or in the man-made fat Caprenin (see below). Behenic acid has a systematic name of docosanoic acid, a shorthand designation of $C_{20:0}$, a melting point of 80.0°C, and a molecular weight of 340.6. (See also Figure 1.11 for graphic)

Bile acids play an important role in the emulsification and digestion of food lipids. Bile acids are manufactured in the liver from cholesterol and stored in the gallbladder. Their secretion into the small intestine is stimulated by the consumption of a fatty meal. Under normal circumstances, most (85 to 90 percent) of the bile acids are recycled and returned to the gallbladder to be combined with the small amount being manufactured (200-500 mg/day).

Butyric acid is a short-chain saturated fatty acid with 4 carbons and no double bonds. It is found in milk fat and butter from ruminant animals at about 3 to 4 percent of the total fat. It has a systematic name of butanoic acid, a shorthand designation of $C_{4:0}$, a melting point of -7.9°C, and a molecular weight of 88.1.

Canola oil is extracted from the seeds of a variety of the species *Brassica napus* or *Brassica campestris*. It is a genetically engineered low erucic acid rapeseed oil and it was developed in Canada. It has been available in the U.S. market since the mid 1980s (see Chapter 4).

Capric acid is a medium-chain saturated fatty acid with 10 carbons and no double bonds. It is found in coconut and palm kernel oils (4 to 6 percent) and milk fat and butter from ruminant animals (about 2 percent). It has a systematic name of decanoic acid, a shorthand designation of $C_{10:0}$, a melting point of 29.6°C, and a molecular weight of

172.3. (See also Figure 1.11 for graphic)

Caproic acid is a short-chain saturated fatty acid with 6 carbons and no double bonds. It is found in milk fat and butter (about 2 percent) and in coconut oil and palm kernel oil in very small amounts (less than 1 percent). It has a systematic name of hexanoic acid, a shorthand designation of $C_{6:0}$, a melting point of -3.3°C, and a molecular weight of 116.2.

Caprylic acid is a medium-chain saturated fatty acid with 8 carbons and no double bonds. It is found in coconut (8 percent), palm kernel oils (4 percent), and milk fat and butter from ruminant animals (about 1 to 2 percent). It has a systematic name of octanoic acid, a shorthand designation of $C_{8:0}$, a melting point of 12.7°C, and a molecular weight of 144.2.

Carbon chains form the backbone of fatty acids (and other structures such as waxes). Carbon is unique in that it will form chains or rings of carbon atoms joined by chemical bonds in which one, two, or three pairs of electrons may be shared. If one pair of electrons is shared, the bond is called a *single bond* and is shown like this, -C-C-. If two pairs are shared, it is called a *double bond* and is shown as -C=C- in pictures of molecular structures. Likewise, the sharing of three pairs gives a *triple bond* and is shown as -C≡C-. A carbon bond which shares only one pair of electrons is called a *saturated bond*, and generally in the case of fats, the other electrons of the carbons are shared by hydrogen atoms when they are not shared by another carbon. A carbon bond which shares more than one pair of electrons is called an *unsaturated bond*. The bonds are attached to each carbon in a particular way so that they form a tetrahedral structure.

Carboxyl group is the acid group of organic compounds. The carboxyl group is found on the carboxyl end of a fatty acid and because of its particular structure it allows the fatty acid to combine with other structures. The carboxyl group is designated by the structure -COOH or -COO⁻ + H⁺ and it is a weak acid.

Cardiovascular disease (CVD) is the term used to designate a variety of diseases of the heart and blood vessels. The terms ischemic heart disease (IHD), coronary artery disease (CAD), coronary heart disease (CHD) are all used interchangeably, and which one is used depends on the particular agency or researcher. There are numerous factors thought to cause or to increase the risk of CVD. The factors that have been reported in the medical literature include (listing not in any particular order of importance): viral (cytomegalovirus) and bacterial (*helicobacter pylori*, *chlamydia*) infections, homocysteinuria, chemical toxins, oxidized LDL cholesterol, hypertension, diabetes, kidney disease, obesity, high uric acid (gout), smoking, *trans* fatty acids, high intake of omega-6 polyunsaturates, blood clotting abnormalities, and familial hyperlipidemias.

Carotenoids are plant pigments that are mainly lipid soluble. The best known carotenoid is beta-carotene. Other important carotenoids are lycopene, lutein, and zeaxanthin. Carotenoids are responsible for the red, orange or yellow colors in plants. They can act as antioxidants or pro-oxidants depending on the particular system.

Catalysts are materials that speed up chemical reactions without becoming part of the final product. In fats and oils processing, catalysts are typically used for hydrogenation processes. Hydrogenation catalysts in the United States are usually made of nickel and sulfur, but they can be made of more expensive minerals such as platinum, palladium, or rhodium. Some of these catalysts have been made of copper chromite.

Cerotic acid is a saturated fatty acid with 26 carbons and no double bonds. The usual food sources of this fatty acid, other than that found in animal brains, are plant and insect waxes. It has a systematic name of hexacosanoic acid, a shorthand designation of $C_{26:0}$, a melting point of 87.7°C, and a molecular weight of 396.7.

Cetoleic acid is a monounsaturated fatty acid with 22 carbons and one *cis* double bond in the n-11 ($\Delta 11$) position. The most common sources of cetoleic acid are fish oils such as herring (23 percent), capelin (20 percent), cod liver (11 percent), sardine (4 percent), and anchovy and menhaden (2 percent). It has a systematic name of *cis*-11-docosenoic acid, a shorthand designation of $C_{22:1n-11}$, and a molecular weight of 338.6.

Cholesterol is a mammalian sterol (a high molecular weight alcohol), which is a structural component of all cell surfaces and all intercellular membranes in concentrations up to 40 percent of the total membrane.

Circulating cholesterol, which is not water soluble, is carried through the blood by lipoproteins, which are water soluble (see also Lipoproteins). Circulating cholesterol exists in a free form (about 30 percent) and in a form esterified to a fatty acid (about 70 percent); the fatty acid is usually the essential fatty acid linoleic acid (C18:2). The myelinated structures of the brain and the central nervous system are especially rich in cholesterol. In these and other membranes, cholesterol is usually found in free form rather than in the esterified form. Cholesterol is also the precursor molecule for steroid hormones (e.g., cortisone, aldosterone), sex hormones (e.g., progesterone, testosterone, estrogen), bile acids (e.g., cholic acid), and vitamin D. Cholesterol also acts as an antioxidant. A lack of cholesterol in tissues has been identified as a factor in malformation of eyes. Cholesterol is synthesized from (18 units of) the two carbon molecule acetyl-CoA, primarily in the liver (90 percent), but nearly every properly functioning cell can manufacture some cholesterol. The molecular weight of cholesterol is 386.7. (See Figure 1.16 for graphic, Figure 2.9 for cholesterol to hormone pathways, and see also Oxidized cholesterol below)

Choline is an important metabolite that is technically named trimethyl amino ethanol. It is important as a source of methyl groups and for its role in acetylcholine where it is part of the neurotransmitter, and its role as a component of phosphatidylcholine (lecithin). The molecular weight is 121.2.

Chylomicrons are lipoproteins that transport triglycerides and other lipids through the lymph system from the intestinal cells following meals. They deliver triglycerides to various tissues other than the liver and the enzyme lipoprotein lipase plays an active role in the uptake of triglycerides into the extra hepatic tissues. Chylomicrons are made in the intestinal cell and are the least dense of the lipoproteins.

Cocoa butter is the fat extracted from the cocoa bean *Theobromo cacao*. It has a unique fatty acid composition and is used mainly for candies and in the pharmaceutical industry (see Chapter 4).

Coconut oil is the oil extracted from the fruit of the coconut palm *Cocus nucifera*. It is a very stable food oil and is a major source (approximately 50 percent) of the antimicrobial fatty acid lauric acid, which is probably a conditionally essential saturated fatty acid. Lauric acid is important in functional foods and in soaps and cosmetics (see Chapter 4).

cis-**Configuration** represents the *cis* geometric placement of those hydrogens attached to the carbons of a double bond. When both hydrogens are on the same side of the double bond they are said to be *cis* to each other. This *cis* configuration forces a bend in the fatty acid chain. In nature, most (but not all) plant and animal unsaturated fatty acids have *cis* double bonds. (See *trans*-configuration and Figure 1.12 for graphics of *cis* fatty acids.)

Cold-pressed is the description given to a food oil that is supposed to have been extracted from a seed or grain without the use of high temperatures or solvents.

Conjugated linoleic acid (CLA) is an 18 carbon fatty acid with two double bonds formed in ruminant animals. The double bonds are on adjacent carbons with only a single bond between rather than being separated from each other by a methyl group as is found in the regular linoleic acid. One of the double bonds is in the *cis* configuration and one of the double bonds is in the *trans* configuration. The most common natural CLA is the *cis*-9, *trans*-11. CLA was first identified about two decades ago by the Australian dairy researcher Peter Parodi and has been given the name alpha-rumenic acid by Dr. Parodi. The most common CLA has a systematic name of *cis*-9, *trans*-11 octadecadienoic acid, a shorthand designation of $C_{18:2ct}$, and a molecular weight of 280.4. (See also Chapter 1 for discussion and graphic of structure)

Cooking oil is the term applied to liquid oils that are stable enough to be used in cooking processes. The category generally used in government documents is salad and cooking oils.

Corn oil is the oil extracted from the germ of corn of the genus *Zea mays* L. Approximately 60 percent of corn oil is the essential fatty acid linoleic acid. Corn oil is used primarily as a salad and cooking oil and in the manufacture of margarines (see Chapter 4).

Cottonseed oil is the oil extracted from the meat of the cottonseed *Gossypium*. It is used as a frying oil in the southern states, especially for frying potato chips, and as a component of shortenings because of its content of palmitic acid (approximately 25 percent)(see Chapter 4).

Cyclooxygenase (COX) is the enzyme that catalyzes the first committed step in the pathways that form prostaglandins and thromboxanes from the omega-6 precursor arachidonic acid (AA), and the omega-3 precursor eicosapentaenoic acid (EPA). These fatty acids are competitive for this enzyme. The prostaglandin PGI_2 and the thromboxane TXA_2 are formed from AA; the prostaglandin PGI_3 and the thromboxane TXA_3 are formed from EPA. There is major research currently underway to characterize various inhibitors to the different forms of the enzyme; they are called COX-1 or COX-2 inhibitors.

Desaturases are the enzymes that introduce the double bond into a fatty acid molecule. Delta-6-desaturase (d-6-d) introduces a double bond between the sixth and seventh carbons counting from the carboxyl end of the fatty acid. This reaction results in the formation of gamma-linolenic acid (18:3n-6) from linoleic acid (18:2n-6) in the omega-6 pathway, or in the omega-3 pathway d-6-d introduces the fourth double bond into the alpha-linolenic acid (18:3n-3) and forms a fatty acid called only by its systematic name octadecatetraenoic acid. Delta-9-desaturase (d-9-d) introduces a double bond between the ninth and tenth carbons counting from the carboxyl end of the fatty acid. This is the desaturase that forms oleic acid (18:1n-9) from stearic acid, or palmitoleic acid (16:1n 9) from palmitic acid. Delta-5-desaturase (d-5-d) introduces a double bond between the fifth and sixth carbons of a 20 carbon fatty acid counting from the carboxyl end. Arachidonic acid (20:4n-6) is formed from dihomo-gamma-linolenic acid (20:3n-6) and eicosapentaenoic acid (EPA) (20:5n-3) is formed from eicosatetraenoic acid (20:4n-3) by the d-5-d enzyme in the omega-3 pathway. See Figures 1.9 and 1.10 for omega-6 and omega-3 pathways. Mammals do not have the delta-12-desaturase or the delta-15-desaturase, so they cannot form linoleic acid or alpha-linolenic acid; only plants have these desaturases. (See Essential fatty acids.)

Desaturation is an oxidative process that results in the introduction of a double bond into a fatty acid by the enzymatic removal of two hydrogens from adjacent carbons. This is the activity performed by desaturases (see above).

DHA see **Docosahexaenoic acid**

Diglycerides are molecules with only two fatty acids attached to the glycerol. The fatty acids can be attached to the two outer hydroxyl groups of the glycerol or they can be attached to one outer and the middle hydroxyl group of the glycerol. A diglyceride is more polar than a triglyceride. In food, diglycerides are used as emulsifiers. In the body, the phospholipids are formed from diglycerides in one of the pathways.

Dihomogamma(γ)-linolenic acid (DGLA) is an omega-6 fatty acid with 20 carbons and 3 double bonds; it is formed by elongation of the 18 carbon fatty acid gamma(γ)-linolenic acid (GLA). DGLA is the precursor molecule to the series-1 eicosanoids (thromboxanes and prostacyclins). It has a systematic name of *cis*-8,*cis*-11,*cis*-14-eicosatrienoic acid, a shorthand designation of $C_{20:3}$, and a molecular weight of 306.5. (See also Figure 1.9 for pathway)

Docosahexaenoic acid (DHA) is an omega-3 (n-3) polyunsaturated fatty acid with 22 carbons and 6 double bonds. This very long-chain omega-3 fatty acid is formed in the body by a series of desaturation and elongation steps starting with alpha(α)-linolenic acid. (See Figure 1.10) DHA is a storage fatty acid that the body shortens (retroconverts) and saturates to form eicosapentaenoic acid (EPA) for prostaglandins or other eicosanoids in the 3 series, or it is a metabolic fatty acid that is used in membranes especially in the brain and the eye. A practical dietary source of DHA is unhydrogenated fish oil and fatty fish. Chicken skin is reported to have trace amounts of DHA, and some algae are being used to produce DHA commercially. DHA has a systematic name of *cis*-4,*cis*-7,*cis*-10,*cis*-13,*cis*-16,*cis*-19-docosahexaenoic acid, a shorthand designation of $C_{22:6\,n-3}$, and a molecular weight of 328.6. (See also Figure 1.10 for pathway and Figure 1.12 for graphic)

Docosapentaenoic acid (DPA) is the name given to two different fatty acids. One is an omega-6 (n-6) polyunsaturated fatty acid with 22 carbons and 5 double bonds, which is the last fatty acid in the omega-6 family. The other is an omega-3 (n-3) polyunsaturated fatty acid called clupanodonic acid with 22 carbons and 5 double bonds, which is formed between EPA and DHA in the omega-3 pathway. This omega-3 fatty acid is found in fish, and it is a precursor to EPA through retroconversion. These two fatty acids have systematic names of *cis*-4,*cis*-7,*cis*-10,*cis*-13,*cis*-16-docosapentaenoic acid and *cis*-7,*cis*-10,*cis*-13,*cis*-16,*cis*-19-docosahexaenoic acid respectively, shorthand designations of $C_{22:5n-6}$ and $C_{22:5n-3}$, and each have a molecular weight of 330.5. (See Figures 1.9 and

1.10 for pathways)

Double bond is the name given in fats and oils terminology to the linkage between two carbons in the fatty acid chain when the two carbons share two links with each other instead of one. A double bond is called an unsaturated bond, and fatty acids that have double bonds are unsaturated fatty acids. The unsaturated bond causes or results in constriction to the movement between the two carbons and alters the shape of the chain. The bonds between carbons and hydrogens in fatty acids are single saturated chemical bonds that are covalent bonds and not ionic bonds. Covalent bonds are stronger than ionic bonds, but double bonds that are covalent and unsaturated are not as strong as single bonds that are covalent and fully saturated. Consequently, the sites of double bonds in fatty acids are potentially reactive and less stable than the sites of single bonds. This is one of the reasons that unsaturated fatty acids are more reactive than saturated fatty acids.

DPA see **Docosapentaenoic acid**

EFA see essential fatty acids

Eicosapentaenoic acid (EPA) is an omega-3 (n-3) polyunsaturated fatty acid with 20 carbons and 5 double bonds. This very long-chain omega-3 fatty acid is formed in the body by a series of desaturation and elongation steps starting with alpha-linolenic acid. (See Figure 1.10) EPA is the immediate precursor to the series 3 prostaglandins and other eicosanoids. (See Figure 2.8) This omega-3 fatty acid is found primarily in fish oils and fatty fish. It has a systematic name of *cis*-5,*cis*-8,*cis*-11,*cis*-14,*cis*-17-eicosapentaenoic acid, a shorthand designation of $C_{20:5\ n-3}$, and a molecular weight of 302.5. (See also Figure 1.12 for graphic)

Eicosanoids is the collective term for the 20-carbon oxygenated fatty acid derivatives formed from the elongated essential fatty acids, which act as local hormones with effects close to their site of synthesis. Eicosanoids include prostacyclins, prostaglandins, thromboxanes, and leukotrienes. See Prostaglandins.

Elaidic acid is the name given to the 18 carbon *trans* fatty acid with a double bond in the Δ9-10 position. It is a major *trans* in partially hydrogenated vegetable fats and oils, and has been studied fairly extensively.

Frequently, researchers refer to *trans* fatty acids as if there was only the $\Delta 9$, but it usually makes up between 15 and 20 percent of the total *trans* fatty acids in a given fat. Elaidic acid has a systematic name of trans-9-octadecenoic acid, a shorthand designation of $C_{18:1t}$, a melting point of 44°C, and a molecular weight of 282.5. (See also Figure 1.11 for graphic)

Elongation is the term given to the enzymatic process of adding two more carbons to a fatty acid chain. Examples: Stearic acid is made in the body from palmitic acid by an elongation reaction; palmitic acid has 16 carbons and stearic acid has 18 carbons. Arachidonic acid is made by the body from linoleic acid by an elongation reaction (as well as two desaturase reactions); linoleic acid has 18 carbons and arachidonic acid has 20 carbons.

Emulsifiers are surface-active agents that facilitate the mixing of fat and water, usually because they contain within their single molecule both a water soluble portion and a lipid (fat) soluble portion. A common emulsifier is the phospholipid lecithin, which has two fatty acids that are lipid soluble and a phosphate and choline group that is water soluble. Foods such as mayonnaise and other salad dressings are oil in water mixtures and they would not maintain their consistency without emulsifiers such as lecithin from egg yolks. Monoglycerides and diglycerides are emulsifiers. Bile acids also act as emulsifiers during the digestive process. The emulsification of food fats and oils is necessary for their digestion; emulsified fats are hydrolyzed in the small intestine into their individual fatty acids and glycerol.

Enzymes in biological systems are protein catalysts whose function is to make chemical reactions happen. They are complex globular protein molecules. Without enzymes nothing would be properly built or properly degraded in the body. Enzymes are usually very specific in the reaction they facilitate. Thus the enzyme lipase that hydrolyzes triglycerides into two free fatty acids and a monoglyceride (or three fatty acids and glycerol) does not hydrolyze a starch molecule into individual maltose and glucose molecules, nor does it hydrolyze protein peptides into amino acids. Lipases only work on (fats and oils) lipids. The names given to enzymes have an ending with -ase as well as wording that describes their action, and all enzymes have been given systematic numbering. The enzyme lipase hydrolyzes lipids and its number is E.C.3.1.1.3, the enzyme amylase hydrolyzes starch and its number is

E.C.3.2.1.1., while the enzyme trypsin (a protease) hydrolyzes protein into peptides and its number is E.C.3.4.21.4. There are special manuals that list all the enzymes by number and give all the known specific information about their individual reactions such as how much substrate they need to be efficient, whether or not there is a feedback effect when too much product is formed, which vitamins or minerals they need as cofactors, at what temperatures they work most efficiently, at what temperatures they are denatured, and whether they work best in acid conditions or alkaline conditions.

EPA *see Eicosapentaenoic acid*

Erucic acid is an omega-9 (n-9) fatty acid with 22 carbons and one *cis* double bond in the $\Delta 13$ position. The most common sources of erucic acid are rapeseed oil (50 to 60 percent), other mustard family seeds, and nasturtium seeds (80 percent). It has a systematic name of *cis*-13-docosenoic acid, a shorthand designation of $C_{22:1n-9}$, a melting point of 34.7°C, and a molecular weight of 338.6. (See also Figure 1.7 for pathway)

Essential fatty acids (EFAs) are fatty acids that the mammalian body cannot make and that must be obtained from the diet because they are needed for certain essential activities in the body. They were first identified in the 1920s and 1930s by the biochemists GO and MM Burr (*JBC* 1929;82:345) and HM Evans and H Lepkoveky (*JBC* 1932;96:157). Without essential fatty acids in the diet, the necessary prostaglandins and other eicosanoids cannot be formed, the brain does not develop properly, and the body does not grow properly. There are two essential fatty acids that are polyunsaturated; they are the omega-6 (n-6) fatty acid linoleic acid and the omega-3 (n-3) fatty acid alpha-linolenic acid. There are a number of other fatty acids that are considered conditionally essential by some researchers. Gamma-linolenic acid is thought to be a conditionally essential fatty acid for some people whose delta-6-desaturase is not functioning adequately. Lauric acid is probably a conditionally essential saturated fatty acid, and palmitoleic acid may be a conditionally essential monounsaturated fatty acid.

Esterification is the chemical action that joins an alcohol and acid together and results in the formation of an ester molecule. The OH part of the alcohol molecule combines with the COOH part of the acid and the molecule HOH (water) is removed. This combining results in an ester linkage. Glycerol needs to combine with three acid groups to be completely esterified. When there is only partial esterification, molecules such as monoglycerides and diglycerides are formed. A triglyceride is a molecule that results from esterification of the alcohol glycerol and three fatty acids. A wax is a molecule that results from esterification of a very long chain alcohol and a very long chain fatty acid.

Expeller pressed is the term used for extraction of oil from seeds. The oil seeds are ground under pressure using a large worm screw mechanism and the oil is "expelled" from the cylindrical chamber through openings in the sides of the cylinder. This type of extraction usually uses no added heat, other than what is generated by the action of the grinding, and is frequently referred to as "cold pressed."

Fat is basically a solid collection of mostly (greater than 95 percent) triglycerides. Fat is solid because the melting properties of most of its individual fatty acids are above ambient temperature.

Fatty acids are carboxylic acids with carbon chain lengths ranging from 3 to 24 carbons (a purist would also include the 2 carbon acetic acid and the 26- and 28-carbon fatty acids found in waxes); the most abundant fatty acids found in foods are 16 and 18 carbons long.

Flax seed oil is extracted from the seed of *Linum usitatissumum* plant. It is also called food grade linseed oil and is a source of the essential fatty acid alpha-linolenic acid (see Chapter 4).

Fractionation is the method by which parts of fats and oils are separated based on melting characteristics as well as well as by chemical means. An example of fractionation might involve the removal of high-melting triglycerides from oils by controlled temperature cooling. This could result in the removal of all of the components that solidify at 32°F (0°C). An oil treated by this method, would be called "winterized."

Free fatty acids are not bound to glycerol. In food fat, free fatty acids are usually removed during deodorization and refining because their presence results in foaming if the fat is being used for frying. In the body, free fatty acids are formed, for example, when the fatty acids are hydrolyzed from triglycerides or formed during fatty acid synthesis. They are carried on albumin in the blood.

Free radical is the name given to a reactive molecule that has an unpaired electron. An unpaired electron seeks a mate, and as a result forms another unpaired electron. Free radicals are unstable intermediates in many reactions. Some of these reactions involve undesirable activity such as lipid oxidation and rancidity, where free radicals are derived from, e.g., the decomposition of unsaturated fatty acids. But free radical activity is also part of normal metabolic function in cells. The formation of prostaglandins involves a free radical intermediate. Ozone-induced reactive free radicals can interact with sulfhydryl groups in proteins as well as with unsaturated fatty acids.

Frying oils are considered to be in two categories, i.e., light duty and high-stability. They are usually more heavily partially hydrogenated for the high stability category than for the light duty category. High stability oils are used in commercial frying operations; light duty oils are usually used in the home.

Gadoleic acid and **Godonic acid** (n-11 and n-9, respectively) are both monounsaturated fatty acids with 20 carbons and 1 double bond. These fatty acids are found in small amounts in various fish fats/oils. They are also found in substantial amounts in rapeseed oil (12 percent), and in small amounts in lard (1.3 percent), oat oil (2.4 percent), and peanut oil (1.4 percent). These fatty acids have systematic names of *cis*-9- and *cis*-11-eicosenoic acid, shorthand designations of $C_{20:1}$, a melting point of about 24°C, and both have a molecular weight of 310.5.

Gamma(γ)-linolenic acid (GLA) is an omega-6 (n-6) polyunsaturated fatty acid with 18 carbons and 3 double bonds. It is an intermediate fatty acid formed from linoleic acid by the delta-6-desaturase enzyme in the pathway to arachidonic acid. GLA is found in several plant oils including borage oil (20 percent), black currant oil (15 to 19 percent), and evening primrose oil (9 percent). It has a systematic name of *cis*-6, *cis*-9, *cis*-12, octadecatrienoic acid, a shorthand designation of $C_{18:3 \text{ n-6}}$, an apparently undetermined melting point below -5°C, and a molecular weight of 278.4. (See also Figures 1.9 for pathway and 1.12 for graphic)

Generally regarded as safe (GRAS) is the category established by the Food and Drug Administration to identify food additives that have been used for a sufficient period and do not require premarket clearance. Some of the foods have been given GRAS status through food industry lobbying and petition.

Genetic engineering is the informal term for recombinant DNA technology. The transfer of different characteristics through the use of *e. coli* as a vector is the most common, and this technology has been used to change characteristics of seeds such as soybeans and rapeseed.

Glycerol is a 3 carbon alcohol molecule. It is the backbone of triglycerides and those phospholipids, which are glycerophospholipids such as phosphatidylcholine, phosphatidylethanolamine, phosphatidylinositol, phosphatidylserine, phosphatidic acid, and cardiolipin. Food grade glycerol is used for maintaining moisture in such items as marshmallows, fudge, and baked goods. Graphics of glycerol are shown in Chapter 1 on page 12.

Glycogen is the storage form of carbohydrate in animal tissues, especially liver and muscle cells. It is a polymer of D-glucose, and is the main storage polysaccharide in animals whereas starch is the storage polysaccharide in plants.

Glycerolipids are membrane lipids that have the glycerol backbone as opposed to sphingolipids, which have the sphingosine backbone. (See Glycerol above and Sphingolipids below)

Glycolipids are membrane lipids that contain sugar molecules. They are found predominantly in the brain and are frequently called cerebrosides. Some glycolipids are derivatives of the sphingolipids known as ceramides. They are found in the red blood cell membrane and are the determinants of the A, B, and O blood grouping. Gangliosides are the most complex of these sphingolipids and problems of the metabolism of these molecules is at the root of some of the genetic lipid storage disorders such as Tay-Sachs, Niemann-Pick, and Gaucher diseases.

Grapeseed oil is extracted from the grapeseeds that are by-products of the wine industry (see Chapter 4).

Groundnut oil See peanut oil.

HDL See high-density lipoproteins.

Heat of combustion is a measure of the amount of energy produced by oxidation. For determining the heat of combustion of foods, the food being studied is burned in a bomb calorimeter. Fats have higher heats of combustion because they have little oxygen and all their carbons and hydrogens give off heat, carbohydrates have many oxygen molecules that combine with their hydrogens to form water and only the carbons produce heat, and the nitrogen in proteins does not produce energy when it is burned. The caloric value of foods (carbohydrates, fats, and proteins) has been calculated using the heat of combustion measurements and certain correction factors. Based on these calculations the values of 4 calories per gram of pure carbohydrate, 9 calories per gram of pure fat, and 4 calories per gram of protein have been established. These are the numbers used for calculating the caloric value of a diet when the proportion of the carbohydrate, fat, and protein are known. The average value for fat is 9 calories per gram of fat, but this is really only correct for the typical 16 to 18 carbon fatty acid. Shorter chain fatty acids have lower and longer chain fatty acids have higher heats of combustion.

Hemp seed oil is extracted from the seed of *Cannabis sativa* (see Chapter 4).

High-density lipoproteins (HDL) are a heterogeneous class of lipoproteins known best as the most dense of the serum lipoproteins. Circulating HDL is reported to function as a carrier of cholesterol away from peripheral cells to the liver through a series of transfer steps. A low level of HDL cholesterol (less than 35 mg/dl) is thought to be a predictive risk for cardiovascular disease.

Hydrogenation of fats and oils is a type of chemical process that adds hydrogen to unsaturated double bonds. Total hydrogenation would turn any unsaturated fatty acid into a saturated fatty acid. Total hydrogenation of an oil such as soybean oil produces a mixture of approximately 10 percent palmitic acid and 90 percent stearic acid with physical properties like wax. Total hydrogenation of canola oil (low erucic acid rapeseed oil) would produce 4 percent palmitic acid and 94-96 percent stearic acid, but total hydrogenation of regular rapeseed oil would only produce 47 percent stearic acid because 13 percent would be arachidic acid (20 carbon saturate) and 35 percent would be behenic acid (22 carbon saturate). (See also partial hydrogenation)

Interesterification is the term usually applied to the rearrangement of the fatty acids on the glycerol molecules in an effort to give new properties to a fat or oil without using hydrogenation. Typically, triglycerides from two different batches of oil are hydrolyzed to free fatty acids and glycerol using an alkaline catalyst such as sodium hydroxide. These two batches are then combined and acid is added to cause the reforming (reesterification) of rearranged triglycerides. The result is a new fat or oil with a restructured composition. In the case of a single oil, the rearranged triglycerides may give a different mixing characteristic. Some interesterification is more complex and accomplished a varying temperatures. Structured lipids are usually formed by interesterification. Use of immobilized plant lipases instead of acid and alkaline catalysts has been actively investigated and found to be successful on a laboratory scale. (See also transesterification)

Iodine value (IV) is a measure of the number of double bonds in a fat or oil. Unprocessed soybean oil has an iodine value of between 125 and 138 while many partially hydrogenated soybean oils range from IV 40 to 90. High linoleic safflower oil has an IV of 138 to 151 whereas high oleic safflower oil has an IV of 85 to 93. The IV for olive oil is 76 to 90, for tallow is 33 to 50, for palm oil is 45 to 56, for butter is 25 to 42, and for coconut oil is 7 to 13.

Isomer is the term given to a molecule with the same chemical composition as another molecule but with a different 3-dimensional structure. With respect to fatty acids, two molecules with the same number of carbons and hydrogens on the chain but with double bonds in a different places or with different geometry of the double bonds would be isomers to each other. The single bonds can wiggle around so that the chain can "wag" above its melting point but the double bonds cannot; they are held in a fixed position. However, the hydrogens (H) attached to the carbons (C) of the double bond can be in one of two arrangements (isomers) relative to each other. Both hydrogens can be on the same side of the bond (both on the head side or both on the feet side) or they can be opposite sides (head:foot). If they are both on the same side they are called *cis* to each other. But if both hydrogens are on opposite sides they are called *trans*. (See also Figure 1.1)

Ketones are molecules that result from the incomplete oxidation of fatty acids. Several amino acids can also be formed into ketones when they are incompletely burned. Ketones are acetone, beta-hydroxybutyric acid, and acetoacetic acid. Excess ketones in the blood induce a condition called ketosis; ketosis can be a result of disease (semi-starvation and uncontrolled diabetes mellitus) or a result of a ketogenic diet. A ketogenic diet, high in fat is used for treating epilepsy in children. Some high protein, high fat diets are known to produce ketosis during dieting.

Lauric acid is a medium-chain saturated fatty acid with 12 carbons and no double bonds. It is found in coconut, palm kernel, and other lauric oils (at levels of 44 to 53 percent of total fatty acids), the new genetically engineered laurate canola (at about 36 percent of the total fat), and milk fat and butter from ruminant animals (about 3 percent of the total fat). Minor amounts (less than half a percent) are found in numerous plant oils. Lauric acid is known to the pharmaceutical industry for its good antimicrobial properties, and the monoglyceride derivative of lauric acid, monolaurin, is known to have even more potent antimicrobial properties against lipid coated RNA and DNA viruses, numerous pathogenic gram positive bacteria, some pathogenic gram negative bacteria, and various pathogenic protozoa. Lauric acid has a systematic name of dodecanoic acid, a shorthand designation of $C_{12:0}$, a melting point of 42.2°C, and a molecular weight of 200.3. (See also Figure 1.11 for graphic)

Lauric oils are oils with lauric acid as their major fatty acid. They include babassu oil, coconut oil, cohune oil, palm kernel oil, tucum oil. The new genetically engineered laurate canola has not been included in the category of lauric oils in literature.

LDL See low density lipoprotein.

Lecithin is the popular name for phosphatidylcholine, a phospholipid containing glycerol, two fatty acids, phosphoric acid, and choline. In the body, lecithin is a part of all the cellular membranes. It is found in egg yolk and as byproduct primarily of soybean oil extraction, it is found in many foods where it acts as an emulsifier. Lecithin is presently used in most chocolate candies where it can replace the lengthy conching procedure formerly used in producing smooth chocolate.

Leukodystrophies are genetic disorders (referred to as inborn errors of metabolism) involving incomplete breakdown and turnover of complex lipids such as sulphatides (metachromatic leukodystrophy) and galactosylceramides (globoid cell leukodystrophy; also called Krabbe disease). These leukodystrophies involve degeneration of brain white-matter and are not compatible with life beyond childhood. (See also adrenoleukodystrophy)

Leukotrienes are eicosanoids originally isolated from leukocytes by researchers expanding the investigation of prostaglandins. Some of the leukotrienes have been identified as the "slow-reacting substances of anaphylaxis" involved in histamine release in anaphylactic shock and other allergic reactions.

Lignoceric acid is a very long chain saturated fatty acid with 24 carbons and no double bonds. It is found in small amounts of 1 percent in rapeseed oil and peanut oil and less in other plant oils. In biological systems it is found in the brain. It has a systematic name of tetracosanoic acid, a shorthand designation of $C_{24:0}$, a melting point of 84.2°C, and a molecular weight of 368.6

Linoleic acid (LA) is an omega-6 (n-6) polyunsaturated fatty acid with 18 carbons and two double bonds. It is one of the two essential polyunsaturated fatty acids and is the precursor to other fatty acids such as gamma-linolenic acid, dihomogamma-linolenic acid, arachidonic acid, and all series 1 and series 2 eicosanoids. Linoleic acid is found in large amounts in unrefined oils such as safflower seed oil (78 percent), sunflower seed oil (68 percent), corn oil (57 percent), cottonseed oil (53 percent), and soybean oil (53 percent). It has a systematic name of *cis*-9,*cis*-12-octadecadienoic acid, a shorthand designation of $C_{18:2}$, a melting point of -5°C, and a molecular weight of 280.5. (See also Figure 1.9 for pathway and Figure 1.12 for graphic)

Linolenic acid See alpha-linolenic acid or gamma-linolenic acid.

Linseed oil See flax seed oil.

Lipid is the generic term that represents many different molecules including: fatty acids, triglycerides, phospholipids, sphingolipids, cholesterol, cholesterol esters, other sterols, prostaglandins, sphingo-myelin, gangliosides, glycolipids, lipoproteins, fat soluble vitamins.

Lipases are the enzymes responsible for the digestion of lipids. For example, pancreatic lipase forms free fatty acids and β-monoglycerides from triglycerides during digestion. Some lipases are nonspecific and will attack any linkage on the fat (triglyceride) molecule, and some lipases are very specific so that only certain linkages of the triglycerides are broken.

Lipidoses is the generic term for lipid storage diseases (also called lysosomal storage disorders and peroxisomal diseases). These diseases are caused by a lack of a key enzyme involved in the breakdown and turnover of a complex lipid (e.g., the sphingolipids, gangliosides, cerebrosides, sphingomyelin). Lipid storage diseases include Tay-Sachs disease (β-hexosaminidase A deficiency), Niemann-Pick disease (sphingomyelinase deficiency), Gaucher's disease (glucocerebrosidase deficiency), Fabry's disease (β-galactosidase deficiency), Zellweger syndrome (multiple reduced peroxisomal enzymes), Refsum's disease (lack of α-oxidation enzyme), and several leukodystrophies (see above).

Lipoic acid is one of five cofactors in the enzyme complex that forms acetyl Co-A from pyruvate. It is a sulfur-containing molecule and it serves both as an electron carrier and as a carrier of an acetyl or other acyl group.

Lipoproteins are a heterogeneous group of conjugated proteins with lipid and some carbohydrate incorporated into their structure. Lipoproteins are found as soluble macromolecules and also as structural macromolecules. The lipoproteins that circulate in the blood are soluble types. They are categorized by their density into chylomicrons, very low density lipoproteins (VLDL), low density lipoproteins (LDL), intermediate density lipoproteins (IDL), high density lipoproteins (HDL), and very high density lipoproteins (VHDL). They are best known for their transport of cholesterol and triglycerides, but drugs are also bound to and carried by the different lipoproteins.

Lipoprotein [a] (Lp[a]) is considered a rather unique lipoprotein for which high plasma levels promote a 2- to 3-fold increase in risk for atherosclerosis. The structure of Lp[a] is similar to LDL, but its density is higher. Lp[a] is thought to be mostly under genetic control, but *trans* fatty acids in the diet increase its levels and saturated fatty acids in the diet decrease its levels.

Lipoxygenase is an enzyme found widely in plants. It is responsible for the formation of hydroperoxides from linoleic acid and linolenic acid. Lipoxygenase is responsible for the enzymatic degradation of linoleic acid to short chain aldehydes.

Low-density lipoproteins (LDL) are a class of lipoproteins known best as the least dense of the serum lipoproteins (next to very low density lipoproteins (VLDL)). These lipoproteins have been implicated in various disease states, but in actuality they are the body's carriers of lipids and cholesterol used for building tissues.

Long-chain fatty acids have between 14 and 24 carbons in their fatty acid chains. They can be saturated, monounsaturated, or polyunsaturated. Long-chain saturated fatty acids are: myristic acid (C14:0), palmitic acid (C16:0), stearic acid (C18:0), arachidic acid (C20:0), behenic acid (C22:0), lignoceric acid (C24:0), and cerotic acid (C26:0). The common long-chain *cis*-monounsaturated fatty acids are: myristoleic acid (C14:1n-9), palmitoleic acid (C16:1n-9 or C16:1n-7), oleic acid (C18:1n-9), vaccenic acid (C18:1n-11), gadoleic acid (C20:1n-11), godonic acid (C20:1n-9), erucic acid (C22:1n-9), and nervonic acid (C24:1n-9). The common long-chain *cis*-methylene interrupted polyunsaturated fatty acids are linoleic acid (C18:2n-6), gamma-linolenic acid (C18:3n-6), alpha-linolenic acid (C18:3n-3), stearidonic acid (C18:4n-3, dihomo-γ-linolenic acid (C20:3n-6), Mead's acid (C20:3n-9), arachidonic acid (C20:4n-6), eicosapentaenoic acid (C20:5n-3), docosapentaenoic acid (C22:5n-6), docosapentaenoic acid (C22:5n-3), and docosahexaenoic acid (C22:6n-3). (See also very long-chain fatty acids)

Margarine is a fat product originally designed as an imitation butter. It is defined as a product containing up to 20 percent water in a water-in-oil mixture. The usual margarine is 80 percent fat. The 20 percent non-fat portion is a combination of water and salts or other solids. A dictionary defines margarine in 1873 as "a food product made usually from vegetable oils churned with ripened skim milk to a smooth emulsion and used like butter." The former president of the Margarine Manufacturers' Association, Dr. S. F. Riepma, wrote in 1970 that "a completely adequate definition, however, should take the following into account: *Margarine is a flavored food that is 80 percent fat, made by blending selected oils and fats with other ingredients, and usually fortified with vitamin A, to provide a spread and cooking fat that serves the purpose of butter but is different in composition* *and certain characteristics."* (his italics) Margarine is usually thought of as being made with partially hydrogenated vegetable oils, and thus a source of *trans* fatty acids. This depends on the kind of fat or oil used in the formulation of margarine. Some of the early margarines were simply blends of animal fats (tallows or lard) with skim milk or buttermilk, or they were blends of oils such a coconut oil that did not require partial hydrogenation to form a solid margarine fat. The original name margarine (or oleomargarine) comes from the fatty acid margaric acid found in lard and tallows. Most of the margarines sold during the period from 1950 to 1990 were made from partially hydrogenated soybean oil, or corn oil in the United States and canola oil in Canada. Newer spreads that are referred to as "imitation margarines" or just as "spreads" sometimes use various processes that avoid partial hydrogenation.

Mead acid (Mead's acid) is an omega-9 (n-9) polyunsaturated fatty acids with 20 carbons and 3 double bonds. It is a marker of essential fatty acid deficiency and is formed from oleic acid when there is inadequate linoleic acid in the diet by the same set of enzymes that form arachidonic acid from linoleic acid. It has a systematic name of *cis*-5, *cis*-8, *cis*-11-eicosatrienoic acid, a shorthand designation of $C_{20:3n-9}$, an apparently unreported melting point, and a molecular weight of 306.5.

Medium-chain fatty acids have between 8 and 12 carbons in their fatty acid chains. They are typically saturated fatty acids. Caproic acid (C6:0) is sometimes listed as a medium-chain fatty acid, but it is preferably put in the category with short-chain fatty acids. Caprylic acid (C8:0), capric acid (C10:0), and lauric acid (C12:0) are the common medium-chain fatty acids.

Medium chain triglyceride (MCT) is the term given to triglycerides that are made up of medium chain fatty acids. A specialty oil called MCT oil is a man-made oil with mostly medium chain fatty acids with 8 carbons and 10 carbons.

Melting point properties of fats and oil determine whether they are solid or liquid at any given temperature. When the temperature is below the point at which the crystal structure of a fat melts, that fat will be solid. When the temperature is above the point at which the fat melts, it will be a liquid. (See Figure 1.4)

Membranes are to mammalian cells and organs what walls are to plants and most bacteria; they hold cells and subcellular components together. Biological membranes have large amounts and widely varied kinds of lipids. Most membranes however are similar and their structures are organized as lipid bilayer matrixes containing phospholipids, cholesterol, glycolipids, and various proteins.

Methyl esters are the combination of the alcohol methanol and a fatty acid. This is a form of fatty acids used for analysis of fats.

Methyl group is the term that designates the carbon with three attached hydrogens.

Methylene interrupted is the term used to designate the double bond system in natural polyunsaturated fatty acids. For example, in linoleic acid there is a double bond between the 9th and 10th carbons, no double bonds between the 10th and 11th carbons and no double bonds between the 11th and 12th carbons but there is a double bond between the 12th and 13th carbons; linoleic acid has two double bonds which are cis-methylene interrupted. (-C=C-C-C=C-)

Milk fat is the lipid portion of mammalian milks and it is sometimes referred to as butterfat. The prototype of milk fat in the United States comes from the dairy cow. The fat in most milk contributes about 48 to 50 percent of the calories in whole milk and almost all of the flavor. Approximately 95 percent of milk fat is in the form of triglycerides. Typical fatty acid classes are 66 percent saturated, 30 percent monounsaturated, and 4 percent polyunsaturated. Milk fat from cows has been shown to have more than 500 different fatty acids and fatty acid derivatives, many of which are found only in trace amounts. Since milk fat is highly emulsified, it is very digestible. All things being equal (e.g., feed, lactation status, temperature), milk fat is higher in the milk from Guernsey and Jersey cows than from Holstein cows.

Monoglycerides are molecules formed by the attachment of one fatty acid molecule to a glycerol molecule. The activity of the monoglyceride depends on the type of fatty acid attached. Monoglycerides such as monolaurin are active antimicrobial molecules. The monoglyceride of palmitoleic is also an antimicrobial, as are the monoglycerides of capric acid, caprylic acid and caproic acid. Other monoglycerides serve as emulsifiers. In biological systems, monoglycerides are generally formed from the digestion of triglycerides by different lipases. The most common monoglyceride of digestion is the β-monoglyceride where the fatty acid is attached to the middle hydroxyl group of glycerol.

Monolaurin is the monoglyceride of lauric acid. It is a combination of one molecule of glycerol and one molecule of lauric acid. This monoglyceride functions as a potent antimicrobial lipid which is known to have antiviral properties (especially against lipid coated viruses), antibacterial properties (against numerous bacteria), and antiprotozoal properties. Monolaurin is formed in the gastrointestinal tract when a source of lauric acid is in the food supply. Sources for lauric acid include lauric oils such as coconut oil (50 percent is lauric acid) and human milk (up to 17 percent has been documented). Commercial monolaurin is available in powder (capsule) form.

Monounsaturated fatty acids are fatty acids that contain one double bond. See also Long-chain fatty acids.

Myelin is an important plasma membrane in the central nervous system. More than three-quarters of the myelin membrane is lipid, and of that lipid about 40 percent is phospholipid. The membrane wrapping on the nerve axon is myelin and diseases such as multiple sclerosis are caused in part by the breakdown of the integrity and composition of the membrane. The lipid composition of normal human myelin is 22 percent cholesterol, 15 percent phosphatidylethanolamine, 10 percent phosphatidylcholine, 8 percent sphingomyelin, 9 percent phosphatidyl-serine, and 28 percent glycolipid.

Myristic acid is a saturated fatty acid with 14 carbons and no double bonds. Some researchers consider it a long-chain fatty acid; some consider it a medium-chain fatty acid. Myristic acid is used in the body's metabolism in important functions involving stabilization of some of the cellular proteins. Myristic acid occurs widely in most animal and vegetable fats. Nutmeg butter is a major source at 70 to 80 percent. Lauric oils usually contain about 16 to 18 percent and milk fats 8 to 12 percent. It has a systematic name of tetradecanoic acid, a shorthand designation of $C_{14:0}$, a melting point of 52.1°C, and a molecular weight of 228.4. (See also Figure 1.11 for graphic)

n-9 see Omega-9

n-7 see Omega-7

n-6 see Omega-6

n-3 see Omega-3

Nervonic acid is a monounsaturated fatty acid with 24 carbons and one *cis* double bond in the Δ15, n-9 position. Nervonic acid is a major fatty acid in many sphingolipids. Honesty seed oil (*Lunaria bennis*) has about 25 percent nervonic acid. This fatty acid has a systematic name of *cis*-15-tetracosenoic acid, a shorthand designation of $C_{24:1n-9}$, a probable melting point of 24°C, and a molecular weight of 380.7.

Nisinic acid is an omega-3 (n-3) polyunsaturated fatty acid with 24 carbons and 6 double bonds. This very-long-chain fatty acid is found in most fish. Nisinic acid has a systematic name of *cis*-6, *cis*-9, *cis*-12, *cis*-15, *cis*-18, *cis*-21-tetracosahexaenoic acid, a shorthand designation of $C_{24:6n-3}$, and a molecular weight of 370.7.

Nut oils are extracted from those various nuts usually used in their whole states as food. They are generally much more expensive than oils extracted from seeds of grains or legumes. (see **Chapter 4**)

Odd-chain fatty acids differ from typical fatty acids by having an odd number of carbons in their chain instead of the usual even number of carbons. For example, they might have 13, 15, 17 or 19 carbons instead of 14, 16, or 18 carbons. These odd-chain fatty acids are made by many microorganisms. Some of them are called branch-chain because they are not straight chains. They are most often found in milk fat and adipose fat from ruminant animals.

Oil used as food is basically a liquid collection of mostly (greater than 95 percent) triglycerides. A collection of triglycerides whose collective melting points are below a certain ambient temperature will be called an oil or a fat depending on the climate. For example, coconut oil and palm kernel oil are always liquid in the tropics where they are produced. They would have been called fats if they had originated in the cold northern or southern climates.

Oleic acid is the monounsaturated fatty acid with 18 carbons and one *cis* double bond in the n-9 position. Oleic acid is found in all animal and vegetable fats. The amounts can be as high as 80 percent of the total fatty acids. Oleic acid is formed from stearic acid by the action of the delta-9-desaturase. It has a systematic name of *cis*-9-octadecenoic acid, a shorthand designation of $C_{18:1n-9}$, a melting point of 16°C, and a molecular weight of 282.5. (See also Figure 1.7 for pathway and Figures 1.1 and 1.12 for graphic structure)

Olestra is an artificial fat made by attaching six to eight fatty acids to a molecule of sucrose. It is not digested by humans or other animals. (See section in Chapter 1 and Figure 1.15 for graphic)

Olive oil is extracted from the fruit of an evergreen tree *Olea europaea*. It is well-known as an oil high in monounsaturated fatty acids. (See Chapter 4)

Omega is the term used to designate the methyl end of the fatty acid chain; the methyl end is opposite to the carboxyl end. (See figure of basic fatty acid in Chapter 1)

Omega 9 (also called n-9) is the family of *cis* monounsaturated fatty acids with the double bond occurring 9 carbons in from the omega end of the fatty acid. The n-9 family would include oleic acid, a minor form of palmitoleic acid that results from chain-shortening of oleic acid, gadoleic acid (20 carbons), erucic acid (22 carbons), and nervonic acid (24 carbons). (See Figure 1.7 of the n-9 family in Chapter 1)

Omega-7 (also called n-7) is the family of *cis* monounsaturated fatty acids with the double bond occurring 7 carbons in from the omega end of the fatty acid. The n-7 family is found primarily in animal tissues and includes one form of palmitoleic that resulted from desaturation of palmitic acid (90 percent of 16:1 is n-7), and an 18 carbon fatty acid called vaccenic acid that is formed by elongating the n-7 palmitoleic acid. (See Figure 1.8 of the n-7 family in Chapter 1)

Omega-6 (also called n-6) is the family of *cis* polyunsaturated fatty acids with the first double bond occurring 6 carbons in from the omega end of the fatty acid. The n-6 family would include linoleic acid (18 carbons, 2 double bonds), gamma-linolenic acid (18 carbons, 3 double bonds), and arachidonic acid (20 carbons, 4 double bonds). It also includes some tissue fatty acids that don't have common names. (See Figure 1.9 of the n-6 family in Chapter 1)

Omega-3 (also called n-3) is the family of *cis* polyunsaturated fatty acids with the first double bond occurring 3 carbons in from the omega end of the fatty acid. The n-3 family would include fatty acids such as alpha-linolenic acid (18 carbons, 3 double bonds), EPA (20 carbons, 5 double bonds), and DHA (22 carbons, 6 double bonds). (See Figure 1.10 of the n-3 family in Chapter 1)

Organelle is the term used to describe a subcellular component that acts like an "organ" to the cell in a similar sense to the way an organ acts to the whole organism. Examples of organelles are lysosomes (which help clean up the cell), microsomes (where a lot of synthesis takes place), and mitochondria (where energy is produced).

Oxidized (oxidation) is the term used for fats and oils when the fatty acids are broken down in a step-by-step process to produce energy. The fatty acids lose electrons and the energy molecule being formed gains the electron charge and is reduced. Burning is a form of oxidation. Rusting is also a form of oxidation. Fats and oils that are oxidized before they are ingested are called rancid and they are not safe to eat.

Oxidized cholesterol occurs in food when careless processing occurs. For example, unnecessary exposure to oxygen during the drying of eggs or milk can result in substantial levels of oxidized cholesterol being formed. Oxidation of cholesterol can also occur in the tissues of animals including humans when the cholesterol is acting as an antioxidant.

Palmitic acid is a saturated fatty acid with 16 carbons and no double bonds. Palmitic acid is called the "stem" fatty acid because it is the basic *de novo* fatty acid made from acetyl-CoA. Lung surfactant is exceptionally rich in palmitic acid making up about 68 percent of the surfactant phospholipids. In foods, palmitic acid ranges from a low of about 3 percent in rapeseed oil to a high of 45 percent in palm oil. Butter fat, chicken fat, cocoa butter, cottonseed oil, lard, and tallow all have approximately 25 to 26 percent palmitic acid. Olive oil has 14 percent, corn and peanut oil about 12 percent, and soybean oil 11 percent; other oils have somewhat lower levels. Human milk fat ranges from 20 to 25 percent palmitic acid. It has a systematic name of hexadecanoic acid, a shorthand designation of $C_{16:0}$, a melting point of 60.7°C, and a molecular weight of 256.4. (See also Figure 1.11 for graphic)

Palmitoleic acid is a monounsaturated fatty acid with 16 carbons and one *cis* double bond. Macadamia nuts have about 23 percent, chicken fat about 6 to 8 percent, most animal fats 2 to 4 percent and other fats and oils lesser amounts of palmitoleic acid. It has a systematic name of cis-9-hexadecenoic acid or cis-7-hexadecenoic acid, a shorthand designation of $C_{16:1}$, a melting point of 0-1°C, and a molecular weight of 254.4. (See also Figure 1.2 for graphic)

Palm oil is extracted from the fruit of the oil palm *Elaeis guineensis*. It is a known source of the antioxidant tocopherols and tocotrienols, and beta-carotene and other carotenoids. (See Chapter 4)

Palm kernel oil is extracted from the nut of the oil palm fruit *Elaeis guineensis*. It is a lauric oil. (See Chapter 4)

Partial hydrogenation is a commercial process whose intended use is for getting rid of double bonds in polyunsaturated fatty acids. Partial hydrogenation of food fats and oils turns polyunsaturated fatty acids into less unsaturated fatty acids, but not necessarily into saturated fatty acids. The formation of *trans* fatty acids is a major effect of partial hydrogenation. (See Figure 1.5)

Peanut oil is extracted from the seed of the legume *Arachis hypogaea*. (See Chapter 4)

Perilla seed oil is extracted from the seed of *Perilla frutescens*. (See Chapter 4)

Peroxide value (PV) represents the amount of hydroperoxides in a fat or oil. Peroxides form as the result of oxidation, and levels above a certain amount indicate that the fat or oil is unstable and more likely to autooxidize and become rancid. PV values are usually included in the spec sheets of commercial fats and oils.

Peroxisomes are small parts of cells that are responsible for oxidizing fatty acids that cannot be metabolized in the mitochondria, such as very-long-chain fatty acids and *trans* fatty acids. Peroxisomes are more likely to produce free radicals.

Petroselenic acid is a monounsaturated fatty acid with 18 carbons and one *cis* double bond. It has been extracted from parsley seed oil and other plant seeds. It has a systematic name of *cis*-6-octadecenoic acid, a shorthand designation of $C_{18:1n-12}$, and a molecular weight of 282.5.

Phospholipids are compounds made up of glycerol plus a phosphate group with a polar base and 2 fatty acids. Phospholipids function principally as structural molecules in physiological membranes (e.g., lipid bilayer), and because they have both water-soluble and lipid-soluble parts they form the communication link between the polar and non-polar substances in the cells and are considered surfactants. They can also act as emulsifiers. Many of their fatty acids are the long-chain polyunsaturates that are substrates for the formation of prostaglandins and leukotrienes. Their polar bases are compounds such as choline, serine, inositol, and ethanolamine. The names for the common phospholipids are: phosphatidylcholine (commonly called lecithin), phosphatidylethanolamine, phosphatidylinositol, phosphatidylserine, sphingomyelin, cardiolipin. Phosphatidic acid is the precursor to the other phospholipids. (See Figure 2.7 for typical phospholipid structures)

Phospholipases are enzymes that aid in the turnover of phospholipids. There are a number of phopholipases that have different names and they degrade different parts of the phospholipid molecule. They include phospholipase A1, phospholipase A2, phospholipase C, phospholipase D, and lysophospholipase (phospholipase B).

Phytanic acid is an important branch chain fatty acid found in the brain. One of the genetic lipid storage diseases is called **Refsum's disease**. In this disease, the enzyme needed to break down this fatty acid by alpha-α-oxidization is missing. This disease can be mitigated by a very strict diet that eliminates precursors to phytanic acid, which are phytols found in green plants and dairy and animal fats, which contain preformed phytanic acid. Enzyme replacement therapy is also used.

Pi-electrons refers to the electrons of a double bond. These electrons spin around the area of the carbon molecules. When they are joined by the electrons of the sigma bond, they collectively have a different area to cover depending on whether or not there are hydrogens on the same side of the double bond or on opposite sides of the double bond.

Plasmalogens are specialized membrane lipids that are similar to phospholipids but one of their fatty acids is attached to the glycerol with an ether linkage instead of an ester linkage

Polymerization is the process that occurs when polyunsaturated fatty acids go through free radical or autooxidation reactions, link with each other at sites of unsaturation, and form polymers (chemically joined).

Polyunsaturated fatty acids (PUFAs) are fatty acids that contain two or more double bonds in their chains. (See Long-chain fatty acids.)

Prostacyclins are one subclass of eicosanoids. (See Prostaglandins)

Prostaglandins (PGs) are one class of the biologically active lipids that play important metabolic roles. They are hormone-like metabolites that act locally and they are eicosanoids. They are formed from essential fatty acids by elongation and desaturation reactions, followed by formation of cyclic endoperoxides. These endoperoxides are further formed into prostacyclins, prostaglandins or thromboxanes . Prostacyclins and thromboxanes usually have opposing effects in the same tissue. There are three families of prostaglandins, referred to as Series I, Series II, and Series III. Series I and II prostaglandins are formed from omega-6 fatty acids and Series III prostaglandins are formed from omega-3 fatty acids. (See Chapter 2 for discussion and Figure 2.8 for the prostaglandin pathways, see also Eicosanoids)

PUFA See polyunsaturated fatty acids

Rancidity is the term used to describe the undesirable breakdown of fats and oils that is somewhat the equivalent of "rusting." The pungent odor and sharp off-flavors of rancid fats are produced by the release of breakdown products from the oxidation of the fatty acids and triglycerides.

Rapeseed oil is extracted from seed of various plants of the mustard family including *Brassica napus, B. rapa, and B. campestris.* (See Chapter 4)

Refsum's Disease (see phytanic acid)

Rice bran oil is extracted from the bran of *Oryza sativa*. (See Chapter 4)

Safflower oil is extracted from the seeds of *Carthamus tinctorius*. (See Chapter 4)

Salad oils are liquid oils belonging to the category of salad and cooking oils. They can be any kind of oil as long as it is appropriately liquid at ambient temperatures. In the United States, the common vegetable oils currently used as salad oils are: unhydrogenated or minimally hydrogenated canola oil, corn oil, cottonseed oil, olive oil, peanut oil, safflower seed oil, unhydrogenated or minimally hydrogenated soybean oil, and sunflower seed oil.

Saponification involves the alkaline hydrolysis of triglycerides to form soaps of fatty acids and glycerol. Saponification value (usually a range of numbers) is the measure of the average length of the carbon chains in the fatty acids that make up the triglycerides. A fat such as coconut oil with a low melting point has a high saponification number (250-264) because it is rich in fatty acids with 12 or fewer carbons. A fat such as rapeseed oil, on the other hand, has a higher melting point and a lower saponification number (168-183) because it is rich in fatty acids with 20 and more carbons.

Saturated fatty acids are fatty acids with no double bonds. They can be short-chain fatty acids (<8 carbons), medium-chain fatty acids (8-12 carbons), long-chain fatty acids (14-22 carbons), and very long-chain fatty acids (>22 carbons). (See Chapter 1)

Sesame oil is extracted from the seeds of the herb *Sesamum indicum*. (See Chapter 4)

SFA see saturated fatty acids

Short-chain fatty acids are less than 8 carbons long. The most common are propionic acid (3 carbons long), butyric acid (4 carbons long), and caproic acid (6 carbons long). These fatty acids are always saturated. (See Chapter 1)

Shortening is the term used to designate a fat in its anhydrous form (anhydrous means that it does not contain any water) generally used for baking. Animal fats that are shortenings are lard and tallow. Most of the shortenings currently in commercial use are partially hydrogenated soybean and cottonseed oil or partially hydrogenated canola oil. These shortenings are usually solid in texture. There are also shortenings used for commercial frying called liquid shortenings that are pourable.

Solid Fat Index (SFI) and Solid Fat Content (SFC) are the technical terms used for a measurements of solids present in a fat or oil at a given series of temperatures. These measurements are used by, e.g., the baking industry to determine whether or not the functional properties of a particular shortening are appropriate for the baking task, or by the industry to determine the melting properties of coating fats. (Stauffer, 1996 has a lengthy discussion of these tests.)

Solvents are generally used in the commercial extraction of most seed oils used for food. Presently these solvents are limited to a form of 'hexane' that is a mixture of hexane and methylpentane. Although some alcohols, and recently supercritical carbon dioxide are being suggested as appropriate, they are not yet being used commercially. Solvents used in the analysis of fats and oils include both non-polar and polar solvents including chloroform, methylene chloride, methanol, sodium methoxide, heptane, and isooctane, among others.

Solvent extracted on the label implies that the fat or oil has been extracted from the tissue or seed using a solvent such as hexane.

Soybean oil is extracted from the seeds (beans) of the legume *Glycine max*. (See Chapter 4)

Sphingolipids are complex membrane lipids whose backbone is the long chain amino alcohol sphingosine instead of glycerol. These lipids occur in all tissues including blood but are most concentrated in the white matter of the central nervous system. Sphingolipids include sphingomyelin and glyco-sphingolipids such as cerebrosides, sulfatides, globosides, and gangliosides. There are a number of sphingolipid storage diseases in man that have been widely written about. They include Tay-Sachs disease, Gaucher's disease, Fabry's disease, and several leukodystrophies. These storage diseases occur when the enzymes that normally process the various sphingolipids are not functioning properly because of a genetic defect. (See Lipidoses and Leukodystrophies above.)

Sphingomyelin is a sphingolipid that is also a phospholipid. It is one of the major structural lipids in the membranes of the nervous tissue. The most common fatty acids in sphingomyelin are the 16, 18, and 24 carbon saturated fatty acids, respectively, palmitic acid, stearic acid, and lignoceric acid, and the 24 carbon monounsaturated fatty acid nervonic acid. The myelin (white matter) has large amounts of lignoceric acid in its sphingomyelin, and the grey matter has mostly stearic acid.

Stearic acid is a saturated fatty acid with 18 carbons and no double bonds. In foods, stearic acid ranges from a low of 1 percent in rapeseed oil to a high of 35 percent in cocoa butter. It has a systematic name of octadecanoic acid, a shorthand designation of $C_{18:0}$, a melting point of 69.6°C, and a molecular weight of 284.5. (See also Figures 1.1 and 1.11)

Surfactants are chemical compounds or molecules that can act at the interface between two (2) phases such as water and oil. Surfactants lower the surface tension and allow a certain amount of mixing of the 2 phases.

TFA see *trans* fatty acids

Thromboxanes are one subclass of eicosanoids. (See Prostaglandins and Eicosanoids)

Timnodonic acid is a polyunsaturated fatty acid with 20 carbons and 5 double bonds. This fatty acid is an isomer of EPA, and the name originally was mistakenly used for EPA. It has a systematic name of *cis-4,cis-8,cis-12,cis-15,cis-18*-eicosapentaenoic acid, a shorthand designation of $C_{20:5}$, and a molecular weight of 302.5.

Tocopherols are fat soluble antioxidants most commonly known as vitamin E. Chemically the tocopherols are alcohols. There are four natural tocopherols, alpha (α), beta (β), gamma (γ), and delta (δ). In the blood, 83% of the vitamin E is α-tocopherol and most of the rest is γ-tocopherol. Synthetic vitamin E, which is listed on vitamin supplement labels as *dl*, is a mixture of 8 isomers of which 7 do not have the same activity as the natural form. Many natural oils are good sources of tocopherols. Refined oils that are stripped of their vitamin E and oils that are solvent extracted have greatly reduced levels of vitamin E. (See Chapter 4)

Tocotrienols are fat soluble antioxidants in the vitamin E family. There are four natural tocotrienols, alpha (α), beta (β), gamma (γ), and delta (δ). Some fats and oils known to be sources of tocotrienols are palm oil, wheat germ oil, rice bran oil, palm kernel oil, coconut oil, and lard. (See Chapter 4)

trans-**Configuration** represents the *trans* geometric placement of the hydrogens attached to the carbons of a double bond. When both hydrogens are on the opposite side of the double bond the bond angle is nearly the same as for a single bond. A *trans* double bond, however, shortens the fatty acid chain very slightly. The distance between, e.g., carbon 8 and carbon 11 of a typical *trans* fatty acid (i.e., one that is 18 carbons long) when there is a *trans* double bond between carbon 9 and carbon 10 is 3.77Å, whereas the distance between the same carbons on a saturated fatty acid of the same length is 3.81Å. (See also Figures 1.1 and 1.14)

Transesterification is the term sometimes applied to an industrial process used to rearrange the distribution of fatty acids on the triglyceride molecules. However, transesterification is also the term usually used for the chemical process of forming derivatives of fatty acids such as the methyl esters used for analysis. Transesterification is accomplished by combining the fat or oil triglycerides with a derivative donor such as methanol in an appropriate solvent at an appropriate temperature for an adequate length of time. This results in hydrolysis of the triglycerides and the end result is then a collection of single fatty acids condensed with single molecules of methanol, which forms methyl esters; if ethanol is used, ethyl esters are formed.

trans **Fatty acid** is the term given to a fatty acid having one or more double bonds in the *trans* geometric configuration (as opposed to the *cis* configuration). In a *trans* fatty acid, the hydrogens attached to the carbons sharing a double bond are on opposite sides of the plane of the carbons. The *trans* fatty acids are formed by a chemical catalytic process called partial hydrogenation or by biohydrogenation in the rumen of ruminant animals. (See also *trans*-Configuration above and Figures 1.1 and 1.14)

***trans*-Vaccenic acid** is an isomer of *cis*-vaccenic acid and it is designated chemically as a monounsaturated fatty acid. It has 18 carbons and one *trans* double bond in the (Δ11) position. This fatty acid is found in small amounts (1-4 percent) in ruminant fats and is a precursor to conjugated linoleic acid. *trans*-Vaccenic acid has a systematic name of *trans*-11-octadecenoic acid, a shorthand designation of $C_{18:1t\Delta11}$, and a molecular weight of 282.5. (See also Figure 1.14 for graphic)

Triglyceride is a molecule made up of three fatty acid molecules attached to a glycerol molecule by ester linkages (see Esterification). Triglycerides (TGs) are space-saving, non-hydrated, less-oxidized molecules (9 kcal/g) compared to carbohydrate or protein molecules (4 kcal/g). Triglycerides are used by the body as fuel storage molecules and for organ padding. They act as carriers for fat soluble vitamins and other fat soluble nutrients. They are also substrate for the synthesis of phospholipids and sphingolipids, and when oxidized to acetyl CoA, they are substrate for cholesterol synthesis. (See Figures 1.2 and 1.3 for graphic)

Ultraviolet (UV) light is the part of the electromagnetic spectrum responsible for changing the cholesterol in the skin into the first form of vitamin D. It is also the part of the sun's spectrum responsible for tanning of the skin, or for burning of the skin on excessive exposure especially in people with fair skin. The wavelength for UV averages about 300 nm, which is between visible light (about 600 nm) and x rays (about 50 nm), and it is invisible to the eye.

Unsaturated fatty acids are fatty acids with one or more double bonds. Unsaturated fatty acid families include all the fatty acids that have their first double bond in the same position counting from the omega end of the molecule. Sometimes these families are referred to as omega-3, omega-6, omega-7, and omega-9, but in technical literature they are referred to as n-3, n-6, n-7, and n-9. These families of fatty acids all have only *cis* double bonds. The *trans* fatty acids are also unsaturated fatty acids, but by convention they do not belong to the above families.

Vaccenic acid is an omega-7 (n-7) monounsaturated fatty acid with 18 carbons and one *cis* double bond in the (Δ11) position. This fatty acid is found in very small amounts in most animal and vegetable fats and oils. Vaccenic acid has a systematic name of *cis*-11-octadecenoic acid, a shorthand designation of $C_{18:1n-7}$, a melting point of 15°C, and a molecular weight of 282.5.

Vanaspati is a butter substitute in India. It is usually made from partially hydrogenated vegetable oils. Occasionally it can be found made from unhydrogenated palm oil.

Very long-chain fatty acids (VLCFA) (see long-chain fatty acids) is a term given by some researchers and writers when they want to refer to fatty acids longer than 20 carbons, sometimes with no distinction being made between saturates, monounsaturates, or polyunsaturates. The term is usually used when researchers are referring to those very long-chain fatty acids, which are longer that 24 carbons, and which are found in higher animals in the brain and myelin, or other specialized tissues such as the retina and spermatozoa. They can be as long as 30 carbons. (See also tables in Appendix D)

Very low density lipoprotein (VLDL) is the major lipoprotein manufactured in the liver and it is the carrier that delivers the endogenously synthesized triglycerides from the liver to the cells outside the liver.

Vitamin A is a retinoid (isoprenoid structure) whose active forms are retinol, retinal, and retinoic acid. The *Merck Index* describes vitamin A as an anti-infective vitamin, and also point out that it occurs in animals but not in plants. Preformed vitamin A for the commercial market is extracted from fish liver oils. Plant carotenoids are converted in the mammalian liver into vitamin A. Vitamin A has a molecular weight of 286.5. (See Chapter 2)

Vitamin D is a fat soluble sterol molecule and is not a true vitamin in the sense that the word vitamin is usually understood. It is, rather, a steroid with hormonal-like activity, which is initially formed using cholesterol in the skin, to make cholecalciferol, which is vitamin D3, from 7-dehydrocholesterol by exposure to ultraviolet radiation. Cholecalciferol, which can be obtained in the diet from certain animal foods, is activated in the liver to 25-hydroxy-cholecalciferol form, and then further activated by being hydroxylated in the kidney to 1,25-dihydroxycholecalciferol.

The active forms of vitamin D mediate intestinal calcium absorption, bone calcium metabolism, and maintenance of plasma calcium homeostasis. The molecular weight of vitamin D is 384.6. (See Chapter 2)

Vitamin E is made up of several fat soluble tocopherol and tocotrienol (alcohol) molecules. This vitamin is known for its antioxidant properties and antisterility properties in the rat. It is found largely in plant materials, especially seed and grains and the unrefined oils extracted from them. The best known of the vitamin E forms is alpha-α-tocopherol. The molecular weight of vitamin E is 430.7. (See Chapter 2, also Tocopherol and Tocotrienol above)

Vitamin K is the general name for a group of naphthoquinone derivatives known to be required for the bioactivation of proteins involved in maintenance of normal blood clotting, and in maintenance of bone matrix calcium. There are three groups of vitamin K compounds: phylloquinone (K1), found in green plants; menaquinones (K2), produced by intestinal bacteria; and menadione (K3), a synthetic form. The molecular weight of the naphthoquinone is 173.2.

APPENDIX B

Acronyms and Abbreviations

There are many abbreviations that are used in discussing the politics and technicalities of food fats and oils as well as the biology and health aspects of lipids. This list of acronyms should be useful as you read this and other books that deal with these topics.

AA	arachidonic acid
ACN	American College of Nutrition
ADA	American Dietetic Association
AHA	American Heart Association
AIDS	acquired immune deficiency syndrome
AJCN	American Journal of Clinical Nutrition
ALA	alpha-linolenic acid
AOCS	American Oil Chemists' Society
ASA	American Soybean Association
BHA	butylated hydroxyanisol
BHT	butylated hydroxytoluene
CE	cholesterol ester
CHD	coronary heart disease
CNS	certified nutrition specialist
COMA	United Kingdom Commission on Medical Aspects of Health
COOH	carboxyl group
CSPI	Center for Science in the Public Interest
CVD	coronary vascular disease or cerebral vascular disease
D6D	delta-6-desaturase
DGLA	dihomo-gamma-linolenic acid
DHA	docosahexaenoic acid
EDTA	ethylene diamine tetraacetic acid

EFA(s)	essential fatty acid(s)
EPA	eicosapentaenoic acid
EPA	Environmental Protection Agency

FA	fatty acid
FAO	Food and Agriculture Organization
FASEB	Federation of American Societies for Experimental Biology
FDA	Food and Drug Administration

| GLA | gamma-linolenic acid |
| GRAS | generally recognized as safe |

HDL	high density lipoprotein
HEAR	high erucic acid rapeseed
HHS	Health and Human Services
HNIS	Human Nutrition Information Service

IDL	intermediate density lipoprotein
IHD	ischemic heart disease
ISEO	Institute of Shortening and Edible Oils

LA	linoleic acid
LCFA	long-chain fatty acid
LDL	low density lipoprotein
LEAR	low erucic acid rapeseed
LNA	linolenic acid
Lp(a)	lipoprotein (a)
LSRO-FASEB	Life Sciences Research Office of the Federation of American Societies for Experimental Biology

MCFA	medium-chain fatty acid
MCT	medium-chain triglycerides
MDR	minimum daily requirement

NAS-NRC	National Academy of Sciences - National Research Council
NEFA	non-esterified fatty acid
NEJM	*New England Journal of Medicine*
NFCS	Nationwide Food Consumption Survey

NHANES	National Health and Nutrition Examination Survey
NIH	National Institutes of Health
NHLBI	National Heart, Lung, and Blood Institute
OA	oleic acid
OH	hydroxy
PA	palmitic acid
PG	prostaglandin
PL	phospholipid
PUFA	polyunsaturated fatty acid
SCFA	short-chain fatty acid
SFA	saturated fatty acid
TG	triglyceride
TXA	thromboxane
UFA	unsaturated fatty acid
UK	United Kingdom (England)
USDA	United States Department of Agriculture
UV	ultraviolet (wavelength)
VLCFA	very long-chain fatty acid
VLDL	very low density lipoprotein

APPENDIX C

Food Composition Tables

Dairy Food
Natural Cheeses
Commonly Used Fruit/ Seed Oils
Less Commonly Used Fruit/Seed Oils
Commonly Used Fats From Animal and Marine Sources
Domestic Meats
Organ Meats
Domestic Poultry
Poultry Livers
Common Game
Variety Meats
Low Fat Fin Fish
Medium Fat Fin Fish
Higher Fat Fin Fish
Popular Seeds
Popular Nuts
Nut Butters
Vegetables and Beans

These tables contain composition data for natural foods that are adequate sources of some or all of the various important fatty acid classes. In addition to the data for total fat, total saturated fatty acids, total monounsaturated fatty acids, and total polyunsaturated fatty acids, the tables include composition data for cholesterol, vitamin E, lauric acid, total omega-3 fatty acids, and total omega-6 fatty acids.

	Energy (kcal)	total fat,g	sat fat,g	mono fat,g	poly fat,g	trans fat,g	chol, mg	vit E, mg	lauric acid,g	omega3 fat,g	omega6 fat,g
Dairy Food											
Whole Milk-3.7% Fat, 8fl oz	157	8.9	5.6	2.6	0.3	0.2	35	0.24	0.25	0.13	0.20
Whole Milk-3.3% Fat, 8fl oz	150	8.1	5.1	2.4	0.3	0.2	33	0.24	0.23	0.12	0.18
2% Fat Milk-w/+VitA 8fl oz	121	4.7	2.9	1.4	0.2	0.1	18	0.17	0.13	0.07	0.10
1% Fat Milk w/+Vit A 8fl oz	102	2.6	1.6	0.8	0.1	0.1	10	0.10	0.07	0.04	0.06
Skim Milk-w/+Vit A 8fl oz	86	0.4	0.3	0.1	0.0	0.0	4	0.10	0.01	0.00	0.01
Buttermilk- skim milk, 8fl oz	99	2.2	1.3	0.6	0.1	0.0	9	0.17	0.06	0.03	0.05
European Kefir, 8fl oz	149	8.2	–	–	–	–	–	–	–	–	–
Kefir-2% Milkfat, 8fl oz	122	4.5	2.9	1.2	0.1	–	10	–	0.15	0.04	0.09
Whole Milk Yogurt-Plain, 1cup	150	8.0	5.1	2.2	0.2	0.2	31	0.22	0.27	0.07	0.16
Low Fat Yogurt-Plain, 1cup	155	3.8	2.5	1.0	0.1	0.1	15	0.10	0.13	0.03	0.08
Cultured Sour Cream, 1cup	492	48.3	29.9	13.9	1.8	–	102	1.50	1.35	0.70	1.09
Cultured Sour Cream, 1tbs	31	3.0	1.9	0.9	0.1	–	6	0.09	0.08	0.04	0.07
Heavy Whipping Cream-fluid, 1cup	821	88.1	54.7	25.5	3.3	–	326	1.50	2.48	1.28	1.98
Heavy Whipping Cream-Fluid, 1tbs	51	5.5	3.4	1.6	0.2	–	20	0.09	0.15	0.08	0.12
Light Cream, 1cup	468	46.3	28.8	13.4	1.7	–	159	0.36	1.30	0.67	1.05
Light Cream, 1tbs	29	2.9	1.8	0.8	0.1	–	10	0.02	0.08	0.04	0.06
Half & Half Cream, 1cup	315	27.8	17.3	8.0	1.0	–	89	0.27	0.78	0.40	0.63
Half & Half Cream, 1tbs	20	1.7	1.1	0.5	0.1	–	6	0.02	0.05	0.02	0.04
Natural Cheeses											
Asiago , 2 oz	213	15.6	10.1	4.1	0.6	–	52	0.28	0.30	0.20	0.35
Blue , 2 oz	200	16.3	10.6	4.4	0.5	–	43	0.36	0.28	0.15	0.30
Brick , 2 oz	210	16.8	10.7	4.9	0.4	–	54	0.28	0.28	0.17	0.28

	Energy (kcal)	total fat,g	sat fat,g	mono fat,g	poly fat,g	trans fat,g	chol, mg	vit E, mg	lauric acid,g	omega3 fat,g	omega6 fat,g
Cheddar , 2 oz	228	18.3	12.0	5.3	0.5	0.5	60	0.20	0.30	0.21	0.33
Cheshire , 2 oz	219	17.4	11.1	4.9	0.5	–	58	0.36	0.28	0.19	0.30
Colby , 2 oz	223	18.2	11.5	5.3	0.5	–	54	0.20	0.24	0.16	0.38
Cottage Cheese, 2 oz											
Cream , 2 oz	198	19.3	12.5	5.6	0.7	0.6	62	0.53	0.26	0.28	0.44
Edam / Ball , 2 oz	202	15.3	10.0	4.6	0.4	–	51	0.43	0.28	0.14	0.24
Elbinger , 2 oz	210	16.3	10.7	4.9	0.4	–	54	0.28	0.27	0.17	0.28
Emmentaler , 2 oz	213	15.5	10.1	4.1	0.6	–	52	0.28	0.30	0.20	0.35
European Emmental , 2 oz	218	16.3	10.5	4.1	0.6	–	52	9.84*	0.31	0.21	0.38
European Gorgonzola , 2 oz	204	17.7	10.8	4.9	1.0	–	49	–	0.73	0.52	0.46
Fontina , 2 oz	221	17.5	10.9	4.9	0.9	–	66	0.20	0.46	0.45	0.49
Goat -Hard , 2 oz	256	20.2	13.9	4.6	0.5	–	60	0.44	0.89	0	0.48
Goat -Semi-Soft, 2 oz	206	16.9	11.7	3.9	0.4	–	45	0.37	0.75	0	0.40
Goat -Soft Type, 2 oz	152	12.0	8.3	2.7	0.3	–	26	0.30	0.53	0	0.28
Gouda , 2 oz	202	15.5	10.0	4.4	0.4	–	65	0.20	0.69	0.22	0.15
Gruyere , 2 oz	234	18.3	10.7	5.7	1.0	–	62	0.20	0.52	0.24	0.74
Havarti , 2 oz	210	16.5	10.7	4.9	0.4	–	54	0.28	0.28	0.17	0.28
Jarlsberg , 2 oz	213	15.6	10.1	4.1	0.6	–	52	0.28	0.30	0.20	0.35
Limburger , 2 oz	185	15.3	9.5	4.9	0.3	–	51	0.36	0.49	0.09	0.19
Monterey Jack , 2 oz	211	17.2	10.8	5.0	0.5	–	50	0.19	0.23	0.15	0.36
Mozzarella -PartSkim, 2 oz	159	9.5	6.2	2.7	0.3	–	31	0.36	0.10	0.08	0.20
Mozzarella -Whole Milk, 2 oz	159	12.2	7.5	3.7	0.4	–	44	0.36	0.39	0.21	0.22
Muenster , 2 oz	209	17.0	10.8	4.9	0.4	–	54	0.26	0.21	0.13	0.24

*value given in data base of 19.84 mg suggests added vitamin E in this product

	Energy (kcal)	total fat,g	sat fat,g	mono fat,g	poly fat,g	trans fat,g	chol, mg	vit E, mg	lauric acid,g	omega3 fat,g	omega6 fat,g
Neufchatel, 2 oz	147	13.3	8.4	3.8	0.4	--	43	0.53	0.16	0.11	0.25
Parmesan -Grated, 2 oz	259	17.0	10.8	4.9	0.4	--	45	0.45	0.56	0.20	0.18
Parmesan -Hard, 2 oz	222	14.6	9.3	4.3	0.3	--	38	0.45	0.48	0.17	0.15
Port Du Salut , 2 oz	200	16.0	9.5	5.3	0.4	--	70	0.28	0.44	0.20	0.21
Provolone , 2 oz	199	15.1	9.7	4.2	0.4	--	39	0.20	0.20	0.16	0.28
Ricotta -Part Skim Milk, 2 oz	78	4.5	2.8	1.3	0.1	--	17	0.36	0.06	0.04	0.11
Ricotta -Whole Milk, 2 oz	99	7.4	4.7	2.0	0.2	--	29	0.37	0.09	0.06	0.15
Romano , 2 oz	219	15.3	9.7	4.4	0.3	--	59	0.41	0.52	0.18	0.16
Roquefort , 2 oz	209	17.4	10.9	4.8	0.7	--	51	0.44	0.74	0.40	0.35
String Stick , 2 oz	144	9.0	5.7	2.6	0.3	--	34	0.36	0.09	0.08	0.19
Swiss -Shredded, 2 oz	213	15.6	10.1	4.1	0.6	--	52	0.28	0.30	0.20	0.35
Tilsit -Whole Milk, 2 oz	193	14.7	9.6	4.0	0.4	--	58	0.40	0.61	0.18	0.23
Yogurt , 2 oz	43	0.1	0.1	0.0	0.0	--	2	0.01	--	--	--
Commonly Used Fruit/Seed Oils											
Canola Oil, 1 tbs	120	13.6	1.0	8.0	4.0	0.0	0	2.90	0	1.3	2.8
Canola Oil ,1 cup	1927	218	15.5	128.4	64.5	0.5	0	45.80	0	20.3	44.2
Cocoa Butter Oil, 1 tbs	120	13.6	8.1	4.5	0.4	0	0	2.71	0	0.01	0.38
Cocoa Butter Oil ,1 cup	1927	218	130.2	71.7	6.5	0	0	43.38	0	0.22	6.10
Coconut Oil, 1 tbs	117	13.6	11.8	0.8	0.2	0	0	0.04	6.01	0	0.25
Coconut Oil ,1 cup	1879	218	188.6	12.6	3.9	0	0	0.61	96.22	0	3.92
Corn Oil, 1 tbs	120	13.6	1.7	3.3	8.0	0	0	11.34	0	0.11	7.90
Corn Oil ,1 cup	1927	218	27.7	52.8	128.0	0	0	181.38	0	1.53	126.44
Cottonseed Oil, 1 tbs	120	13.6	3.5	2.4	7.1	0	0	8.88	0	0.03	7.03
Cottonseed Oil ,1 cup	1927	218	56.5	38.8	113.1	0	0	142.14	0	0.44	112.49

	Energy (kcal)	total fat,g	sat fat,g	mono fat,g	poly fat,g	trans fat,g	chol, mg	v t E, IU,g	lauric acid,g	omega3 fat,g	omega6 fat,g
Extra Virgin Olive Oil, 1 tbs	126	14	2.0	10.8	1.3	0	0	1.74	--	0.10	1.12
Extra Virgin Olive Oil, 1 cup	2016	224	31.4	172.5	20.2	0	0	27.78	--	1.57	17.92
Palm Oil, 1 tbs	120	13.6	6.7	5.0	1.3	0	0	5.23	0.01	0.03	1.24
Palm Oil, 1 cup	1927	218	107.5	80.7	20.3	0	0	83.71	0.22	0.44	19.84
Palm Kernel Oil, 1 tbs	117	13.6	11.1	1.6	0.2	0	0	0.84	6.40	0	0.22
Palm Kernel Oil, 1 cup	1879	218	177.7	24.8	3.5	0	0	13.49	102.46	0	3.49
Peanut Oil, 1 tbs	119	13.5	2.3	6.2	4.3	0	0	3.38	0	0	4.32
Peanut Oil ,1 cup	1909	216	36.5	99.8	69.1	0	0	54.00	0	0	69.12
Poppyseed Oil, 1 tbs	120	13.6	1.8	2.7	8.5	0	0	5.97	0	0	8.50
Poppyseed Oil, 1 cup	1927	218	29.4	43.0	136.0	0	0	95.48	0	0	136.03
Safflower Oil Hi Linoleic, 1 tbs	120	13.6	1.2	1.6	10.2	0	-	5.87	0	0.05	10.10
Safflower Oil Hi Linoleic, 1 cup	1927	218	19.8	26.4	162.4	0	-	93.96	0	0.87	161.54
Safflower Oil Hi Oleic, 1 tbs	120	13.6	0.8	10.2	1.9	0	0	4.68	0	0	1.93
Safflower Oil Hi Oleic ,1 cup	1924	217.6	13.3	163.8	30.9	0	0	74.85	0	0	30.90
Sesame Oil, 1 tbs	120	13.6	1.9	5.4	5.7	0	0	3.96	0	0.04	5.63
Sesame Oil, 1 cup	1927	218	31.0	86.5	90.9	0	0	63.44	0	0.65	90.03
Soybean Oil (eg,Wesson), 1 tbs	120	13.6	2.0	3.2	7.9	0	0	12.77	0	0.93	6.95
Soybean Oil (eg,Wesson),1 cup	1927	218	31.4	50.8	126.2	0	0	204.27	0	14.82	111.18
Sunflower Oil Hi Linoleic,1 tbs	120	13.6	1.4	2.7	9.0	0.1	0	8.56	0	0	8.95
Sunflower Oil Hi Linoleic, 1cup	1927	218	22.4	42.5	143.3	1.1	0	138.65	0	0	143.23
Sunflower Oil-Hi Oleic, 1 tbs	124	14	1.4	11.7	0.5	0	0	--	0	0.03	0.50
Sunflower Oil-Hi Oleic, 1 cup	1980	224	21.8	187.3	8.5	0	0	--	0	0.43	8.08

	Energy (kcal)	total fat,g	sat fat,g	mono fat,g	poly fat,g	trans fat,g	chol, mg	vit E, mg	lauric acid,g	omega3 fat,g	omega6 fat,g
Less Commonly Used Fruit/Seed Oils											
Almond Oil, 1 tbs	120	13.6	1.12	9.52	2.4	0	0	5.46	0	0	2.37
Almond Oil, 1 cup	1927	218	17.9	152.4	37.9	0	0	87.42	0	0	37.93
Avocado Oil, 1 tbs	124	14	1.62	9.9	1.9	-	-	0.16	0	0.13	1.75
Avocado Oil, 1 cup	1980	224	26.0	158.1	30.2	-	-	2.62	0	2.14	28
Linseed/Flaxseed Oil, 1 tbs	120	13.5	1.3	2.3	9.3	0	--	0.28	0	7.52	1.82
Linseed/Flaxseed Oil, 1 cup	1913	216.5	20.9	37.4	149.5	0	--	4.57	0	120.33	29.16
Grapeseed Oil, 1 tbs	120	13.6	1.3	2.2	9.5	0	0	8.42	0	0.01	9.48
Grapeseed Oil, 1 cup	1927	218	20.9	35.1	152.4	0	0	135	0	0.22	151.73
Hazelnut Oil, 1 tbs	120	13.6	1.0	10.6	1.4	0	0	6.43	0	0	1.38
Hazelnut Oil, 1 cup	1927	218	16.1	170.0	22.2	0	0	102.90	0	0	22.02
Rice Bran Oil, 1 tbs	120	13.6	2.7	5.4	4.8	0	0	6.95	0	0.22	4.55
Rice Bran Oil, 1 cup	1927	218	43.0	85.7	76.3	0	0	111.18	0	3.49	72.81
Walnut Oil, 1 tbs	120	13.6	1.2	3.1	8.6	0	0	4.37	0	1.42	7.21
Walnut Oil, 1 cup	1927	218	19.8	49.7	138.0	0	0	69.98	0	22.67	115.32
Wheat Germ Oil, 1 tbs	120	13.6	26	2.0	8.4	0	0	26.11	0	0.94	7.45
Wheat Germ Oil, 1 cup	1924	217.6	40.9	32.9	134.3	0	0	417.79	0	15.01	119.24
Commonly Used Fats from Animal and Marine Sources											
Butter-Unsalted, 1 tbs	102	11.5	7.2	3.3	0.4	0	31	0.22	0.32	0.17	0.26
Butter-Unsalted, 1 cup	1628	184.1	114.6	53.1	6.8	0	497	3.59	5.17	2.68	4.15
Butter Oil (Ghee), 1 tbs	112	12.8	7.9	3.8	0.5	0	33	0.38	0.36	0.18	0.29
Butter Oil (Ghee),1 cup	1796	204.0	126.9	58.8	7.6	0	525	6.15	5.70	2.96	4.60

	Energy (kcal)	total fat,g	sat fat,g	mono fat,g	poly fat,g	trans fat,g	chol, mg	αt E, mg	lauric acid,g	omega3 fat,g	omega6 fat,g
Rendered Chicken Fat, 1 tbs	115	12.8	3.8	5.7	2.7	0.00	11	0.3	0.01	0.13	2.5
Rendered Chicken Fat ,1 cup	1845	204.6	61.1	91.6	42.8	0.02	174	6.1	0.20	2.05	40.18
Duck Fat, 1 tbs	115	12.8	4.3	6.3	1.6	--	13	0.3	0	0.13	1.53
Duck Fat, 1 cup	1845	204.6	68.1	101.1	26.4	--	205	6.1	0	2.03	24.42
Goose Fat, 1 tbs	115	12.8	3.5	7.3	1.4	--	13	0.4	0	0.06	1.26
Goose Fat, 1 cup	1845	204.6	56.8	116.2	22.6	--	205	6.2	0	1.02	20.09
Domestic Meats											
Beef Steak-Club-1/4"Trim-Broiled 3.5 oz	205	9.3	3.6	3.8	0.3	--	75	0.1	0.01	0.02	0.28
Beef Roast-Bottom Round-1/4"Trim 3.5 oz	273	16.8	6.3	7.3	0.6	0.75	95	0.4	0.04	0.17	0.47
Beef Chuck-Pot-Roast-1/4"Trim 3.5 oz	214	8.2	3.0	3.4	0.3	--	100	0.1	0.01	0.02	0.30
Veal Loin Chop-Lean-Braised 3.5 oz	224	9.1	2.5	3.2	0.8	--	124	0.4	0.02	0.04	0.77
Veal Sirloin-Roasted-3.5 oz	200	10.4	4.5	4.0	0.7	--	101	0.4	0.03	0.07	0.60
Veal Shoulder-Whole-Lean-Roasted 3.5 oz	169	6.6	2.5	2.4	0.5	--	113	0.5	0.02	0.04	0.49
Lamb Loin Chop-1/4"Trim-Broiled 3.5 oz	314	22.9	9.8	9.6	1.7	0	99	0.3	0.10	0.35	1.32
Lamb Leg-Whole-1/8"Trim-Roasted 3.5 oz	240	14.3	5.9	6.1	1.0	0	91	0.1	0.06	0.19	0.82

	Energy (kcal)	total fat,g	sat fat,g	mono fat,g	poly fat,g	trans fat,g	chol, mg	vit E, mg	lauric acid,g	omega3 fat,g	omega6 fat,g
Lamb Shoulder Roast-1/4"Trim 3.5 oz	274	19.8	8.4	8.1	1.6	0	91	0.14	0.08	0.34	1.27
Pork Steak-Blade-Lean-Broiled 3.5 oz	225	12.4	4.4	5.6	1.1	0	93	0.41	0.01	0.04	0.97
Pork Roast Center Loin, Bone-in, Lean 3.5 oz	198	8.9	3.3	4.0	0.7	0	78	0.46	0.01	0.02	0.65
Fresh Pork Ham(Leg)-Roasted 3.5 oz	271	17.5	6.4	7.8	1.7	0	93	0.30	0.01	0.05	1.58
Organ Meats											
Beef Liver-Fried 3.5 oz	215	8.0	2.7	1.6	1.7	--	478	1.61	0	0.29	1.33
Veal Liver-Braised 3.5 oz	164	6.9	2.6	1.5	1.1	--	557	0.35	0	0.08	1.00
Lamb Liver-Braised 3.5 oz	218	8.8	3.4	1.8	1.3	0	497	0.32	0	0.12	1.19
Pork Liver-Braised 3.5 oz	164	4.4	1.4	0.6	1.0	0	352	0.57	0	0.07	0.94
Domestic Poultry											
Chicken Breast-Roasted 3.5 oz	196	7.7	2.2	3.0	1.7	--	83	0.57	0.01	0.10	1.48
Chicken Thigh-Roasted 3.5 oz	245	15.4	4.3	6.1	3.4	--	92	1.14	0.03	0.20	3.11
Turkey-White-Roasted 3.5 oz	196	8.3	2.3	2.8	2.0	--	75	--	0.01	0.13	1.80
Turkey-Dark-Roasted 3.5 oz	219	11.4	3.5	3.6	3.1	--	88	--	0.01	0.19	2.84
Goose-Roasted 3.5 oz	303	21.7	6.8	10.2	2.5	0	90	2.56	0.04	0.18	2.24
Duck-Roasted 3.5 oz	334	28.2	9.6	12.8	3.6	0	83	1.27	0.04	0.29	3.34

	Energy (kcal)	total fat,g	sat fat,g	mono fat,g	poly fat,g	trans fat,g	chol, mg	vit E, mg	lauric acid,g	omega3 fat,g	omega6 fat,g
Poultry Livers											
Chicken Livers-Simmered 3.5 oz	156	5.4	1.8	1.3	0.9	--	626	1.69	0	0.11	0.73
Turkey Livers-Simmered 3.5 oz	168	5.9	1.9	1.5	1.1	--	621	3.18	0	0.01	0.99
Goose Liver-Raw 3.5 oz	132	4.3	1.6	0.8	0.3	--	511	1.43	0	0.01	0.25
Common Game											
Deer/Venison-Roasted 3.5 oz	157	3.2	1.2	0.9	0.6	0	111	0.25	0	0.09	0.53
Elk Meat-Roasted 3.5 oz	145	1.9	0.7	0.5	0.4	0	72	0.03	0	0.06	0.34
Bison Meat-Roasted 3.5 oz	142	2.4	0.9	0.9	0.2	0	81	0.14	0	0.04	0.20
Beefalo Meat-Roasted 3.5 oz	186	6.3	2.7	2.7	0.2	0	58	0.18	0.01	0.06	0.14
Goat Meat-Roasted 3.5 oz	142	3.0	0.9	1.4	0.2	0	74	0.05	0	0.02	0.21
Wild Rabbit Meat-Stewed 3.5 oz	172	3.5	1.0	0.9	0.7	0	122	0.78	0	0.14	0.54
Squirrel Meat-Roasted 3.5 oz	172	4.6	0.8	1.3	1.4	0	120	0.74	0	0.12	1.32
Variety Meats											
Beef Salami-cooked 2oz	148	11.7	5.1	5.4	0.6		37	0.38	0.03	0.13	0.45
Pork Salami-Dry/Hard 2 oz	231	19.1	6.7	9.1	2.1		45	0.16	0	0.16	1.94
Beef Bologna 2 oz	177	16.2	6.9	8.0	0.6	0.9	33	0.28	0.02	0.14	0.48
Pork Bologna 2 oz	140	11.3	3.9	5.6	1.2		33	0.28	0.01	0.16	1.04
Liverwurst Sausage-Pork 2 oz	185	16.2	6.0	7.5	1.5	0.1	90	0.39	0	0.08	1.39
Italian Pork Sausage-Cooked 2 oz	183	14.6	5.2	6.8	1.9	0.1	44	0.18	0.03	0.25	1.61
Polish Sausage-Pork 2 oz	185	16.3	5.9	7.7	1.7	0.1	40	0.16	0.04	0.16	1.58
Pepperoni Sausage-Beef&Pork 2 oz	282	24.9	9.1	12.0	2.5	0.2	45	0.21	0	0.23	2.20

	Energy (kcal)	total fat,g	sat fat,g	mono fat,g	poly fat,g	trans fat,g	chol, mg	vit E, mg	lauric acid,g	omega3 fat,g	omega6 fat,g
Variety Meats (cont'd)											
Beef Bacon-Cured -Cooked 2 oz	255	19.5	8.2	10.0	0.9		67	0.12	0.05	0.19	0.71
Pork Bacon-Cured-Cooked 2 oz	327	27.9	9.9	13.5	3.3	0	48	0.33	0.04	0.45	2.85
Canadian Bacon-Cured-Pork 2 oz	105	4.8	1.6	2.3	0.5	0	33	0.19	0.01	0.07	0.40
Low Fat Fin Fish											
Atlantic Cod Filt-Bkd/Brld, 3.5oz	104	0.8	0.2	0.1	0.3	0	55	1.29	0	0.16	0.03
Pacific Cod Filt-Bkd/Brld, 3.5oz	104	0.8	0.1	0.1	0.3	0	47	0.34	0	0.28	0.03
Sole/Flounder Filt-Bkd/Brld, 3.5oz	116	1.5	0.4	0.2	0.6	0	67	2.28	0	0.51	0.06
Grouper Fillet-Bkd/Brld, 3.5oz	117	1.3	0.3	0.3	0.4	0	47	0.62	0	0.26	0.07
Haddock Fillet-Bkd/Brld, 3.5oz	111	0.9	0.2	0.1	0.3	0	73	1.19	0	0.24	0.04
Atl Ocean Perch Filt-BkdBrld, 3.5oz	120	2.1	0.3	0.8	0.5	0	54	1.62	0.0	0.44	0.04
Mix Spec Perch Filt-Bkd/Brld, 3.5oz	116	1.2	0.2	0.2	0.5	0	114	1.50	0	0.34	0.08
Northern Pike Filt-Bkd/Brld, 3.5oz	112	0.9	0.1	0.2	0.3	0	50	0.24	0.0	0.16	0.08
Walleye Pike Filt-Bkd/Brld, 3.5oz	118	1.5	0.3	0.4	0.6	0	109	0.29	0	0.41	0.11
Sea Bass Filt-Mix-Bkd/Brld, 3.5oz	123	2.5	0.6	0.5	0.9	0	53	0.62	0	0.76	0.03
Snapper Filt-Mxd-Bkd/Brld, 3.5oz	127	1.7	0.4	0.3	0.6	0	47	0.82	0	0.32	0.07
Skipjack Tuna Filt-Bkd/Brld, 3.5oz	131	1.3	0.4	0.2	0.4	0	60	1.25		0.33	0.05
Whiting Filt-Mxd-Bkd/Brld, 3.5oz	115	1.7	0.4	0.4	0.6	0	83	0.38	0	0.53	0.04
Medium Fat Fin Fish											
FreshwaterBassFilt-Bkd/Brld, 3.5oz	145	4.7	1.0	1.8	1.3	0	86	0.99	0	0.90	0.29
Striped Bass Filt-Bkd/Brld, 3.5oz	123	3.0	0.6	0.8	1.0	0	102	0.60	0	0.88	0.08
Bluefish Fillet-Bkd/Brld, 3.5oz	158	5.4	1.2	2.3	1.3	0	75	0.99	0	0.82	0.06

	Energy (kcal)	total fat,g	sat fat,g	mono fat,g	poly fat,g	trans fat,g	chol, mg	vit E, mg	lauric acid,g	omega3 fat,g	omega6 fat,g
Carp Fillet-Fish-Bk/Br, 3.5oz	161	7.1	1.4	3.0	1.8	0	83	1.06	0.05	0.79	0.85
Channel Catfish-Wild-Bk/Br, 3.5oz	104	2.8	0.7	1.1	0.6	0	71	-	0	0.33	0.23
Farm Channel Catfish-Bk/Br, 3.5oz	151	8.0	1.8	4.1	1.4	0	64	1.31	0	0.24	1.01
Atlantic Croaker Fillet-Raw, 3.5oz	103	3.1	1.1	1.1	0.5	0	61	0.99	0	0.23	0.14
Atl/Pac HalibutFillet-Bk/Br, 3.5oz	130	2.9	0.4	1.0	0.9	0	41	0.99	0	0.55	0.22
Atl Herring Fillet-Bk/Br, 3.5oz	201	11.5	2.6	4.8	2.7	0	76	1.33	0.01	2.13	0.24
Pickled Atlantic Herring-Piece, 20g	52	3.6	0.5	2.4	0.3	0	3	0.32	0	0.28	0.04
King Mackerel Fillet-Bk/Br, 3.5oz	133	2.5	0.5	1.0	0.6	0	67	1.72	0.00	0.39	0.08
Spanish Mackerel Fil-Bk/Br, 3.5oz	157	6.3	1.8	2.1	1.8	0	72	1.14	0.01	1.33	0.26
Striped Mullet Fillet-Bk/Br, 3.5oz	149	4.8	1.4	1.4	0.9	0	62	1.21	0.00	0.36	0.19
Atl Salmon Fil-Wild-Bk/Br, 3.5oz	181	8.1	1.2	2.7	3.2	0	70	1.25	–	2.20	0.56
Sockeye Salmon-Can-Draind, 3.5oz	152	7.3	1.6	3.1	1.9	0	44	1.59	0	1.24	0.45
Pink Salmon Fillet-Bk/Br, 3.5oz	148	4.4	0.7	1.2	1.7	0	66	1.25	0	1.32	0.16
Chum Salmon-Canned-Drnd,3.5oz	140	5.5	1.5	1.9	1.5	0	39	1.59	0	1.21	0.13
Seatrout Fillet-Mix-Bk/Br, 3.5oz	132	4.6	1.3	1.1	0.9	0	105	0.25	0	0.48	0.33
Rainbow Smelt-Bk/Br, 3.5oz	123	3.1	0.6	0.8	1.1	0	89	0.62	0.00	0.94	0.13
Swordfish-Bk/Br, 3.5oz	154	5.1	1.4	2.0	1.2	0	50	0.62	0	1.08	0.12
Fresh Bluefin Tuna-Bk/Br, 3.5oz	183	6.2	1.6	2.0	1.8	0	49	1.25	0	1.49	0.12
Light Tuna/Water-Can-Drnd, 165g	191	1.4	0.4	0.3	0.6	0	50	0.87	0	0.45	0.07
White Tuna/Water-Can-Drnd, 172g	220	5.1	1.4	1.3	1.9	0	72	2.73	0	1.60	0.18
Whitefish Fillet-Mx-Bk/Br, 3.5oz	171	7.4	1.2	2.5	2.7	0	76	0.25	0	1.84	0.63

Higher Fat Fin Fish

	Energy (kcal)	total fat,g	sat fat,g	mono fat,g	poly fat,g	trans fat,g	chol, mg	vit E, mg	lauric acid,g	omega3 fat,g	omega6 fat,g
Pacific Herring Fillet-Bk/Br, 3.5oz	248	17.7	4.1	8.7	3.1	0	98	1.29	0.02	2.18	0.37
Atlantic Mackerel Fil-Bk/Br, 3.5oz	260	17.7	4.1	7.0	4.3	0	74	1.84	0.02	1.30	0.20

	Energy (kcal)	total fat,g	sat fat,g	mono fat,g	poly fat,g	trans fat,g	chol, mg	vit E, mg	lauric acid,g	omega3 fat,g	omega6 fat,g
Higher Fat Fin Fish (Cont'd)											
Pac/Jack Mackerel Fil-Bk/Br,3.5oz	199	10.0	2.9	3.3	2.5	0	60	1.70	0.01	1.90	0.25
Sablefish Fillet-Bk/Br, 3.5oz	248	19.4	4.1	10.2	2.6	0	62	0.62	0.01	1.89	0.34
Sockeye Salmon Filt-Bk/Br, 3.5oz	214	10.9	1.9	5.2	2.4	0	86	1.25	0	1.28	0.14
Chinook Salmon Fil-Bk/Br, 3.5oz	229	13.3	3.2	5.7	2.6	0	84	1.70	0	1.83	0.33
Farm Atl Salmon Fil-Bk/Br, 3.5oz	204	12.3	2.5	4.4	4.4	0	62	0.88	0	2.14	1.83
Fish Eggs											
Roe-Mixed Species-Bkd/Brld, 3.5oz	202	8.2	1.9	2.1	3.4	0	475	8.43	0	2.99	0.27
Sturgeon Roe, 3.5oz	250	17.8	4.0	4.6	7.4	0	583	6.95	0	6.51	0.58
Crustaceans and Mollusks											
AlaskaKingCrab Leg-Stm, 134g	130	2.1	0.2	0.2	0.7	0	71	1.21	0.00	0.57	0.08
Blue Crab-Steamed/Boiled, 48g	49	0.8	0.1	0.1	0.3	0	48	0.48	0	0.24	0.05
WholeDungenessCrab-Stm, 127g	140	1.6	0.2	0.3	0.5	0	96	1.54	0	0.50	0
Blue Crab Cakes, each, 60g	93	4.5	0.9	1.7	1.4	—	90	0.90	0	0.32	1.00
Northern Lobster-Stm/Boil, 3.5oz	97	0.6	0.1	0.2	0.1	0	71	1.44	0	0.08	0.00
Dried Octopus-Cooked, 3.5oz	182	2.7	0.7	0.2	1.0	0	460	2.37	0	0.68	0.21
Octopus-Steamed/Boiled, 3.5oz	163	2.1	0.4	0.3	0.5	0	95	2.28	0	0.31	0.10
Prawns/Lg Shrimp-Stmd/Boil,3.5oz	98	1.1	0.3	0.2	0.4	0	193	0.74	0	0.32	0.09
Small Shrimp-Mix-Stmd/Boil,3.5oz	98	1.1	0.3	0.2	0.4	0	193	0.74	0	0.32	0.09
Squid/Calamari-Baked, 3.5oz	137	4.7	1.0	1.5	1.6	0	279	1.91	–	–	–
Large Clams-Mix-Stmd/Boil, 3.5oz	147	1.9	0.2	0.2	0.5	0	66	1.94	0	0.29	0.11
Blue Mussels-Steam/Boil, 3.5oz	171	4.4	0.8	1.0	1.2	0	56	1.44	0	0.82	0.17
EastOysters-Wld-Stmd-Md, 3.5oz	136	4.9	1.5	0.6	1.9	0	104	1.59	0	1.21	0.27

	Energy (kcal)	total fat,g	sat fat,g	mono fat,g	poly fat,g	trans fat,g	chol, mg	vit E, mg	lauric acid,g	omega3 fat,g	omega6 fat,g
PacOysters-Stmd/Boil-Med, 3.5oz	162	4.6	1.0	0.7	1.8	0	99	1.76	0	1.43	0.14
Scallops-Steamed/Boiled, 3.5oz	106	3.1	0.5	1.1	1.0	0	32	1.34	0	0.77	0.10
Popular Seeds											
Chia Seeds-dried 0.5 oz	67	3.7	0.5	1.0	1.0	0	0	—	0	0.55	0.46
Flax Seeds 2 tbs	95	6.9	0.6	1.3	4.3	0	0	0.97	0	3.51	0.84
Dry Pumpkin Seeds 2 tbs	93	7.9	1.5	2.5	3.6	0	0	1.88	0.01	0.03	3.57
Popular Nuts											
Dried Acorn Nuts 1 oz	144	8.9	1.2	5.6	1.7	0	0	—	0	0	1.72
Dried Almond Nuts -2 tbs	105	9.3	0.9	6.0	1.9	0	0	4.35	0.00	0.07	1.86
Dried Brazilnuts-shelled 2 tbs	115	11.6	2.8	4.0	4.2	0	0	1.35	0	0.01	4.16
Dried Butternuts 0.5 oz	87	8.1	0.2	1.5	6.0	0	0	0.50	0	1.24	4.78
Dry Roasted Cashew Nuts-2 tbs	98	7.9	1.6	4.7	1.3	0	0	1.88	0.13	0.03	1.31
Fresh Coconut-shredded 0.5 cup	142	13.4	12.0	0.6	0.1	0	0	0.25	5.96	0	0.15
Dried Coconut-0.5 cup(unsweet)	257	25.2	22.5	1.1	0.3	0	0	0.53	11.15	0	0.28
Coconut Milk-canned 0.5 cup	223	24.1	21.6	1.0	0.3	0	0	0.73	10.69	0	0.26
Filberts/Hazelnuts-chpd 2 tbs	91	9.0	0.7	7.1	0.9	0	0	3.44	0	0.02	0.84
Dried Macadamia Nuts 2 tbs	118	12.3	1.8	9.7	0.2	0	0	0.07	0	0	0.21
Dried Pecans-2 tbs	99	10.0	0.8	6.3	2.5	0	0	0.47	0	0.10	2.38
Dried Pine Nuts (Pignolia) 2 tbs	96	8.6	1.3	3.2	3.6	0	0	0.60	0	0.11	3.51
Dried Pistachio Nuts 2 tbs	92	7.7	1.0	5.2	1.2	0	0	0.82	0	0.04	1.12
Black Walnuts-chpd 2 tbs	95	8.8	0.6	2.0	5.9	0	0	0.41	0	0.52	5.23
English Walnuts-chpd 2 tbs	96	9.3	0.9	2.1	5.9	0	0	2.94	0	1.02	4.77

	Energy (kcal)	total fat,g	sat fat,g	mono fat,g	poly fat,g	trans fat,g	chol, mg	vit E, mg	lauric acid,g	omega3 fat,g	omega6 fat,g
Nut Butters											
Peanut Butter-smooth 2tbs	190	16.3	3.3	7.8	4.4	–	0	3.20	0.01	0.02	4.38
Almond Butter-plain 2tbs	203	18.9	1.8	12.3	4.0	0	0	7.68	0.00	0.14	3.81
Cashew Butter 2tbs	188	15.8	3.1	9.3	2.7	0	0	0.50	0.26	0.05	2.61
Sunflower Seed Butter 2tbs	185	15.3	1.6	2.9	10.1	0	0	15.36	0	0.02	10.05
Sesame Butter (Tahini) 2tbs	190	16.3	2.3	6.1	7.1	0	0	0.73	0	0.12	7.01
Vegetables and Beans (total fat > 1 gram per typical serving)											
Tomatoes-boiled 1 cup	65	1.0	0.1	0.2	0.4	0	0	2.76	0	0.01	0.39
Soybeans- green- boiled 0.5 cup	127	5.8	0.7	1.1	2.7	0	0	0.01	0	0.32	2.39
Avocado-Calif-pureed-1 cup	407	39.8	6.0	25.8	4.7	0	0	3.08	0	0.26	4.43
Avocado-Florida-pureed-1 cup	258	20.4	4.0	11.2	3.4	0	0	3.08	0	0.20	3.21

– no data available

Data in the above tables are from ESHA Food Processor and U.S.D.A. Handbook 8.

APPENDIX D

Tables

Table D.1   Composition of Fats And Oils: Fatty Acid Classes in Food Fats Ranked by Long-chain Saturates

Typical "Animal" Fats (Unhydrogenated)	%Sat	%Mono	%Poly
Lamb tallow	58	38	2
Beef tallow	49-54	42-48	3-4
Butter	14* + 52	30	4
Human milk fat	48	33	16
Lard	44	45	11
Prawns	43	25	29
Tuna	41	28	30
Chicken fat	30-32	48-50	18-23
Calf bone marrow	31	63	6
Salmon	17-28	37-49	23-45
Sardines	30	26	42
Herring	20	59	16

Typical "Vegetable" Fats (Unhydrogenated)			
Cocoa butter	60	38	2
Palm oil	49	40	10
Cottonseed oil	29	18	52
Coconut oil	63* +28	6	3
Palm kernel oil	56* +27	18	1
Peanut oil	16	56	26
Olive oil	15	73	10
Soybean oil	15	22	62
Corn oil	14	27	59
Sunflower seed oil	13	18	69
Safflower oil	9	11	80
High Oleic Safflower oil	9	80	11
Canola oil (low erucic acid rapeseed)	7	65	28

* Short and medium chain fatty acids 12 carbons and less, caloric content and metabolism of the shortest (C6, C8 and C10) is closer to carbohydrates.

Table D.1 (Continued)

Typical Hydrogenated Vegetable Fats

	%Sat	%Mono	%Poly
Hard (stick) margarines			
(A)	39	51**	10**
(B)	18	65**	17**
Soft (tub) margarines			
(A)	31	53**	16**
(B)	23	55**	22**
Vegetable shortenings			
(A)	22-32	22-33**	44-55**
(B)	15-40	45-76**	2-30**

Sat = saturated; Mono = monounsaturated; Poly = polyunsaturated

** Contains *trans* fatty acids, which cannot properly be termed monounsaturated or polyunsaturated for purposes of labeling, but which are chemically monounsaturated or polyunsaturated.

Data from Food Fats and Oils, Institute of Shortening and Edible Oils, Inc. August 1974; Nutrition Quarterly, September 1977; Masson, L., *Journal of the American Oil Chemists' Society* 58:249-255 (1981); Egan *et al, Pearson's Chemical Analysis of Foods*, 8th Edition, 1981; Enig *et al, Journal of the American Oil Chemists' Society* 60:1788-1795 (1983).

Table D.2　　**Composition and Sources of the Most Common Dietary Fatty Acids**

Fatty Acid	Carbon Length	Saturation[1,2,3]	Most Common Food Sources
Butyric	4	Saturated	Butter (~4%)
Caproic	6	Saturated	Butter (~2%), coconut and palm kernel oils (<1%)
Caprylic	8	Saturated	Coconut (8%) and palm kernel (4%) oils, butter (1%)
Capric	10	Saturated	Coconut and palm kernel oils (4-6%), butter (2%)
Lauric	12	Saturated	Coconut and palm kernel oils (48-50%), butter (3%)
Myristic	14	Saturated	Nutmeg butter (87%), coconut and palm kernel oils (16-18%), butter (12%), animal tallows (3-5%)
Palmitic	16	Saturated	Palm oil (45%), cocoa butter (25%), chicken fat (23%), butterfat (26%), animal tallows (~25%), cottonseed oil (25%), other temperate seed oils (~10-12%)
Palmitoleic	16	Monounsaturated *cis* $\Delta 7$, *cis* $\Delta 9$	Marine animal oils, chicken fat, ruminant tallows, lard, butterfat, olive oil
Stearic	18	Saturated	Cocoa butter (35%), animal tallows (20-25%), butterfat and lard (12.5%), chicken fat (6%), seed oils (2-5%)

Table D.2   (Continued)

Fatty Acid	Carbon Length	Saturation[1,2,3]	Most Common Food Sources
Oleic (omega-9)	18	Monounsaturated *cis* Δ9	All animal and vegetable fats and oils; olive (~70%), hybrid safflower and sunflower (~80%), canola (~64%), animal tallows and butterfat (30-50%), peanut oil (~50%), palm oil (40%), other temperate seed oils (15-30%)
Vaccenic (omega-7)	18	Monounsaturated *cis* Δ11	All animal/vegetable fats and oils in small amounts
Oleic" isomers	18	Monounsaturated *cis* Δ4-8, Δ10, Δ12-16	Partially hydrogenated vegetable fats and oils (6-10%)
Elaidic	18	Monounsaturated *trans* Δ9	Partially hydrogenated vegetable fats and oils (2-6%)
trans Vaccenic	18	Monounsaturated *trans* Δ11	Ruminant fats (1-4%), and partially hydrogenated vegetable and marine fats and oils (3-10%)
"Elaidic" isomers	18	Monounsaturated *trans* Δ4-8, Δ10, Δ12-16	Partially hydrogenated vegetable and marine fats and oils (10-50%)
Linoleic (omega-6)	18	Diunsaturated *cis* Δ9,12	All vegetable and animal fats and oils (2-80%); safflower oil (80%), sunflower oil (68%), corn oil (57%), soybean and cottonseed oil (53%), peanut oil (46%), lard, olive, and palm oil (10%), animal tallows and butterfat (2-4%)

Table D.2   (Continued)

Fatty Acid Sources	Carbon Length	Saturation[1,2,3]	Most Common Food
Linoleic isomers	18	Diunsaturated *cis* Δ8,12	Partially hydrogenated vegetable and marine oils
"Linolelaidic" isomers	18	Diunsaturated *trans,trans; cis,trans; trans,cis;* Δ9,11; 9,12; 9,13; 9,14; 9,15; 10,15; 8,12	Partially hydrogenated vegetable and marine oils
Linolenic (α) (omega-3)	18	Triunsaturated *cis* Δ9,12,15	Soybean and rapeseed oils (7-10%), flax seed oil, purslane
Linolenic (γ) (omega-6)	18	Triunsaturated *cis* Δ6,9,12	Evening primrose oil (9%), black current seed oil (15-19%), borage oil (~20%), and animal fats
Stearidonic (omega-3)	18	Tetraunsaturated *cis* Δ6,9,12,15	Black current seed oil (2-3%), some fish oils (1-2%)
Arachidic	20	Saturated	Peanut oil
Gadoleic and Gondoic	20	Monounsaturated *cis* Δ9, Δ11	Rapeseed oil, fish oils (unhydrogenated)
Gadoleic isomers	20	Monounsaturated Δ? *trans* and *cis*	Partially hydrogenated fish oils
Arachidonic (omega-6)	20	Tetraunsaturated *cis* Δ5,8,11,14	Lard and other animal and fish fats
Eicosapentanoic (EPA)(omega-3)	20	Pentaunsaturated *cis* Δ5,8,11,14,17	Fish oils (unhydrogenated) and some animal tissues
Timnodonic isomer of EPA	20	Pentaunsaturated *cis* Δ4,8,12,15,18	?Fish oils

Table D.2   (Continued)

Fatty Acid	Carbon Length	Saturation[1,2,3]	Most Common Food Sources
Behenic	22	Saturated	Peanut oil, Caprenin[4]
Cetoleic	22	Monounsaturated *cis* Δ11	Fish oils (unhydrogenated)
Erucic	22	Monounsaturated *cis* Δ13	Rapeseed oil
Erucic isomers	22	Monounsaturated Δ? *trans* and *cis*	Partially hydrogenated fish and rapeseed oils
Docosapentaenoic (DPA)(omega-3)	22	Pentaunsaturated *cis* Δ7,10,13,16,19	Fish oils
Docosahexaenoic (DHA)(omega-3) (Cervonic)	22	Hexaunsaturated *cis* Δ4,7,10,13,16,19	Fish oils (unhydrogenated)
Lignoceric	24	Saturated	Peanut oil
Nervonic	24	Monounsaturated *cis* Δ15	Honesty seed oil, (animal nerve tissue, eg, brain)
Nisinic (omega-3)	24	Hexaunsaturated *cis* Δ6,9,12,15,18,21	Fish oils
Cerotic	26	Saturated	Plant and insect waxes
Montanic	28	Saturated	Plant waxes
Melissic	30	Saturated	Waxes

[1] Saturated = no double bonds
[2] Monounsaturated = one double bond
[3] Di = two double bonds, tri = three, tetra = four, penta = five, and hexa = six; these are commonly categorized as "polyunsaturated" fatty acids
[4] Structured lipid manufactured by The Procter & Gamble Co.

Table D.3　　Fatty Acid Nomenclature: Common, Systematic, and
　　　　　　　Shorthand Names; Molecular Weights of the Most
　　　　　　　Common Dietary Fatty Acids

Common Name	Systematic Name	Shorthand Name	Molecular Weight
Butyric	butanoic	4:0	88.108
Caproic	hexanoic	6:0	116.162
Caprylic	octanoic	8:0	144.216
Capric	decanoic	10:0	172.270
Lauric	dodecanoic	12:0	200.324
Myristic	tetradecanoic	14:0	228.378
Palmitic	hexadecanoic	16:0	256.432
Palmitoleic	*cis*-9-hexadecenoic *cis*-7-hexadecenoic	16:1	254.432
Stearic	octadecanoic	18:0	284.486
Oleic	*cis*-9-octadecenoic	c18:1	282.486
Vaccenic	*cis*-11-octadecenoic	c18:1	282.486
"Oleic" isomers	*cis*-5...8,10-octadecenoic *cis*-12...16-octadecenoic	c18:1	282.486
Elaidic	*trans*-9-octadecenoic	t18:1	282.486
trans Vaccenic	*trans*-11-octadecenoic	t18:1	282.486
"Elaidic" isomers	*trans*-4...8,10-octadecenoic *trans*-12...16-octadecenoic	t18:1	282.486
Linoleic	*cis*-9,*cis*-12-octadecadienoic	18:2	280.486
Linoleic isomers	*cis*-8,*cis*-12-octadecadienoic	18:2	280.486

Table D.3 · (Continued)

Common Name	Systematic Name	Shorthand Name	Molecular Weight
"Linolelaidic"	*trans*-9,*trans*-12-octadecadienoic *cis*-9,*trans*-12-octadecadienoic; *trans*,9,*cis*-12-octadecadienoic; *trans*-9,*trans*-11-octadecadienoic; also 8,12; 9,13; 9,14; 9,15; 10,15; etc. isomers	18:2	280.486
Linolenic (α)	*cis*-9,*cis*-12, *cis*-15-octadecatrienoic	18:3	278.486
Linolenic (γ)	*cis*-6,*cis*-9,*cis*-12-octadecatrienoic	18:3	278.486
Stearidonic	*cis*-6,*cis*-9,*cis*-12,*cis*-15-octadecatetraenoic	18:4	276.486
Arachidic	eicosanoic	20:0	312.540
Gadoleic and Godonic	*cis*-9-eicosenoic *cis*-11-eicosenoic	20:1	310.540
Gadoleic isomers	*trans*-? or *cis*-?-eicosenoic	20:1	310.540
Arachidonic	*cis*-5,*cis*-8,*cis*-11,*cis*-14-eicosatetraenoic	20:4	304.540
Eicosapentanoic (EPA)	*cis*-5,*cis*-8,*cis*-11,*cis*-14,*cis*-17-eicosapentaenoic	20:5	302.540
Behenic	docosanoic	22:0	340.594
Cetoleic	*cis*-11-docosaenoic		
Erucic	*cis*-13-docosaenoic	22:1	338.594
Erucic isomers	*trans*-? or *cis*-?-docosaenoic	22:1	338.594
Docosapentanoic	*cis*-7,*cis*-10,*cis*-13,*cis*-13, *cis*-19-docosapentaenoic	22:5	330.5
Docosahexanoic (DHA)	*cis*-4,*cis*-7,*cis*-10,*cis*-13,*cis*-16, *cis*-19- docosahexaenoic	22:6	328.594
Lignoceric	tetracosanoic	24:0	368.648
Nervonic	cis-15-tetracosenoic	24:1	370.7
Nisinic	*cis*-6,*cis*-9,*cis*-12,*cis*-15-*cis*-18,*cis*-21-tetracosahexaenoic	24:6	360.6

Table D.3   (Continued)

Common Name	Systematic Name	Shorthand Name	Molecular Weight
Cerotic	n-hexacosanoic	26:0	396.7
Montanic	n-octacosanoic	28:0	424.7
Melissic	triacontanoic	30:0	452.8

Table D.4   Melting Points* of the Most Common Fatty Acids

Saturated Fatty Acids	Melting Point °C/°F
Butyric	-8/17.6
Caproic	-3.3/25.9
Caprylic	12.7-16.7/54.9-62.1
Capric	29.6-31.6/85.3-88.9
Lauric	42.2-44.8/108.0-112.6
Myristic	52.1-54.4/125.8-129.9
Palmitic	60.7-62.9/141.3-145.6
Stearic	69.6-70.1/157.3-158.2
Arachidic	75.4-76.1/167.7-169.0
Behenic	80.0/176.0
Lignoceric	84.2/183.6
Cerotic	87.7/189.9
Montanic	90.0/194.0
Melissic	93.6/200.5

Monounsaturated Fatty Acids	
Palmitoleic	0-1/32.0-33.8
Oleic	16.0-16.3/60.8-61.3
Vaccenic (cis)	15.0/59.0
Gadoleic and Godonic	~24.0-25.0/75.2-77.0
Erucic	34.7/94.5
Nervonic	43.0/109.4

Polyunsaturated Fatty Acids	
Linoleic	-5.0/23.0
Linolenic (α)	-11.0/12.2
Arachidonic	-49.5/-57.1

Trans Fatty Acids	
Elaidic (*trans* Δ9)	45.0/113.0
Vaccenic (*trans* Δ11)	44.0/111.2
CLA	22.0/71.6

* Different sources use different values; the values in this table are given as single values when only one value is in most of the literature, as an average value when two values that are almost identical are given, and as ranges when there are several different values in the analytical references. (The reasons for varying values may sometimes be related to different forms of the fatty acids (e.g., β) or impurities in the sample.)

Table D.5   Selected Web Sites for Fats and Oils Information

Government*

U.S. Department of Agriculture   www.usda.gov
U.S. Food and Drug Administration   www.fda.gov
National Institutes of Health   www.nih.gov
* search for "fats and oils" in search boxes

Informational

Trans Fat Alert   www.transfatalert.com

Nonprofit

American Oil Chemist Society   www.aocs.org
Celiac Disease Foundation   www.celiac.org
Center for Research on Lauric Oils, Inc. www.lauric.org
International Food Information Council   www.ific.net
Weston A. Price Foundation   www.westonaprice.org

Trade Associations

American Meat Institute   www.meatami.org
American Soybean Association   www.oilseeds.org
Canola Council of Canada   www.canola.org.
Corn Refiners Association   www.corn.org
National Association of Margarine
          Manufacturers   www.margarine.org
National Cottonseed Products
          Association   www.cottonseed.com
National Dairy Council   www.ndc.org
National Milk Producers Federation   www.nmpf.org

The above web sites include some of the better known sites from the
food industry and government sources

CHAPTER NOTES

Notes to Chapter 1.

Selected Texts

Bailey's Industrial Oil & Fat Products, 5th Edition (ed: YH Hui) John Wiley & Sons, Inc. New York. 1996. (The 5 volume set sells for $895)

G.J. Brisson. *Lipids in Human Nutrition: An Appraisal of Some Dietary Concepts.* Jack K. Burgess, Inc. Englewood, NJ, 1981. (This book may be out of print, but it should be available in most large libraries that carry medical books.)

M.I. Gurr & J.L. Harwood, *Lipid Biochemistry: An Introduction, 4th Edition,* Chapman and Hall, 1990. (If this text is not available, the 2nd (1975) or 3rd edition (authors are MI Gurr & AT James) may be around. They are also published by Chapman and Hall.)

J.M. deMan. Chapter 2, Lipids, in *Principles of Food Chemistry*, 2nd Edition. AVI Van Nostrand Reinhold, New York, 1990.

The Role of Fats in Human Nutrition, 2nd Edition, (A.J. Vergroesen, M. Crawford, eds.) Academic Press, 1989.

M.C. Linder, *Nutritional Biochemistry and Metabolism with Clinical Applications*, Elsevier, 1985; 2nd Edition, Appleton & Lange, Norwalk CT, 1991.

Fatty Acids in Food and Their Health Implications, (C.K. Chow, ed.), Marcel Dekker, Inc. 1992. (37 chapters)

Trans Fatty Acids in Human Nutrition (J.L. Sebedio and W.W. Christie, eds) Volume 9 in the Oil Press Lipid Library. The Oily Press, Dundee, Scotland, 1998

CE Stauffer, *Fats and Oils*, Eagan Press Handbook Series, Eagan Press, St. Paul MN, 1996.

Selected Journals/Series References

Chin SF, Liu W, Storkson JM, Ha YL, Pariza MW. 1992. Dietary sources of conjugated dienoic isomers of linoleic acid, a newly recognized class of anticarcinogens. *Journal of Food Composition and Analysis* 5:185-197.

Enig, M.G., Pallansch, L.A., Sampugna, J. and Keeney, M. 1983. "Fatty Acid Composition of Fat of Selected Food Items with Emphasis on *Trans* Components." *Journal of the American Oil Chemists Society.* 60:1788-1795.

Enig, M.G., Budowski, P. and Blondheim, S.H. 1984. "*Trans* Unsaturated Fatty Acids in Margarines and Human Subcutaneous Fat in Israel." *Human Nutrition: Clinical Nutrition.* 38C:223-230.

Enig, M.G., Atal, S., Keeney, M. and Sampugna, J. 1990. "Isomeric *Trans* Fatty Acids in the U.S. Diet." *Journal of the American College of Nutrition*. 9:471-486.

Enig, M.G., Atal, S., Keeney, M. and Sampugna, J. "Responses to: Drs. Applewhite and Hunter; Drs. De Villiers, Grundy, Holub, and Kummerow; Dr. Katan" 1991. *Journal of the American College of Nutrition* 10:512-514, 517-518, 519-521.

Enig, M.G. 1992. "Products of Partial Hydrogenation of Vegetable Oils." *Food Safety Notebook* 3:41-42.

Enig, M.G. 1993. Research Review: Trans Fatty Acids - An Update. *Nutrition Quarterly* 17(4): 79-95.

Enig, M.G. 1996. Trans Fatty Acids in Diets and Data Bases. *Cereal Foods World* 41(2):58-63.

Hodgson JM, Wahlqvist ML, Boxall JA, and Balazs ND. 1993. Can linoleic acid contribute to coronary artery disease? *American Journal of Clinical Nutrition* 58:228-234.

Kinsella, J.E. Food lipids and fatty acids: importance in food quality, nutrition, and health. The 1988 W.O. Atwater Memorial Lecture, *Food Technology*. October 1988.

Ratnayake, W.M.N., Hollywood, R., O'Grady, E. and Pelletier, G. 1993. Fatty Acids in Some Common Food Items in Canada. *Journal of the American College of Nutrition* 12:651-660.

Sampugna, J., Pallansch, L.A., Enig, M.G., Keeney, M. 1982. Rapid analysis of *trans* fatty acids on SP-2340 Glass capillary columns. *Journal of Chromatography* 249:245-255.

Smith, L.M., Dunkley, W.L, Franke, A., and Dairiki, T. 1978. Measurement of *trans* and other isomeric unsaturated fatty acids in butter and margarine. *Journal of the American Oil Chemists Society* 55:257-261.

Wahle, K.W.J. and James W.P.T. 1993. Isomeric fatty acids and human health. *European Journal of Clinical Nutrition* 47:828-839.

Wood, R. 1983. Geometrical and positional monoene isomers in beef and several processed meats. In: *Dietary Fats and Health* E.G. Perkins and W.J. Visek (Eds.) p. 341-358. American Oil Chemists' Society, Champaign, IL.

Notes to Chapter 2.

General texts

Coronary Heart Disease: The Dietary Sense and Nonsense. GV Mann, ed. Janus Publishing, London, 1993. (Proceedings of the Veritas Society,)

E.R. Pinckney & C. Pinckney, *The Cholesterol Controversy*, Sherbourne Press, Los Angeles CA, 1973.

Principles of Biochemistry, 2nd Edition, A.L. Lehninger, D.L. Nelson, M.M. Cox, Worth Publishers, New York, 1993.

R.L. Smith. *The Cholesterol Conspiracy*. Warren H. Green, Inc. St. Louis MO, 1991.

Textbook of Biochemistry with Clinical Applications, 2nd Edition, T.M. Devlin, ed. A Wiley Medical Publication, John Wiley and Sons, New York, 1986.

Selected Journals/Series Articles

Alam SQ et al. 1989. Effect of dietary trans fatty acids on some membrane-associated enzymes and receptors in rat heart. *Lipids* 24:39-44.

Clevidence BA, Judd JT, Schaefer EJ, Jenner JL, Lichtenstein AH, Muesing RA, Wittes J, Sunkin ME. 1997. Plasma lipoprotein (a) levels in men and women consuming diets enriched in saturated, cis-, or trans-monounsaturated fatty acids. *Arterioscler Thromb Vasc Biol* 17:1657-1661.

Devi MA and Das NP. 1994 Antiproliferative effect of polyunsaturated fatty acids and interleukin- 2 on normal and abnormal human lymphocytes. *Experientia* 15;50(5):489-92.

Enig, M.G. "Diet, Serum Cholesterol, and Coronary Heart Disease." Chapter 3 in the *Coronary Heart Disease--The Dietary Sense and Nonsense* (Ed. GV Mann). (Proceedings of the Veritas Society Meeting, Washington, D.C. 13 November 1991). Janus Press, London, 1993 pp 36-60.

Enig, M.G. 1993. Research Review: Trans Fatty Acids - An Update. *Nutrition Quarterly* 17(4): 79-95.

Enig, M.G., Budowski, P. and Blondheim, S.H. 1984. "*Trans* Unsaturated Fatty Acids in Margarines and Human Subcutaneous Fat in Israel." *Human Nutrition:Clinical Nutrition*. 38C:223-230.

Ewertz, M. and Gill, C. 1990. Dietary factors and breast-cancer risk in Denmark. *International Journal of Cancer* 46:779-784.

Gurr, M.I. 1983. *Trans*-fatty acids: metabolic and nutritional significance. International Dairy Federation Bulletin, Document 166. pages 5-18.

Hanis, T., Zedik, V., Sachova, J., et al. 1989. Effects of dietary *trans*-fatty acids on reproductive performance of Wistar rats. *British Journal of Nutrition* 61:519-529.

Hodgson JM, Wahlqvist ML, Boxall JA, and Balazs ND. 1993. Can linoleic acid contribute to coronary artery disease? *American Journal of Clinical Nutrition* 58:228-234.

Hogan, M.L. and Shamsuddin, A.M. 1984. Large intestinal carcinogenesis. I. Promotional effect of dietary fatty acid isomers in the rat model. *Journal of the National Cancer Institute* 73:1293-1296.

Hopewell JW, Robbins ME, van den Aardweg GJ, Morris GM, Ross GA, Whitehouse E, Horrobin DF, Scott CA. 1993. The modulation of radiation-induced damage to pig skin by essential fatty acids. *British Journal of Cancer* 68(1):1-7.

Hunter, J.E. and Applewhite, T.H. 1986. Isomeric fatty acids in the US diet: levels and health perspectives. *American Journal of Clinical Nutrition* 44:707-717.

Jones, D. 1993. *Trans* fatty acids and dieting (Letter) *Lancet* 341:1093

Jones, P.J.H.. 1997. Regulation of cholesterol biosynthesis by diet in humans, *American Journal of Clinical Nutrition* 66:438-446.

Judd, J.T., Clevidence, B.A., Muesing, R.A., Wittes, J., Sunkin, M.E., and Podczasy, J.J. 1996. Dietary *Trans* Fatty Acids: Effects on Plasma Lipids and Lipoproteins of Healthy Men and Women. *American Journal of Clinical Nutrition* 59:861-868.

Khosla, P. and Hayes, K.C. 1996. Dietary Trans-Monounsaturated Fatty Acids Negatively Impact Plasma Lipids in Humans: Critical Review of the Evidence. *Journal of the American College of Nutrition* 15:325-339.

Koletzko, B. and M:uller, J. 1990. *Cis-* and *trans*-isomeric fatty acids in plasma lipids of newborn infants and their mothers. *Biology of the Neonate* 57:172-178.

Koletzko, B. 1991. Supply, metabolism and biological effects of *trans*-isomeric fatty acids in infants. *Die Nahrung* 35:229-283.

Koletzko, B. 1992. *Trans* fatty acids may impair biosynthesis of long-chain polyunsaturates and growth in man. *Acta Paediatrica* 81:302-306.

Kuller, L.H. 1993. *Trans* fatty acids and dieting (Letter) *Lancet* 341:1093-1094.

Kummerow, F.A., Zhou, Q., Mahfouz, M.M. 1999. Effect of trans fatty acids on calcium influx into human arterial endothelial cells. *American Journal of Clinical Nutrition* 70(5):832-838.

Kummerow, F.A. 1979. Effects of isomeric fats on animal tissue, lipid classes, and atherosclerosis. In: *Geometrical and Positional Fatty Acid Isomers*. E.A. Emken and H.J. Dutton (Eds.) p. 151-180. American Oil Chemists' Society, Champaign, IL.

Lagrost, L. 1992. Differential effects of *cis* and *trans* fatty acid isomers, oleic and elaidic acids, on the cholesteryl ester transfer protein activity. *Biochimica Biophysica Acta* 1124:159-162.

Lawson, L.D. and Kummerow, F.A. 1979. β-oxidation of the coenzyme A esters of vaccenic, elaidic, and petroselaidic acids by rat heart mitochondria. *Lipids* 14:501-503.

Mantey, S. 1985. The effect of *trans* fatty acids on some murine T and B cell functions. Master's Thesis, University of Maryland, College Park, MD.

Mensink, R.P. and Katan, M.B. 1990. Effect of dietary *trans* fatty acids on high-density and low-density lipoprotein cholesterol levels in healthy subjects. *New England Journal of Medicine* 323:439-445.

Mensink, R.P., Zock, P.L., Katan, M.B., and Hornstra, G. 1992. Effect of dietary *cis* and *trans* fatty acids on serum lipoprotein [a] levels in humans. *Journal of Lipid Research* 33:1493-1501.

Nelson, G.J. 1998. Dietary fat, *trans* fatty acids, and risk of coronary heart disease. *Nutrition Reviews* 56:250-252.

Nestel, P., Noakes, M., Belling, B., et al 1992. Plasma lipoprotein and Lp[a] changes with substitution of elaidic acid for oleic acid in the diet. *Journal of Lipid Research* 33:1029-1036.

Ohlrogge, J.B., Emken, E.A., and Gulley, R.M. 1981. Human tissue lipids: occurrence of fatty acid isomers from dietary hydrogenated oils. *Journal of Lipid Research* 22:955-960.

Ohlrogge, J.B., Gulley, R.M., and Emken, E.A. 1982. Occurrence of octadecenoic fatty acid isomers from hydrogenated fats in human tissue lipid classes. *Lipids* 17:551-557.

Ostlund-Lindqvist, A.M., Albanus, L., and Croon, L.B. 1985. Effect of dietary *trans* fatty acids on microsomal enzymes and membranes. *Lipids* 20:620-624.

Pan, D. and Storlein, L. 1993. Dietary lipid profile is a determinate of tissue phospholipid fatty acid composition and rate of weight gain in rats. *Journal of Nutrition* 123:512-519.

Pfohl M, Schreiber I, Liebich HM, Haring HU, Hoffmeister HM. 1999. Upregulation of cholesterol synthesis after acute myocardial infarction--is cholesterol a positive acute phase reactant? *Atherosclerosis* 142:389-393.

Ponder, D.L. and Green, N.R. 1985. Effects of dietary fats and butylated hydroxytoluene on mutagen activation in rats. *Cancer Research* 45:558-560.

Ravnskov, U. 1995. Quotation bias in reviews of the diet-heart idea. *Journal of Clinical Epidemiology* 48:713-719.

Sadeghi, S., Wallace, F.A., Calder, P.C. 1999. Dietary lipids modify the cytokine response to bacterial lipopolysaccharide in mice. *Immunology* 96(3):404-410.

Schoenherr, W.D., Jewell, D.E. 1997. Nutritional modification of inflammatory diseases. *Semin Vet Med Surg* (Small Anim) 12(3):212-222.

Siguel, E.N. and Lerman, R.H. 1993. Trans-fatty acid patterns in patients with angiographically documented coronary artery disease. *American Journal of Cardiology* 71:916-920.

Smedman, A.E., Gustafsson, I-B., Berglund, L.G.T., Vessby, B.O.H. 1999. Pentadecanoic acid in serum as a marker for intake of milk fat: relations between intake of milk fat and metabolic risk factors. *American Journal of Clinical Nutrition* 69:22-29.

Strauss E. Developmental Biology: One-Eyed Animals Implicate Cholesterol in Development. *Science* 280:1528-1529;1998.

Teter, B.B., Sampugna, J., and Keeney, M. 1990. Milk fat depression in C57Bl/6J mice consuming partially hydrogenated fat. *Journal of Nutrition* 120:818-824.

Troisi, R., Willett, W.C., and Weiss, S.T. 1992. *Trans*-fatty acid intake in relation to serum lipid concentrations in adult men. *American Journal of Clinical Nutrition* 56:1019-1024.

Van't Veer, P., Kok, F.J., Brants, H.A.M. et al. 1990. Dietary fat and the risk of breast cancer. *International Journal of Epidemiology* 19:12-18.

Vartak S, McCaw R, Davis CS, Robbins ME, Spector AA. 1998. Gamma-linolenic acid (GLA) is cytotoxic to 36B10 malignant rat astrocytoma cells but not to 'normal' rat astrocytes. *British Journal of Cancer* 77(10):1612-1620.

Vartak S, Robbins ME, Spector AA. 1997. Polyunsaturated fatty acids increase the sensitivity of 36B10 rat astrocytoma cells to radiation-induced cell kill. *Lipids* 32(3):283-292.

Wahle, K.W.J. and James W.P.T. 1993. Isomeric fatty acids and human health. *European Journal of Clinical Nutrition* 47:828-839.

Willett, W.C., Stampfer, M.J., Manson, J.A. et al. 1992. Consumption of *trans*-fatty acids in relation to risk of coronary heart disease among women. Society for Epidemiology Research. June 1992.

Willett, W.C., Stampfer, M.J., Manson, J.A. et al. 1993. Intake of *trans* fatty acids and risk of coronary heart disease among women. *Lancet* 341:581-585.

Wood, R. 1992. Effect of butter, mono- and polyunsaturated fatty acid-enriched butter, *trans* fatty acid margarine, and zero *trans* fatty acid margarine on serum lipids and lipoproteins in healthy men. *J Lipid Res* 33:

Zurier RB.1993. Fatty acids, inflammation and immune responses. *Prostaglandins Leukotrienes and Essential Fatty Acids* 48(1):57-62.

Notes to Chapter 3

Selected Texts

Food: The Yearbook of Agriculture 1959. The United States Department of Agriculture. GPO

F.T. Proudfit. *Nutrition and Diet Therapy: A Textbook of Dietetics, 8th Edition*, The Macmillan Company, 1942.

K. Mitchell. *Food in Health and Disease*. FA Davis Company, Philadelphia, 1942.

A.H. Ensminger, M.E. Ensminger, J.E. Konlande, and J.R.K. Robson. *Foods and Nutrition Encyclopedia, 2nd Edition*. Volumes 1 & 2. CRC Press, Boca Raton, Florida 1994.

Selected Journals/Series References

Finley, D.A., Lonnerdal, B., Dewey, K.G., Grivetti, L.E. 1985. Breast milk composition: fat content and fatty acid composition in vegetarians and non-vegetarians. *American Journal of Clinical Nutrition* 41:787-800.

Koletzko, B. 1991. Supply, metabolism and biological effects of *trans*-isomeric fatty acids in infants. *Die Nahrung* 35:229-283.

Lifschitz, F. 1996. Considerations about Dietary Fat Restrictions for Children. J Nutr 126(4 Suppl):1031S-1041S.

Lloyd, L.E. and Cronier, C. 1989. Dietary guidelines: Implications for agriculture. In: *Diet, Nutrition, & Health*. K.K. Carroll. (Ed.) p. 260. McGill-Queen's University Press, Montreal, Quebec.

Olson, R.E. 1995. The dietary recommendations of the American Academy of Pediatrics. *American Journal of Clinical Nutrition* 61:271-273.

van den Reek, M.M., Craig-Schmidt, M.C., Weete, J.D., and Clark, A.J. 1986. Fat in the diets of adolescent girls with emphasis on isomeric fatty acids. *American Journal of Clinical Nutrition* 43:530-537.

Zlotkin S.H.. 1996. A Review of the Canadian "Nutrition Recommen-dations Update: Dietary Fat and Children.". *Journal of Nutrition* 126(4 Suppl):1022S-1027S.

Notes to Chapter 4

Selected Texts

Bailey's Industrial Oil & Fat Products, 5th Edition (ed: YH Hui) John Wiley & Sons, Inc. New York. 1996. (The 5 volume set sells for $895)

J.M. deMan. Chapter 2, Lipids, in *Principles of Food Chemistry*, 2nd Edition. AVI Van Nostrand Reinhold, New York, 1990.

A.H. Ensminger, M.E. Ensminger, J.E. Konlande, and J.R.K. Robson. *Foods and Nutrition Encyclopedia*, 2nd *Edition*. Volumes 1 & 2. CRC Press, Boca Raton, Florida 1994.

F. Gunstone. *Fatty Acid and Lipid Chemistry*. Blackie Academic & Professional; An Imprint of Chapman & Hall, London, 1996.

F. Gunstone (with J.L. Harwood and F.B. Padley). *The Lipid Handbook*, Chapman and Hall, first edition 1986, second edition 1994. (2nd Edition sells for $539.95.)

C.E. Stauffer. *Fats and Oils*, Eagan Press Handbook Series, Eagan Press, St. Paul MN, 1996.

Biochemistry of Lipids, Lipoproteins and Membranes, edited by D.E. Vance and J. Vance.

Elsevier, New York NY, 1991.

Composition of Foods: Fats and Oils, Raw, Processed, and Prepared, Agriculture Handbook 8-4, 1979, 1989; Composition of Foods: Nut and Seed Products, Agriculture Handbook 8-12, 1984,1989. U.S. Department of Agriculture.

Selected Journals/Series References

Information about the sources and composition of different fats and oils can be found in the many research papers to be found in journals such as the *Journal of Agriculture and Food Chemistry* and the *Journal of the American Oil Chemists Society*, as well as British and Canadian journals.

Notes to Chapter 5

Selected Texts

A.L. Forbes. National Nutrition Policy, Food Labeling, and Health Claims, Chapter 94 in Modern Nutrition in Health and Disease, 8th Edition, M. Shils, J. Olson, and M. Shike, eds. Volume 2. Lea and Febiger, Philadelphia PA, 1994.

E.R. Pinckney and C Pinckney. *The Cholesterol Controversy*. Sherbourne Press, Los Angeles CA 1973. (This book is out of print, but it should be available in any large library.)

R.L. Smith. *The Cholesterol Conspiracy*. Warren H. Green, Inc. St. Louis MO, 1991.

Selected Journals/Series References

L.E. Dickey and C.R. Caughman. Fatty Acid Profiles including *trans* Isomers of 123 Food Sources Presented as Grams of Fatty Acid per 100 Grams of Food. U.S. Department of Agriculture 1994 Document.

Dickey, L.E. *trans* Fatty acid isomer content of food sources. *Inform* 6:484 (Abstract) 1995.

Enig, M.G. *Trans* Fatty Acids in Diets and Data Bases. *Cereal Foods World* 41(2):58-63;1996.

Mattson FH.1989. A changing role for dietary monounsaturated fatty acids. *J Am Diet Assoc* 89(3):387-391.

Notes to Chapter 6

General References

Dietary Goals for the United States - Supplemental Views and Dietary Goals for the United States, 1st and 2nd Editions. Committee Prints from the Select Committee on Nutrition and Human Needs, United States Senate. U.S. Government Printing Office,

Washington 1977.

A.L. Forbes. National Nutrition Policy, Food Labeling, and Health Claims, Chapter 94 in *Modern Nutrition in Health and Disease*, 8th Edition, M. Shils, J. Olson, and M. Shike, eds. Volume 2. Lea and Febiger, Philadelphia, Pennsylvania, 1994.

Lloyd, L.E. and Cronier, C. 1989. Dietary guidelines: Implications for agriculture. In: *Diet, Nutrition, & Health*. K.K. Carroll. (Ed.) p. 268. McGill-Queen's University Press, Montreal, Quebec.

Peterkin, B.P., Shore, C.J., and Kerr, R.l. 1979. Some diets that meet the dietary goals for the United States. *Journal of the American Dietetic Association* 74:423-430.

F.T. Proudfit. *Nutrition and Diet Therapy: A Textbook of Dietetics, 8th Edition*, The Macmillan Company, 1942.

Notes to Chapter 7

General references

Enig, M.G., Atal, S., Keeney, M. and Sampugna, J. 1990. "Isomeric *Trans* Fatty Acids in the U.S. Diet." *Journal of the American College of Nutrition*. 9:471-486.

Enig, M.G. 1996. Trans Fatty Acids in Diets and Data Bases. *Cereal Foods World* 41(2):58-63.

Howard BV, Hannah JS, Heiser CC, Jablonski KA, Paidi MC, Alarif L, Robbins DC, Howard WJ. 1995 *American Journal of Clinical Nutrition* 62:392-402.

Mensink, R.P. and Katan, M.B. 1990. Effect of dietary *trans* fatty acids on high-density and low-density lipoprotein cholesterol levels in healthy subjects. *New England Journal of Medicine* 323:439-445.

Strauss E. Developmental Biology: One-Eyed Animals Implicate Cholesterol in Development. *Science* 280:1528-1529;1998.

Stubbs RJ, Harbron CG, Murgatroyd PR, Prentice AM. 1995. Covert manipulation of dietary fat and energy density: effect on substrate flux and food intake in men eating ad libitum. *American Journal of Clinical Nutrition* 62(2):316-329

Stubbs RJ, Ritz P, Coward WA, Prentice AM. 1995. Covert manipulation of the ratio of dietary fat to carbohydrate and energy density: effect on food intake and energy balance in free-living men eating ad libitum. *American Journal of Clinical Nutrition* 62(2):330-337.

Index

About the Author

Dr. Mary G. Enig, received an M.S. and Ph.D. in Nutritional Sciences, from the University of Maryland, College Park. Dr. Enig is the Director of the Nutritional Sciences Division of Enig Associates, Inc. in Silver Spring, Maryland; she has served as President of the Maryland Nutritionists Association and is a Fellow of the American College of Nutrition. Dr. Enig, a consulting nutritionist/biochemist of international renown, is an expert in fats and oils analysis and metabolism, food chemistry and composition, and nutrition and dietetics. She has many years of experience as a lecturer, and has taught graduate-level courses for the Nutritional Sciences Program at the University of Maryland where she was a Faculty Research Associate in the Lipids Research Group, Department of Chemistry and Biochemistry, University of Maryland, College Park.

Dr. Enig, a consultant on nutrition to individuals, industry, and state and federal governments, is certified by the Certification Board for Nutrition Specialists and is licensed in the State of Maryland and the District of Columbia. She maintains a private clinical practice in Silver Spring, Maryland, providing nutritional consultation and assessment, from which her real-life experience with patients brings into sharper focus the connection between nutrition in general and fats and oils in particular and health.

She was appointed by the Governor to the Maryland State Advisory Council on Nutrition (1986-1988) and served as a Contributing Editor of the scientific journal Clinical Nutrition (1989) and as a Consulting Editor of the Journal of the American College of Nutrition (1993). Dr. Enig has authored numerous journal publications, mainly on fats and oils research and nutrient/drug interactions, is a well-known invited lecturer at technical meetings, and also a popular interviewee on radio and television. At various times she has been certified as an expert witness on nutrition in a number of federal district courts.

Well known for her research on trans fatty acids, Dr. Enig has published a comprehensive review of the availability and consumption of trans fatty acids in the U.S. One of her early papers describes the first comprehensive analysis of trans fatty acid (TFA) components of the fat content of over 200 foods; approximately 300 more foods have been analyzed, the results of which will be published. Her finding is that the amounts of TFAs in the U.S. diet from partially hydrogenated vegetable fats and oils are much higher than the edible oil industry will admit. The recent scientific and media attention on the possible adverse health effects of TFAs has brought increased attention to her work.

Dr. Enig has been a vocal member of a small but growing minority of nutritional scientists who have maintained that the evidence allegedly supporting the saturated fat/coronary heart disease relationship is illusionary, and that the potential health threat of *trans* fatty acids (TFAs) has been deliberately minimized by the edible oil industry and governmental and quasi-governmental organizations. The books by T. Moore and R. Smith in the 1980s and a recent series of scientific papers, starting with Mensink and Katan in 1990 and Harvard University researchers beginning in 1993, are now rearranging the scientific landscape by demonstrating that her concerns about TFAs are correct.

www.bethesdapress.com

special offer to registered readers

place
postage
here

Bethesda Press
12501 Prosperity Drive
Suite 340
Silver Spring, Maryland 20904-1689

Bethesda
Press

Do you need nutritional consultation and assessment? For an appointment,

Bethesda Press

Call Dr. Enig's office at (301)680-8600 or email to info @ enig.com

special offer to registered readers

www.bethesdapress.com

↰ fold and tear along this edge first

Register your copy today!

Registered owners of **Know Your Fats** will receive a *<user id>* and *<password>* to access Dr. Mary's knowyourfats.com web site. Benefits include:

● discounted online access to *Ask Dr. Mary* ™

● discounted prices on future titles by Dr. Enig

● free access to expanded FAQs

● book feedback submission form

keep this stub for your records

Please write your serial number here for your own records.

affix serial number here

↰ fold and tear along this edge second

Fill out the required information below:

Name (Last, First, MI)

Address (1)

Address (2)

City   State   Zip Code

Email

URL *(optional)*

ISBN 0-9678126-0-7

9 780967 812601

52995

Serial No. 30161

affix serial number here

Where did you purchase **Know Your Fats** *(optional)*?

☐ bethesdapress.com
☐ amazon.com
☐ borders.com
☐ barnes&noble.com
☐ Borders Books & Music (store)
☐ Barnes & Noble (store)
☐ health food store
☐ catalog
☐ other ____

Where did you learn about **Know Your Fats** *(optional)*?

☐ internet review
☐ NYTimes/WSJ/Washington Post (circle)
☐ television program
☐ radio show interview
☐ book club
☐ health/nutrition web site
☐ physician's/nutritionist's/dietitian's recommendation
☐ other ____